Fu Qingzhu's
OBSTETRICS AND GYNECOLOGY

【汉英对照】
[Chinese-English Edition]

傅青主女科

编译　赵雪丽

Translator & Compiler　Zhao Xueli

英文校审　Tim Harvey, L.Ac., Dipl. OM

Translation Editor　Tim Harvey, L.Ac., Dipl. OM

U0300406

PMPH　PEOPLE'S MEDICAL PUBLISHING HOUSE
·北 京·

图书在版编目（CIP）数据

傅青主女科：汉英对照 / 赵雪丽编译. —北京：
人民卫生出版社，2024.10
ISBN 978-7-117-34159-2

Ⅰ. ①傅… Ⅱ. ①赵… Ⅲ. ①中医妇产科学－中国－
清代－汉、英 Ⅳ. ①R271

中国版本图书馆 CIP 数据核字（2022）第 226875 号

| 人卫智网 | www.ipmph.com | 医学教育、学术、考试、健康，购书智慧智能综合服务平台 |
| 人卫官网 | www.pmph.com | 人卫官方资讯发布平台 |

傅青主女科（汉英对照）
Fu Qingzhu Nüke（Han-Ying Duizhao）

编　　译：赵雪丽
出版发行：人民卫生出版社（中继线 010-59780011）
地　　址：北京市朝阳区潘家园南里 19 号
邮　　编：100021
E - mail：pmph @ pmph.com
购书热线：010-59787592　010-59787584　010-65264830
印　　刷：三河市尚艺印装有限公司
经　　销：新华书店
开　　本：710×1000　1/16　印张：23
字　　数：438 千字
版　　次：2024 年 10 月第 1 版
印　　次：2024 年 11 月第 1 次印刷
标准书号：ISBN 978-7-117-34159-2
定　　价：169.00 元

打击盗版举报电话：010-59787491　E-mail：WQ @ pmph.com
质量问题联系电话：010-59787234　E-mail：zhiliang @ pmph.com
数字融合服务电话：4001118166　E-mail：zengzhi @ pmph.com

·《傅青主女科》汉英对照版编译说明·

　　本书以清代傅山著、欧阳兵据清同治八年（1869）湖北崇文书局刻本整理、人民卫生出版社2006年10月版《傅青主女科》为基础编辑翻译。

　　本书包括带下、血崩、调经、种子、妊娠、小产、正产、产后、产后篇（上卷）、产后篇（下卷）和补集共11部分，书中提及的中药和方剂的汉英对照汇总表以附录形式附后。

　　本书依据实用性原则，对原著进行了部分删节调整。如《鬼胎》和《妊娠中恶》，因带有浓厚的封建迷信色彩，并未收录于本书；随着现代医学的发展，在难产发生时已经可以采用手术等多重手段医治，因此本书中《难产》部分和产后篇中的《横产》《盘肠产》《死产》《断脐》《误破尿胞》等亦未收录；《产后肝萎》叙述不符合逻辑，容易造成误解，亦未收录。为了统一格式体例，产后篇的《骨蒸》和《虚劳》后移到补集中。

　　对原文的准确诠释和理解，是正确翻译的关键所在。编译者参阅了多个版本的《傅青主女科》《傅青主女科校释》和《临产须知简体释文》等书籍，在严谨校勘和正确诠释的基础上进行翻译，力求通过简洁明了的语言，原汁原味地传达医学信息和思想文化内涵。

　　对原著中在现代医学有对应名称的病症，尽量采用现代医学名词翻译，以便于读者理解。如：将产后篇《产后血崩》中"断不可轻于一试，以重伤其门户"句中的"门户"，译为"the neck of the uterus"，原文中的"门户"指的是子宫颈，是一种形象说法，如果直译为"the gate"，则读者难以理解。又如：在产后篇《产后诸症治法》的《血崩》里，"乃当去其败血也"中"败血"指的是瘀血、坏血、因病损而郁积的血，此处即瘀积的产后恶露，应译为"lochiostasis"。美国版本直译为"vanquished blood（战败的血）"，则为误译，词不达意。

　　对于原著中带有思想文化内涵的表达，努力在诠释其内涵的基础上，找到符合目的语地道表达的方法翻译。如：产后篇（下卷）的《泻》中"若脉浮弦，按之不鼓，即为中寒，此盖阴先亡而阳欲去，速宜大补气血……"。此处"中寒"指真阳素虚，阴寒内盛，一得外寒，则直中三阴，而为中寒之症。不能简单理解为

"cold in center（中部寒冷）"，译为"cold attack"更准确。又如：产后诸症治法《妄言妄见》中"若非厚药频服"，"厚药"指性味浓烈浓厚的药物。"Rich"可以指食物是油腻的，但是并不能用来修饰"medicine"或者"formula"，用"potent"修饰"formula"才比较贴切。再如：产后篇（下卷）的《霍乱》中"冷热不调，邪正相搏，上下为霍乱"，"上下为霍乱"指的是"清气不升，浊气不降，生成霍乱"。"上下"直译为"above and below"或者"up and down"，读者无法理解。译为"the clear can not go upward, and the turbid cannot go downward, resulting in sudden turmoil disorder"才能使读者真正理解原文所传递的信息。

书中的计量单位均用汉语拼音斜体，1 *jin* =16 *liang*, 1 *liang* ≈ 30g, 1 *qian* ≈ 3g,1 *fen* ≈ 0.3g。

美国针灸执业医师、美国针灸医师协会会员、加利福尼亚州东方医学会会员、东方医学医师、中医学硕士 Tim Harvey 先生对本书全部译文进行了认真审核，撰写了英文简介，并从西方读者的角度提出了很多宝贵的建议，感谢 Tim Harvey 先生在翻译过程中的悉心指导！

感谢山西省中医药研究院中医基础理论研究所赵怀舟老师、山西中医药大学中医各家学说教研室张俐敏博士和山西中医药大学第一临床学院妇科教研室宗惠博士为本书的校勘诠释给予无私帮助！

感谢山西中医药大学党委书记刘星教授、校长郝慧琴教授、副校长张桓虎教授、中医药博物馆馆长刘润兰老师、傅山文化研究中心主任张维骏教授、研究生学院院长杨继红老师在本书课题立项、翻译和出版过程中给予的大力支持和无私帮助！

编译工作较为浩繁，囿于学力，难免阙谬，敬请方家指正。

赵雪丽

2022 年 10 月

Chinese-English Edition of *Fu Qingzhu's Obstetrics and Gynecology*—an Introduction

This book is compiled and translated based on the book *Fu Qingzhu's Obstetrics and Gynecology* written by *Fu Shan* in the Qing Dynasty, compiled by *Ouyang Bing* according to the book engraved by Hubei Chongwen Book Bureau in the eighth year of *Tongzhi* in the Qing Dynasty (1869) and published by People's Medical Publishing House in October 2006.

This book consists of 11 Volumes, including the following: *Vaginal Discharge Diseases*, *Profuse Uterine Bleeding*, *Menstruation Regulating*, *Conception Promoting*, *Pregnancy*, *Miscarriage*, *Normal Delivery*, *After Delivery*, *Postpartum Disorders* (I), *Postpartum Disorders* (II), *Addendum*, and summary tables of the Chinese and English cross-references to the herbs and formulas mentioned in the book are attached as appendixes.

The book is based on the principle of practicality, with some abridgments and adjustments made to the original text. What has been deleted in this version are those conveying strong feudal superstition and those that are illogical and easily misunderstood. Some contents in the chapters *Difficult Birth* and *Postpartum* are also deleted, as modern medicine has relatively safer methods to solve those difficulties. In order to unify the format and style, *Steaming Bone* and *Consumptive Disease* in the postpartum chapter have been moved to *Addendum*.

An accurate interpretation and understanding of the original text is the key to correct translation. The editor and translator consulted several editions of *Fu Qingzhu's Obstetrics and Gynecology*, *Interpretation of Fu Qingzhu's Obstetrics and Gynecology*, and the *Simplified Interpretation of the Instructions for the Postpartum Period*, and made the translation on the basis of rigorous proofreading and correct interpretation, striving to convey the medical information and ideological and cultural connotations in a simple and clear language.

For those diseases that have corresponding names in modern medicine, we try to translate them with modern medical terms to facilitate readers' understanding. For example, the term "门户" in the phrase "断不可轻于一试，以重伤其门户" (......it is inadvisable to try sexual intercourse, which may cause new damage to the neck of the uterus) in Chapter Sixty-two *Postpartum Profuse Uterine Bleeding* refers to the cervix of the uterus, which is a figurative expression, is translated as "the neck of the uterus", rather than directly as "gate". Another example is that in Chapter Seventy-seven *Profuse Uterine Bleeding*, the word "败血" in the sentence "乃当去其败血也 (......,it is necessary to remove the lochiostasis)" refers to stagnant blood, bad blood, blood that has accumulated due to illness and damage, and here is the stagnant lochia, which should be translated as "lochiostasis". The American version as "vanquished blood" is a mistranslation and does not make sense.

For the expressions with ideological and cultural connotations in the original, we tried to find a translation method that meets the authentic expressions of the target language on the basis of interpreting their connotations. For example, in the Chapter Ninety-three *Diarrhea*, "若脉浮弦，按之不鼓，即为中寒，此盖阴先亡而阳欲去，速宜大补气血……(If the pulse is floating and wiry and does not beat with force when pressed, this is a cold attack. This is a case of yin collapsing first and yang being on the verge of departure. It is proper then to supplement qi and blood greatly and immediately)", "中寒" refers to the yang deficiency and excess internal yin-cold, a condition where an external cold directly attacks the three yin. It should not be simply understood as "cold in center", but should be translated as "cold attack". Another example is the translation of *hou yao* in the expression "若非厚药频服"(Unless potent formulas are administered in quick succession) in Chapter Seventy-nine *Wild Talk and Hallucinations*. Here, "厚药" refers to medicines with strong and thick flavor. Translated as "rich medicine" is not proper, for "rich" should be used to modify food that is greasy instead of modifying medicine or formulas, so it is more appropriate to use "potent formulas". Still another example. In Chapter Ninety-six *Sudden Turmoil Disorder*, "上下为霍乱" means that the clear qi does not rise and the turbid qi does not fall, generating turmoil disorder. Here, the direct translation of "上下", "above and below" or "up and down" is incomprehensible to the reader. While the translation "the clear can not go upward, and the turbid cannot go downward, resulting in sudden turmoil disorder" can make the reader truly understand the message conveyed by the original text.

The units of measurement in the book are italicized in Hanyu Pinyin, 1 *jin* = 16 *liang*, 1 *liang* ≈ 30g, 1 *qian* ≈ 3g, and 1 *fen* ≈ 0.3g.

Thanks go to Mr. Tim Harvey, a practicing American acupuncturist, a member of the American Association of Acupuncturists, a member of the California Oriental Medical Association, a physician in Oriental medicine, and a master of Chinese medicine. He has carefully reviewed all the translations, written the English introduction, and made many valuable suggestions from the perspective of western readers.

Deep sense of gratitude should go to Mr. Zhao Huaizhou, Prof. of the Institute of Basic Theory of Traditional Chinese Medicine, Shanxi Provincial Academy of Traditional Chinese Medicine, Dr. Zhang Limin of the Teaching and Research Department of Various Doctrines of Chinese Medicine, Shanxi University of Chinese Medicine(SUCM), and Dr. Zonghui of the Teaching and Research Department of Gynecology, School of Traditional Chinese Medicine, SUCM. They have rendered their selfless help in the proofreading and interpretation of this book.

I'm extremely grateful to Prof. Liu Xing, Prof. Hao Huiqin, Prof. Zhang Huanhu, Prof. Liu Runlan, Prof. Zhang Weijun, and Prof. Yang Jihong of Shanxi University of Chinese Medicine for their genuine support and selfless help during the research, translation and publication of this book.

Every effort has been made to provide the most accurate translation of the original text possible. However, throughout the reading, you may find that certain words or phrases are not as precise in their translation as they could be. We sincerely apologise in advance for any discrepancies.

Zhao Xueli

October，2022

序

傅山,字青主,号真山、公之它、丹崖子、石道人、松侨老人等。生于明万历三十五年(1607),卒于清康熙二十三年(1684),山西阳曲(今太原市)人。傅山是明清之际伟大的思想家、书画家、医学家,他不仅对哲学、历史、文学、艺术有着深入研究,而且精于中医,擅内、妇、外、幼诸科,著有《傅青主女科》《傅青主男科》《青囊秘诀》等,其中《傅青主女科》影响尤其巨大,是几百年来流传的中医妇科学的经典著作。

傅山的医学思想不仅是《黄帝内经》、张仲景《伤寒杂病论》等古典医学著作理论的传承,而且经过长期实践验证。《傅青主女科》共有 83 个处方,其中有 19 个被引用到第五版中医高等院校教材《中医妇科学》中,占到该教材所引方剂的八分之一;《中国百科全书·中医妇科分册》从 100 多种方书中援引了 383 个处方中,引用《傅青主女科》的有 45 个,占援引处方的 11%,居诸家之首;而近年出版的《吴大真解读经典〈傅青主女科〉》和《中医古籍临床名著评注系列——傅青主女科》等,对《傅青主女科》进行了深入研究导读,足见《傅青主女科》是中医妇产科学中极具影响、不可或缺的重要文献。

《傅青主女科》在国内目前没有英译本出版,国外有由 Yang Shouzhong 和 Liu Dawei 翻译,由美国 BLUE POPPY PRESS 于 1995 年出版发行(ISBN 0-936185-35-X, ISBN 978-0-936185-35-4)的版本。美国版《傅青主女科》于 1995 年到 2018 年进行了 16 次印刷,但存在一些遗漏和错译:漏掉了原著上卷中的"种子"部分从"身瘦不孕"到"便涩腹胀足浮肿不孕"共 10 篇的内容,编译者经过求证,还认为有 20 余处由于对原文理解有偏差而产生的不恰当翻译。

编译者赵雪丽是我校国际交流合作处处长、世界中医药学会联合会翻译专业委员会常务理事、中华中医药学会翻译分会常务委员、山西省高等院校外语教学研究会副会长,是一位有中医学基础的英语教师,常年从事医学英语教学、中医药翻译和国际教育工作。在编译过程中,参阅了多个版本的《傅青主女科》《傅青主女科校释》和《临产须知简体释文》等书籍,求真求源,在严谨校勘和正确诠释的基础上进行翻译,力求通过简洁明了的语言,原汁原味地传达《傅青主女科》中的医学信息和思想文化内涵。

中医是中华优秀传统文化的一部分。中华优秀传统文化是中华民族的文化根脉,其蕴含的思想观念、人文精神、道德规范,不仅是我们中国人思想和精神的内核,对解决人类问题也有重要价值。但传播文化的过程是不易的。英国著名人类学家爱德华·泰勒的代表作《原始文化》于1871年出版,学术界对其评价甚高,认为它开辟了文化史学的新学科,但到1992年才出版中文译本,晚了120余年;雷蒙·阿隆1955年出版的《知识分子的鸦片》作为知识社会学的名著,50年后才有了吕一民、顾杭译注的中文版本。中国拥有大量的中医典籍,在医学界和思想文化界都有重要的地位,而现今把它们系统地翻译出来、在国际上传播,更是晚了数百年。这是一项任重而道远的事业。

希望本书的出版可以为推动中医药文化的传播奉献一份力量,为实现中医医学价值国际传播效果的最大化提供一些思考方向。

刘　星

山西中医药大学党委书记

2022年10月

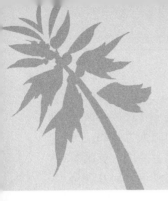

· Preface ·

Fu Shan, known by literary name as Qingzhu, and by courtesy name as Zhenshan, Gongzhi Ta, Danyazi, Shi Daoren, and Songqiao Laoren , was born in 1607 (the 35th year of Wangli in Ming Dynasty) in Yangqu (now Taiyuan City), Shanxi and died in 1684 (the 23rd year of Kangxi in Qing Dynasty). A great thinker, calligrapher and painter, he has a profound knowledge in philosophy, history, literature and art, and is especially proficient in Chinese medicine, an outstanding expert in internal medicine, surgery, gynecology and pediatrics. He has also authored several renowned books such as *Fu Qingzhu's Obstetrics and Gynecology, Fu Qingzhu's Andrology, Fuqingzhu's Formulas(Qing Nang Mi Jue)*, etc., among which *Fu Qingzhu's Obstetrics and Gynecology,* the classic work of gynecology worshiped for centuries, is the most influential.

Fu Shan's medical ideas evolve from the theories of classical medical works such as *Huangdi's Canon of Medicine (Huangdi Neijing)* and *Treatise on Cold Damage and Various Diseases(Shanghan Zabing Lun)* by Zhang Zhongjing, and have been verified by long-term medical practice. There are 83 formulas in his book, 19 of which are quoted in the fifth edition of the textbook *Chinese Medicine Gynecology*, accounting for one-eighth of the total formulas in it. In *Chinese Encyclopedia - Chinese Medicine Gynecology Branch*, 45 out of the 383 formulas collected from more than 100 formula books are from *Fu Qingzhu's Obstetrics and Gynecology*, accounting for 11 percent of the quoted formulas. In recent years, with the publication of *Wu Dazhen's Interpretation of Fu Qingzhu's Obstetrics and Gynecology* and *Commentary Series on Ancient Chinese Medical Clinical Masterpiece—Fu Qingzhu's Obstetrics and Gynecology* etc., in-depth introduction and research is carried further, showing that the book is an influential and indispensable literature of vital significance in Chinese medicine obstetrics and gynecology.

No English version of the book has been found in China yet, though. There is an edition translated by Yang Shouzhong and Liu Dawei and published by BLUE POPPY PRESS in 1995 (ISBN 0-936185-35-X, ISBN 978-0-936185-35-4) and it had been printed and reprinted 16 times from 1995 to 2018. Yet, there exist some omissions and mistranslations in it. For example, ten chapters in the *Promoting Conception* volume, from *Infertility Due to Emaciation* to *Infertility with Difficult Urination*, *Abdominal Distention, and Dropsy (Edema) of Feet* were left out. The editor and translator has been confirmed in her belief that there are more than 20 inappropriate translations caused by misunderstanding.

Mrs. Zhao Xueli, the editor and translator, is the director of International Communication and Cooperation Office of Shanxi University of Chinese Medicine, the executive member of the Translation Committee of the World Federation of Chinese Medicine Societies, the executive member of the Translation Branch of the China Association of Chinese Medicine, and the vice president of the Foreign Language Teaching Research Association of Shanxi Province Higher Education Institutions. She now works as an English teacher with a solid foundation in Chinese medicine and has been committed to teaching medical English, to translating Chinese medicine and to international education. In the process of editing and translating, she has consulted diverse editions of *Fu Qingzhu's Obstetrics and Gynecolog*, *Interpretation of Fu Qingzhu's Obstetrics and Gynecology*, and *the Simplified Interpretation of the Instructions for the Postpartum Period*, seeking the source and seeking the truth, and based her translation on rigorous proofreading and correct interpretation, striving to convey the medical information and ideological and cultural connotations in this book in its original flavor through simple and clear language.

Chinese medicine is a part of the excellent Chinese traditional culture, the cultural root of the Chinese nation. The ideology, humanistic spirit and moral code it contains not only are the core of our Chinese thoughts and spirits, but are also of crucial value for solving problems facing human. Yet, the process of culture spreading is not easy. *Primitive Culture,* the masterpiece of Edward Taylor, eminent British anthropologist, was published in 1871 and spoken highly of by the academic community as opening up a new discipline of cultural history, but its Chinese version did not come until one hundred and twenty years later in 1992; *Opium of the Intellectuals by* Raymond Aron, a masterpiece of the knowledge sociology, was published in 1955, but its Chinese version, translated and annotated by Lyu Yimin and Gu Hang, did not come until fifty years later. China boasts large numbers of classics in Chinese medicine, which have an important place in the medical and intellectual culture, and now, it is our long and arduous mission to translate them systematically and disseminate them internationally.

I hope that the publication of this book can contribute to the dissemination of Chinese medicine culture and provide some perspectives for reflection upon how to maximize the effect of worldwide dissemination of the value of Chinese medicine.

Liu Xing
Secretary of the Party Committee
of Shanxi University of Chinese Medicine
October, 2022

《傅青主女科 汉英对照》简介

《傅青主女科》由清代傅山所著，成书于 1673 年，1827 年在中国首次正式出版。人民卫生出版社基于清同治八年（1869）湖北崇文书局刻本整理后出版的《傅青主女科》，从 2006 年首次出版到 2017 年，历经 15 次印刷。《傅青主女科（汉英对照）》以人民卫生出版社 2006 年出版的版本为蓝本编译而成。作者傅山，字青主，是明清之际伟大的思想家、诗人、学者、书法家和爱国者，是非常著名的妇产科医生。

本书不仅可供中医专业人员使用，也可以供中医爱好者当作妇产科常见病的传统治疗实用参考书。在翻译时，译者力求将文字和概念放入一个更现代的语境中，以帮助西方读者理解作者在中国 17 世纪所表达的内容。

许多妇女一生中都患有不同的妇科疾病。这本书试图给经常使用对抗疗法的医生和医院提出一种可替代现代医学的、更顺应自然的技术——使用中草药来治疗许多不同的妇科疾病。也许这对他们来说并不容易接受，但这也是对传统医学的一次展现。读者会发现，根据疾病的不同性质，治疗方法也是从简单到复杂。

由于这本书是几百年前写的一本书的编译本，一些方剂可能会使用在我们这个时代不常用的成分。但是，它仍可以作为从业者和爱好者的宝贵的参考指南，有助于进一步了解过去中医是如何认识妇科疾病的，并为了解当时的医生如何看待当时的世界提供一个窗口。

从历史和医学的角度来看，这本书让读者深入了解一些与妇科相关的中医的起源和概念。任何有经验的医生都知道，这本书中的许多治疗方法已经证明有很好的疗效。通读整本书，你将从由浅入深、由简单到复杂的内容编排中了解许多曾经只有中国少数特权阶层才知道的方法和概念。希望这个译本也能为西方的从业者提供宝贵的精神财富，并进一步增进他们对中国传统妇产医学的认识、理解和欣赏。

美国针灸师协会会员
加州东方医学协会会员
美国针灸和东方医学协会会员
本书英文校审
Tim Harvey, L.Ac., Dipl. OM
July 2024

Introduction
from the View of Translation Editor

Fu Qingzhu's Obstetrics and Gynecology was derived from a treatise written by Fu Qingzhu, was passed down from the Qing dynasty, and was completed in 1673. It remained relatively unknown to the general public until it was first published in China in 1827. This version is a translation of the book that was published in 2006 and is based on the 1869 publication by Hubei Chongwen Publishing House. There have been 15 other printings between 2006 and 2017. Fu Qingzhu, in his day, was a very famous doctor who specialized in Obstetrics and Gynecology. He was also an ideologist, poet, scholar, calligrapher, and patriot. The people knew him as Shan, and he styled himself as Qingzhu.

The book is for both experienced and new practitioners of traditional Chinese medicine. It is also a practical manual for the layperson to reference the many traditional treatment methods of gynecology's common ailments. In editing the translation, it became necessary to put the words and concepts into a more modern context to facilitate understanding of what the author was expressing back in the 17th century.

Many women suffer from different gynecological ailments throughout their lives. The book attempts to present an alternative to the modern medical techniques often used by allopathic doctors and hospitals, which may be considered too invasive or harsh. Instead, it gives the reader a more natural way, using Chinese herbal remedies to treat many of the causes of different gynecological conditions. The reader will find the treatment for various diagnoses to run from simple to complex depending upon the nature of the problem at hand. Since this book is a translation of a book written many years ago, some herbal remedies may use ingredients that are impractical to use in this day and age. It will, however, serve as an invaluable reference guide to both practitioners and the layperson alike. For both, it will give added insight as to how gynecological conditions were viewed in the past and offer a window onto how doctors of that time viewed the world of their day.

From both a historical and medical perspective, the book promises to give the reader a fascinating look into some of the origins and concepts of traditional Chinese medicine as they relate to gynecology. As any experienced practitioner already knows, many of the treatment methods in this book have proven results. Each chapter builds upon the previous one going from simple conditions to more complicated. If one reads through the entire book, it will reveal many methods and concepts once only known to the privileged few in China. It is hoped that this translation will also serve as a valuable asset to practitioners in the west and further expand their knowledge, understanding, and appreciation of gynecology in traditional Chinese medicine.

Tim Harvey, L.Ac., Dipl. OM
Member of American Society of Acupuncturists,
California State Oriental Medical Association
American Association of Acupuncture and Oriental Medicine
July 2024

目 录

Table of Contents

Volume One ···1

Vaginal Discharge Diseases (Leukorrheal Diseases) ·············1

带下 ··1

　Chapter One　　Whitish Vaginal Discharge ·····················2

　白带下 ···2

　Chapter Two　　Bluish Vaginal Discharge ·······················5

　青带下 ···5

　Chapter Three　Yellowish Vaginal Discharge ··················7

　黄带下 ···7

　Chapter Four　　Blackish Vaginal Discharge ··················10

　黑带下 ···10

　Chapter Five　　Reddish Vaginal Discharge ···················13

　赤带下 ···13

Volume Two ··17

Uterine Bleeding (Metrorrhagia)···17

血崩 ··17

　Chapter Six　　Uterine Bleeding (Metrorrhagia) with Faiting ·······18

　血崩昏暗 ···18

　Chapter Seven　Uterine Bleeding (Metrorrhagia) of Older Women ········20

　年老血崩 ···20

　Chapter Eight　Uterine Bleeding (Metrorrhagia) of Young Married Woman ·····22

　少妇血崩 ···22

　Chapter Nine　Bleeding Due to Sexual Intercourse ········25

　交感出血 ···25

Chapter Ten   Uterine Bleeding (Metrorrhagia) Due to Melancholia ·············28
郁结血崩·············28
Chapter Eleven   Uterine Bleeding (Metrorrhagia) Due to Falling and Strain ·····30
闪跌血崩·············30
Chapter Twelve   Uterine Bleeding Due to Excessive Heat in the Sea of
Blood ·············32
血海太热血崩·············32

Volume Three·············35
Menstruation Regulating ·············35
调经 ·············35
Chapter Thirteen   Earlier Onset of Menstruation (Hypermenorrhea)·············36
经水先期（而多）·············36
Chapter Fourteen   Menstruation Behind Schedule ·············39
经水后期·············39
Chapter Fifteen   Irregular Menstruation ·············41
经水先后无定期·············41
Chapter Sixteen   Intermittent or Irregular Menstruation ·············44
经水数月一行·············44
Chapter Seventeen   Recommencement of Menstruation in Older Women·············46
年老经水复行·············46
Chapter Eighteen   Menstruation Comes Intermittently with Intermittent Pain ·····48
经水忽来忽断时疼时止·············48
Chapter Nineteen   Abdominal Pain Ahead of Menstruation ·············50
经水未来腹先疼·············50
Chapter Twenty   Menstruation Followed by Lower Abdominal Pain ·············52
行经后少腹疼痛·············52
Chapter Twenty-one   Abdominal Pain and Vomiting of Blood Before
Menstruation·············54
经前腹疼吐血·············54
Chapter Twenty-two   Aching and Pain Below the Navel Before the Period Is
About to Come ·············57
经水将来脐下先疼痛·············57
Chapter Twenty-three   Excessive menstruation ·············59
经水过多·············59

Chapter Twenty-four   Watery Discharge Prior to Menstruation ·····················62

经前泄水·······················62

Chapter Twenty-five   Hemafecia Prior to Menstruation ·····················64

经前大便下血·······················64

Chapter Twenty-six   Premature Menopause ·····················68

年未老经水断·······················68

Volume Four ·······················71

Promoting Conception ·····················71

种子 ·······················71

Chapter Twenty-seven   Infertility Due to Emaciation ·····················72

身瘦不孕·······················72

Chapter Twenty-eight   Infertility with Chest Fullness and No Appetite···········75

胸满不思食不孕·······················75

Chapter Twenty-nine   Infertility with Ice-Cold at Lower Abdomen ···········78

下部冰冷不孕·······················78

Chapter Thirty   Infertility with Chest Fullness and Poor Appetite ···········80

胸满少食不孕·······················80

Chapter Thirty-one   Sterility with Tense Feeling at the Lower Abdomen·········83

少腹急迫不孕·······················83

Chapter Thirty-two   Infertility due to Depression ·····················86

嫉妒不孕·······················86

Chapter Thirty-three   Infertility Due to Obesity ·····················88

肥胖不孕·······················88

Chapter Thirty-four   Infertility Due to Bone Steaming and Fever at Night ·······91

骨蒸夜热不孕·······················91

Chapter Thirty-five   Infertility with Aching Lumbus and Abdominal
                       Distention ·····················94

腰酸腹胀不孕·······················94

Chapter Thirty-six   Infertility with Difficult Urination，Abdominal Distention，
                      and Dropsy (Edema) of Feet ·····················97

便涩腹胀足浮肿不孕·······················97

Volume Five ···101

Pregnancy ···101

妊娠 ···101

Chapter Thirty-seven   Malign Obstruction in Pregnancy (Morning Sickness) ·····102

妊娠恶阻···102

Chapter Thirty-eight   Edema during pregnancy ···106

妊娠浮肿···106

Chapter Thirty-nine   Lower Abdominal Pain During Pregnancy ·········109

妊娠少腹疼···109

Chapter Forty   Dry Mouth and Sore Throat During Pregnancy ·········111

妊娠口干咽疼···111

Chapter Forty-one   Vomiting, Diarrhea, and Abdominal Pain During
Pregnancy ···113

妊娠吐泻腹疼···113

Chapter Forty-two   Distention in Chest and Hypochondriac Pain in
Pregnancy ···116

妊娠子悬肋疼···116

Chapter Forty-three   Impact Injury During Pregnancy ···119

妊娠跌损···119

Chapter Forty-four   Vaginal Bleeding During Pregnancy ···121

妊娠胎漏···121

Chapter Forty-five   Fetal Crying in Pregnancy ···123

妊娠子鸣···123

Chapter Forty-six   Lumber and Abdominal Pain, Thirst, Sweating, and
Mania During Pregnancy ···125

妊娠腰腹疼渴汗躁狂···125

Chapter Forty-seven   Abortion due to excessive anger during pregnancy ·······128

妊娠多怒堕胎···128

Volume Six ···131

Miscarriage···131

小产 ···131

Chapter Forty-eight   Miscarriage Due to Sexual Intercourse ···········132

行房小产···132

Chapter Forty-nine   Miscarriage Due to Wrenching and Contusion ···········134

跌闪小产···134

Chapter Fifty   Miscarriage with constipation ················136

大便干结小产 ················136

Chapter Fifty-one   Miscarriage with Aversion to Cold and Abdominal Pain ···139

畏寒腹疼小产 ················139

Chapter Fifty-two   Miscarriage Due to Rage ················141

大怒小产 ················141

Volume Seven ················143
Normal Delivery ················143

正产 ················143

Chapter Fifty-three   Normal Delivery but the Placenta Does not Descend ······144

正产胞衣不下 ················144

Chapter Fifty-four   Normal Delivery But with qi Deficiency, Blood Fainting ······148

正产气虚血晕 ················148

Chapter Fifty-five   Normal Delivery But Blood Fainting & Inability to Speak ·····150

正产血晕不语 ················150

Chapter Fifty-six   Normal Delivery But Lochiostasis Surging the Heart

Causing Fainting and Mania ················152

正产败血攻心晕狂 ················152

Chapter Fifty-seven   Normal Delivery But Intestinal Prolapse ················155

正产肠下 ················155

Volume Eight ················157
After Delivery (Postpartum Disorders) ················157

产后 ················157

Chapter Fifty-eight   Postpartum Lower Abdominal Pain ················158

产后少腹痛 ················158

Chapter Fifty-nine   Postpartum Dyspnea ················161

产后气喘 ················161

Chapter Sixty   Postpartum Aversion to Cold and Body Shivering ·······164

产后恶寒身颤 ················164

Chapter Sixty-one   Postpartum Nausea, Retching and Vomiting ················166

产后恶心呕吐 ················166

Chapter Sixty-two   Postpartum Profuse Uterine Bleeding ················169

产后血崩 ················169

Chapter Sixty-three   Postpartum Incessant Dribbling of Blood Due to the
                       Uterus Damaged by Hand ·············172
产后手伤胞胎淋漓不止·············172
Chapter Sixty-four   Postpartum Swelling and Edema of the Four Limbs ·······174
产后四肢浮肿·············174
Chapter Sixty-five   Discharge of Fleshy Fiber After Delivery ·············177
产后肉线出·············177
Chapter Sixty-six   Postartum Agalactosis Due to qi and Blood Deficiency ·····179
产后气血两虚乳汁不下·············179
Chapter Sixty-seven   Galactostasis due to Postpartum Depression·············181
产后郁结乳汁不通·············181

Volume Nine·············183
Postpartum Disorders Ⅰ·············183
产后篇 上卷·············183
Chapter Sixty-eight   An Overview of Postpartum Disorders ·············184
产后总论·············184
Chapter Sixty-nine   Indications and Contraindications of Antenatal &
                       Postpartum Disorders Ⅰ·············189
产前后方证宜忌 一·············189
Chapter Seventy   Indications and Contraindications of Antenatal &
                   Postpartum Disorders Ⅱ·············191
产前后方证宜忌 二·············191
Chapter Seventy-one   Indications and Contraindications of Antenatal &
                       Postpartum Disorders Ⅲ·············193
产前后方证宜忌 三·············193
Chapter Seventy-two   Indications and Contraindications of Antenatal &
                       Postpartum Disorders Ⅳ·············198
产前后方证宜忌 四·············198
Chapter Seventy-three   Indications and Contraindications of Antenatal &
                         Postpartum Disorders Ⅴ·············201
产前后方证宜忌 五·············201
Chapter Seventy-four   Treatment Methods for Various Postpartum
                        Symptoms Ⅰ·············204
产后诸症治法 一·············204

Chapter Seventy-five　Treatment Methods for Various Postpartum

　　Syndrome Ⅱ ··208

产后诸症治法　二···208

Chapter Seventy-six　Treatment Methods for Various Postpartum

　　Symptoms Ⅲ ··213

产后诸症治法　三···213

Chapter Seventy-seven　Treatment Methods for Various Postpartum

　　Symptoms Ⅳ ···216

产后诸症治法　四···216

Chapter Seventy-eight　Treatment Methods for Various Postpartum

　　Symptoms Ⅴ ···220

产后诸症治法　五···220

Chapter Seventy-nine　Treatment Methods for Various Postpartum

　　Symptoms Ⅵ ···223

产后诸症治法　六···223

Chapter Eighty　Treatment Methods for Various Postpartum Symptoms Ⅶ·····227

产后诸症治法　七···227

Chapter Eighty-one　Treatment Methods for Various Postpartum

　　Symptoms Ⅷ ···230

产后诸症治法　八···230

Chapter Eighty-two　Treatment Methods for Various Postpartum

　　Symptoms Ⅸ···233

产后诸症治法　九···233

Chapter Eighty-three　Treatment Methods for Various Postpartum

　　Symptoms Ⅹ ···236

产后诸症治法　十···236

Chapter Eighty-four　Treatment Methods for Various Postpartum

　　Symptoms Ⅺ···239

产后诸症治法　十一···239

Chapter Eighty-five　Treatment Methods for Various Postpartum

　　Symptoms Ⅻ ···243

产后诸症治法　十二···243

Chapter Eighty-six　Treatment Methods for Various Postpartum

　　Symptoms ⅩⅢ···246

产后诸症治法　十三···246

Chapter Eighty-seven　Treatment Methods for Various Postpartum
　　　　　　　　　　　Symptoms XIV ···248

产后诸症治法 十四···248

Chapter Eighty-eight　Treatment Methods for Various Postpartum
　　　　　　　　　　　Symptoms XV ···252

产后诸症治法 十五···252

Chapter Eighty-nine　Treatment Methods for Various Postpartum
　　　　　　　　　　　Symptoms XVI ···254

产后诸症治法 十六···254

Chapter Ninety　Treatment Methods for Various Postpartum Symptoms XVII ·····256

产后诸症治法 十七···256

Volume Ten ··257

Postpartum Disorders II ··257

产后篇 下卷 ···257

Chapter Ninety-one　Treatment Methods for Various Postpartum
　　　　　　　　　　 Symptoms XVIII ···258

产后诸症治法 十八···258

Chapter Ninety-two　Treatment Methods for Various Postpartum
　　　　　　　　　　 Symptoms XIX ··260

产后诸症治法 十九···260

Chapter Ninety-three　Treatment Methods for Various Postpartum
　　　　　　　　　　　Symptoms XX ··261

产后诸症治法 二十···261

Chapter Ninety-four　Treatment Methods for Various Postpartum
　　　　　　　　　　 Symptoms XXI ··265

产后诸症治法 二十一···265

Chapter Ninety-five　Treatment Methods for Various Postpartum
　　　　　　　　　　 Symptoms XXII ···268

产后诸症治法 二十二···268

Chapter Ninety-six　Treatment Methods for Various Postpartum
　　　　　　　　　　Symptoms XXIII ··272

产后诸症治法 二十三···272

Chapter Ninety-seven　Treatment Methods for Various Postpartum
　　　　　　　　　　　Symptoms XXIV ···275

产后诸症治法 二十四···275

Chapter Ninety-eight   Treatment Methods for Various Postpartum

                       Symptoms XXV ···278

产后诸症治法 二十五···278

Chapter Ninety-nine   Treatment Methods for Various Postpartum

                       Symptoms XXVI ··281

产后诸症治法 二十六···281

Chapter One Hundred   Treatment Methods for Various Postpartum

                       Symptoms XXVII ···284

产后诸症治法 二十七···284

Chapter One Hundred and One   Treatment Methods for Various Postpartum

                       Symptoms XXVIII ··287

产后诸症治法 二十八···287

Chapter One Hundred and Two   Treatment Methods for Various Postpartum

                       Symptoms XXIX ··291

产后诸症治法 二十九···291

Chapter One Hundred and Three   Treatment Methods for Various Postpartum

                       Symptoms XXX ···294

产后诸症治法 三十···294

Chapter One Hundred and Four   Treatment Methods for Various Postpartum

                       Symptoms XXXI ··296

产后诸症治法 三十一···296

Chapter One Hundred and Five   Treatment Methods for Various Postpartum

                       Symptoms XXXII ···298

产后诸症治法 三十二···298

Chapter One Hundred and Six   Treatment Methods for Various Postpartum

                       Symptoms XXXIII ···300

产后诸症治法 三十三···300

Chapter One Hundred and Seven   Treatment Methods for Various Postpartum

                       Symptoms XXXIV ··302

产后诸症治法 三十四···302

Chapter One Hundred and Eight   Treatment Methods for Various

                       Postpartum Symptoms XXXV ·······························304

产后诸症治法 三十五···304

Chapter One Hundred and Nine   Treatment Methods for Various

                       Postpartum Symptoms XXXVI ··························306

产后诸症治法 三十六···306

Chapter One Hundred and Ten　Treatment Methods for Various
　　　Postpartum Symptoms XXXVII ·············308

产后诸症治法 三十七·············308

Chapter One Hundred and Eleven　Treatment Methods for Various
　　　Postpartum Symptoms XXXVIII ·············311

产后诸症治法 三十八·············311

Chapter One Hundred and Twelve　Treatment Methods for Various
　　　Postpartum Symptoms XXXIX ·············315

产后诸症治法 三十九·············315

Chapter One Hundred and Thirteen　Treatment Methods for Various
　　　Postpartum Symptoms XL ·············316

产后诸症治法 四十·············316

Addendum·············319

补集 ·············319

Chapter One Hundred and Fourteen　Postpartum Constipation·············320

产后大便不通·············320

Chapter One Hundred and Fifteen　Postpartum Chicken's Claw Wind·············321

治产后鸡爪风·············321

Chapter One Hundred and Sixteen　Bǎo Chǎn Wú Yōu Sǎn (Safe Pregnancy
　　　Without Worry Powder) ·············322

保产无忧散·············322

Chapter One Hundred and Seventeen　Generalized Edema·············323

治遍体浮肿·············323

Chapter One Hundred and Eighteen　Bǎo Chǎn Shén Xiào Fāng (Child-birth
　　　Protecting Magic Formula)·············324

保产神效方·············324

Chapter One Hundred and Nineteen　Herbal Formulas and Variations for
　　　Various Symptoms Steaming Bone ·············326

骨蒸·············326

Chapter One Hundred and Twenty　Consumptive Disease·············329

虚劳·············329

附录1　中药汇总表·············331
附录2　方剂汇总表·············335

Volume One

Vaginal Discharge Diseases (Leukorrheal Diseases)

带下

白带下

　　夫带下俱是湿症。而以"带"名者,因带脉不能约束,而有此病,故以名之。盖带脉通于任、督,任、督病而带脉始病。带脉者,所以约束胞胎之系也。带脉无力,则难以提系,必然胎胞不固。故曰:带弱则胎易坠,带伤则胎不牢。然而带脉之伤,非独跌闪挫气已也。或行房而放纵,或饮酒而颠狂,虽无疼痛之苦,而有暗耗之害,则气不能化经水,而反变为带病矣。故病带者,惟尼僧、寡妇、出嫁之女多有之,而在室女则少也。况加以脾气之虚,肝气之郁,湿气之侵,热气之逼,安得不成带下之病哉!故妇人有终年累月下流白物,如涕如唾,不能禁止,甚则臭秽者,所谓白带也。夫白带乃湿盛而火衰,肝郁而气弱,则脾土受伤,湿土之气下陷。是以脾精不守,不能化荣血以为经水,反变成白滑之物,由阴门直下,欲自禁而不可得也。治法宜大补脾胃之气,稍佐以舒肝之品,使风木不闭塞于地中,则地气自升腾于天上,脾气健而湿气消,自无白带之患矣。方用完带汤。

　　Leukorrhea that presents with whitish vaginal discharge belongs to dampness syndrome. We name it "*dai*" because the disease's basic pathogenesis is the malfunction of *dai mai* and the decrease of its power of restriction. *Dai mai* communicates with *ren mai* and *du mai*. The abnormality of *ren mai* and *du mai* will affect *dai mai* and cause disease of *dai mai*. *Dai mai* has the function of holding and controlling the embryo. The decrease in its power of restriction will result in fetal instability. Therefore, the weakness of the "*dai*" makes it challenging to maintain embryo stability and thus cause miscarriage.

　　Some causes of impairment of *dai mai* may be a fall from a high place that causes a sudden sprain in the lumbar region. Excessive sexual intercourse and overindulging in alcohol may also impair *dai mai*. Pain may not be immediately upon injury, but the injury is present and leads to qi not being transformed into menstruation. Moreover, coupled with spleen qi deficiency, the stagnation of liver qi, the invasion of dampness, and heat pressure, lead to leukorrheal disease.

Whitish vaginal discharge (that is clear and thin like nasal discharge or saliva, even filthy, smelly, and can be profuse and ceaseless throughout the year) results from excessive dampness and debilitation of fire, stagnation of liver, and weakness of spleen qi.

The spleen qi starts to sag, and its essence cannot be held to nourish blood and transform into menstruation, and so it turns into a white and slippery material and flows out from the vulva spontaneously.

The appropriate treatment is to replenish and restore spleen and stomach qi, soothe the liver by relieving stagnation. This will result in the spleen qi being strengthened and the dampness removed, and so the whitish vaginal discharge disappears naturally. *Wán Dài Tāng* (完带汤, Discharge-Ceasing Decoction) is recommended.

白术（一两，土炒）	山药（一两，炒）
人参（二钱）	白芍（五钱，酒炒）
车前子（三钱，酒炒）	苍术（三钱，制）
甘草（一钱）	陈皮（五分）
黑芥穗（五分）	柴胡（六分）

bái zhú (white atractylodes rhizome), 1 *liang* (dry-fried with earth)

shān yào (common yam rhizome), 1 *liang* (dry-fried)

rén shēn (ginseng), 2 *qian*

bái sháo (white peony root), 5 *qian* (dry-fried with millet wine)

chē qián zǐ (plantago seed), 3 *qian* (dry-fried with millet wine)

cāng zhú (atractylodes rhizome), 3 *qian* (prepared)

gān cǎo (licorice root), 1 *qian*

chén pí (aged tangerine peel), 5 *fen*

hēi jiè suì (charred schizonepeta spike), 5 *fen*

chái hú (bupleurum), 6 *fen*

水煎服。二剂轻，四剂止，六剂则白带全愈。此方脾、胃、肝三经同治之法，寓补于散之中，寄消于升之内。开提肝木之气，则肝血不燥，何至下克脾土。补益脾土之元，则脾气不湿，何难分消水气。至于补脾而兼以补胃者，由里以及表也。脾非胃气之强，则脾之弱不能旺，是补胃正所以补脾耳。

This formula is decocted in water and is taken orally. If two *ji* is taken, the patient feels relieved, if four *ji* is taken, the vaginal discharge stops and if 6 *ji* is taken, it is cured.

Functions: This prescription treats spleen, stomach and liver meridians simultaneously, holds supplement in dispersion and rests elimination on rising. It promotes liver qi and liver blood, replenishes stomach.

When the spleen earth is replenished, the spleen qi is no longer overcome by dampness and can disperse water. Regarding replenishing the stomach simultaneously, we are applying the theory of "from the interior to exterior". Without the strengthening of stomach qi, the function of the spleen cannot be improved. Therefore, replenishing the stomach helps to strengthen the spleen.

Chapter Two
Bluish Vaginal Discharge

青带下

妇人有带下而色青者，甚则绿如绿豆汁，稠黏不断，其气腥臭，所谓青带也。夫青带乃肝经之湿热。肝属木，木色属青，带下流如绿豆汁，明明是肝木之病矣。但肝木最喜水润，湿亦水之积，似湿非肝木之所恶，何以竟成青带之症？不知水为肝木之所喜，而湿实肝木之所恶，以湿为土之气故也。以所恶者合之所喜必有违者矣。肝之性既违，则肝之气必逆。气欲上升，而湿欲下降，两相牵掣，以停住于中焦之间，而走于带脉，遂从阴器而出。其色青绿者，正以其乘肝木之气化也。逆轻者，热必轻而色青；逆重者，热必重而色绿。似乎治青易而治绿难，然而均无所难也。解肝木之火，利膀胱之水，则青绿之带病均去矣。方用加减逍遥散。

Some women have leucorrhea with a bluish color. It can also be green and viscous with a stinking smell. The bluish vaginal discharge is caused by dampness and heat of the liver meridian. The liver belongs to the wood element. Green is the color associated with wood.

The leucorrhea flows down like mung bean juice which is evidently the disease of the liver wood. The liver wood is fond of the moistening of water, and dampness is the accumulation of water. It is supposed that liver should be fond of dampness, how could it develop into bluish vaginal discharge? People know that the liver wood is fond of water, while they don't know it is disgusted with dampness because that the dampness is the qi of spleen earth. Use what the liver disgusted to match what it likes, which will inevitably violate the physiological characteristic of the liver. The violation will result into the qi-counter.

Liver-qi ascends typically, while the nature of dampness is to descend. The ascending and the descending impede each other and stagnate at middle *jiao*, then stream into the *dai mai* and flow out from the vagina. The bluish color of the leucorrhea is due to qi counterflow and presents only in mild cases. In severe cases, there is a fever, and the leucorrhea is green.

Pathogenesis:

The stagnated liver-qi, dampness, and heat detain at the liver meridian. The stagnated liver-qi will result in an up-ward invasion of liver-qi.

Treatment:

Clear heat from the liver meridian and drain water from the bladder. This will disperse both the bluish and greenish discharge.

Jiā Jiǎn Xiāo Yáo Sǎn (加减逍遥散，Variant Free Wanderer Powder) is recommended.

茯苓（五钱）	白芍（酒炒，五钱）
甘草（生用，五钱）	柴胡（一钱）
茵陈（三钱）	陈皮（一钱）
栀子（三钱，炒）	

fú líng (poria), 5 *qian*

bái sháo (white peony root), 5 *qian* (dry-fried with millet wine)

gān cǎo (licorice root), 5 *qian* (raw)

chái hú (bupleurum), 1 *qian*

yīn chén (virgate wormwood herb), 3 *qian*

chén pí (aged tangerine peel), 1 *qian*

zhī zǐ (gardenia), 3 *qian* (dry-fried)

水煎服。二剂而色淡，四剂而青绿之带绝，不必过剂矣。夫逍遥散之立法也，乃解肝郁之药耳，何以治青带若斯其神与？盖湿热留于肝经，因肝气之郁也。郁则必逆，逍遥散最能解肝之郁与逆。郁逆之气既解，则湿热难留，而又益之以茵陈之利湿，栀子之清热，肝气得清，而青绿之带又何自来！此方之所以奇而效捷也。倘仅以利湿清热治青带，而置肝气于不问，安有止带之日哉！

This formula is decocted in water and is taken orally. If 2 *ji* is taken, the leukorrhea's color turns light; if 4 *ji* is taken, the bluish leukorrhea stops. There is no need to take more.

Functions: Disperses stagnated liver qi and relieves depression. Soothes liver qi. Drains dampness, clears heat.

Indications: Liver qi stagnation, leukorrhea that is bluish or green.

Xiāo Yáo Sǎn (逍遥散，Free Wanderer Powder) is especially good at soothing the liver qi. When the stagnated qi is soothed, dampness and heat disappear soon after. *Yīn chén* (茵陈，virgate wormwood herb) is added for draining dampness, *zhī zǐ* (栀子，gardenia) for clearing heat. This combination turns the liver qi clear, and the blue or green discharge will be dispersed. This formula is effective because it drains dampness and clears heat, and soothes the liver qi.

黄带下

妇人有带下而色黄者，宛如黄茶浓汁，其气腥秽，所谓黄带是也。夫黄带乃任脉之湿热也。任脉本不能容水，湿气安得而入，而化为黄带乎？

Yellowish vaginal discharge looks like thick yellow tea water with rotten smell, and is called yellow leukorrhea. The yellowish vaginal discharge is caused by dampness and heat of *ren mai*. *Ren mai* cannot accept water by nature. How can dampness find its way in and change into yellow leukorrea?

不知带脉横生，通于任脉，任脉直上走于唇齿。唇齿之间，原有不断之泉，下贯于任脉以化精，使任脉无热气之绕，则口中之津液尽化为精，以入于肾矣。

The *dai mai* goes transversely and communicates with the *ren mai*. The *ren mai* goes upward and reaches lips and teeth. Primarily, there is spring water (saliva) orignated between lips and teeth comes downward, pours into *ren mai* and melts into essence, therefore, there's no heat invasion of *ren mai*, all fluid from the mouth melts into essence and goes into kidneys.

惟有热邪存于下焦之间，则津液不能化精，而反化湿也。夫湿者，土之气，实水之侵；热者，火之气，实木之生。水色本黑，火色本红，今湿与热合，欲化红而不能，欲返黑而不得，煎熬成汁，因变为黄色矣。

Only when pathogenic heat is stranded in the lower *jiao*, does body fluid transform into dampness instead of essence. As for the dampness, it is the pathogenic qi from earth, while there is invasion of water. As for the heat, it is the pathogenic qi from fire. The dampness and heat together are stewed into thick yellow liquid.

此乃不从水火之化，而从湿化也。所以世之人有以黄带为脾之湿热，单去治脾而不得痊者，是不知真水、真火合成丹邪、元邪，绕于任脉、胞胎之间，而化此黔色也，单治脾何能痊乎！法宜补任脉之虚，而清肾火之炎，则庶几矣。方用易黄汤。

The yellow leukorrhea is not caused by dampness and heat of spleen alone. It is also caused by the fluid and fire in the kidneys and together they transform into *dan* (erysipelas) pathogen and *yuan* (original) pathogen, which is spread around the *ren mai* and embryo and transform into yellowish fluid.

Treatment: Tonifying the deficiency of *ren mai* and clearing the fire inflammation of the kidneys. *Yì Huáng Tāng* (易黄汤, Yellow-Transforming Decoction) is recommended here.

山药（一两，炒）　　　　　芡实（一两，炒）
炒黄柏（二钱，盐水炒）　　车前子（一钱，酒炒）
白果（十枚，碎）

shān yào (common yam rhizome), 1 *liang* (dry-fried)
qiàn shí (euryale seed), 1 *liang* (dry-fried)
huáng bǎi (amur cork-tree bark), 2 *qian* (dry-fried with salt water)
chē qián zǐ (plantago seed), 1 *qian*, (dry-fried with millet wine)
bái guǒ (ginkgo nut), 10 pieces (pound to pieces)

水煎。连服四剂，无不全愈。此不特治黄带方也，凡有带病者，均可治之，而治带之黄者，功更奇也。盖山药、芡实专补任脉之虚，又能利水，加白果引入任脉之中，更为便捷，所以奏功之速也。至于用黄柏清肾中之火也，肾与任脉相通以相济，解肾中之火，即解任脉之热矣。

This formula is decocted in water and taken orally. If 4 *ji* is taken continuously, it is relieved. This formula could be used to relieve all leukorrheal diseases. For yellowish leukorrhea, it can have a remarkable effect.

In the formula, *shān yào* (山药, common yam rhizome), *qiàn shí* (芡实, euryale seed), are used to tonify the deficiency of the *ren mai* and alleviate water retention. *Bái guǒ* (白果, ginkgo nut) is a guiding herb that leads the medicine into *ren mai*, for a faster effect. Since the kidneys are connected with *ren mai* and nourish each other, *huáng bǎi* (黄柏, amur cork-tree bark) is used to clear away the fire in kidneys, and clear heat in *ren mai*.

（凡带症多系脾湿。初病无热，但补脾土兼理冲任之气，其病自愈。若湿久生热，必得清肾火而湿始有去路，方用黄柏，车前子妙。山药，芡实尤能清热生津。）

[Generally, leukorrheal diseases are related to spleen dampness. At the initial stage, there's no heat syndrome. So it is proper to tonify spleen (earth) and regulate qi of the *chong mai* and *ren mai*. If retained for a long time, the dampness will generate pathogenic heat. To alleviate it, we must clear away the heat in kidneys and the dampness in the lower *jiao*. *Huáng bǎi* (黄柏, amur cork-tree bark), *chē qián zǐ* (车前子, plantago seed), *shān yào* (山药, common yam rhizome), *qiàn shí* (芡实, euryale seed) are all used to clear heat and promote fluid production.]

Chapter Four
Blackish Vaginal Discharge

黑带下

妇人有带下而色黑者，甚则如黑豆汁，其气亦腥，所谓黑带也。夫黑带者，火热之极也。或疑火色本红，何以成黑？谓为下寒之极或有之。殊不知火极似水，乃假象也。其症必腹中疼痛，小便时如刀刺，阴门必发肿，面色必发红，日久必黄瘦，饮食必兼人，口中必热渴，饮以凉水，少觉宽快。此胃火太旺，与命门、膀胱、三焦之火合而煎熬，所以熬干而变为碳色，断是火热之极之变，而非少有寒气也。此等之症，不至发狂者，全赖肾水与肺金无病，其生生不息之气，润心济胃以救之耳。所以但成黑带之症，是火结于下而不炎于上也。治法惟以泄火为主，火热退而湿自除矣。方用利火汤。

Black leukorrhea is caused by extreme heat and fire. The discharge is as black as black soybean and has a strong foul smell. Black leukorrheal is caused by extreme fire hot. Some doctors will ask that the natural color corresponding to fire is red, how could it looks black? People hardly realize that the extreme state of fire hot is like water. (The natural color corresponding to water is black.) This is a false impression. The blackish vaginal discharge is due to the fire being compacted at the lower *jiao*, burning the fluid to an extreme state.

The patient may suffer from a sharp stabbing abdominal pain upon urination. There is swelling of the vaginal orifice and a reddish complexion. As time goes by, the patient looks thin with a yellowish complexion, has an excellent appetite, feels thirsty, has a craving for cold drinks, and feels slightly refreshed after drinking some cold water. All these symptoms result from the excessive flourishing of stomach fire, which integrates with fire in *mìng mén* (gate of vitality), the urinary bladder and *sanjiao*, and boiled into the color of carbon. Surly it is the change caused by the extreme fiery hot, not because there's a little cold syndrome. The patient's not going mad can only attribute to the sound of kidney water and lung metal. The kidney qi and lung qi grow constantly, nourish the heart, moisten the stomach, and prevent the patient from going mad. Therefore, the blackish vaginal discharge is due to the fire being compacted at the lower energizer and not flaming up.

Treatment: The primary treatment should be to purge fire. Once the fire is purged, the dampness will be removed.

Lì Huǒ Tāng (利火汤, Fire Discharging Decoction) is recommended.

大黄（三钱）	白术（五钱，土炒）
茯苓（三钱）	车前子（三钱，酒炒）
王不留行（三钱）	黄连（三钱）
栀子（三钱，炒）	知母（二钱）
石膏（五钱，煅）	刘寄奴（三钱）

dà huáng (rhubarb root and rhizome), 3 *qian*

bái zhú (white atractylodes rhizome), 5 *qian* (dry-fried with earth)

fú líng (poria), 3 *qian*

chē qián zǐ (plantago seed), 3 *qian* (dry-fried with millet wine)

wáng bù liú xíng (cowherb seed), 3 *qian*

huáng lián (coptis rhizome), 3 *qian*

zhī zǐ (gardenia), 3 *qian* (dry-fried)

zhī mǔ (common anemarrhena rhizome), 2 *qian*

shí gāo (gypsum), 5 *qian* (calcined)

liú jì nú (artemisia), 3 *qian*

水煎服。一剂小便疼止而通利，二剂黑带变为白，三剂白亦少减，再三剂全愈矣。或谓此方过于迅利，殊不知火盛之时，用不得依违之法，譬如救火之焚，而少为迁缓，则火势延燃，不尽不止。今用黄连、石膏、栀子、知母，一派寒凉之品，入于大黄之中，则迅速扫除，而又得王不留行与刘寄奴之利湿甚急，则湿与热俱无停住之机。佐白术以辅土，茯苓以渗湿，车前以利水，则火退水进，便成既济之卦矣。

This formula is decocted in water and is taken orally. If one *ji* is taken, urinary pain is relieved, and the urine turns clear. After the second *ji* is taken, the black leukorrheal turns white, and the third *ji*, the white leukorrhea, reduces. Another three *ji* and the patient should be symptom-free. This formula is quite potent and has powerful purging actions. It is very cold in nature. However, the very cold nature of the formula is necessary to treat the disease's fire and heat effect to prevent it from getting entirely out of control. So it should be used only in this extreme circumstance.

The cold herbs *huáng lián* (黄连, coptis rhizome), *shí gāo* (石膏, gypsum), *zhī zǐ* (栀子, gardenia), *zhī mǔ* (知母, common anemarrhena rhizome) with *dà huáng* (大黄, rhubarb root and rhizome) added clear heat and purge fire quickly. *Wáng bù liú xíng* (王不留行, cowherb seed) and *liú jì nú* (刘寄奴, artemisia) drain dampness quickly. *Bái zhú* (白术, white atractylodes rhizome) is used to tonify the spleen. *Fú líng* (茯苓, poria) to drain dampness, tonify spleen, and clear heat. *Chē qián zǐ* (车前子, plantago seed) to induce diuresis. When the fire retreats, the water can come back and the fire and water may meet each other.

（病愈后当节饮食，戒辛热之物，调养脾土。若恃有此方，病发即服，必伤元气矣，慎之！）

[After recovering, the patient should have a light diet and avoid hot (spicy) food. The patient can consume warm food and drink to recuperate the spleen.

If the patient's condition relapses and has she not done anything to help the spleen recover and then starts to take this formula again for the condition, her original qi will be hurt. Patients should be cautious!]

• Chapter Five •
Reddish Vaginal Discharge

赤带下

  妇人有带下而色红者，似血非血，淋沥不断，所谓赤带也。夫赤带亦湿病，湿是土之气，宜见黄白之色，今不见黄白而见赤者，火热故也。火色赤，故带下亦赤耳。惟是带脉系于腰脐之间，近乎至阴之地，不宜有火。而今见火症，岂其路通于命门，而命门之火出而烧之耶？不知带脉通于肾，而肾气通于肝。妇人忧思伤脾，又加郁怒伤肝，于是肝经之郁火内炽，下克脾土，脾土不能运化，致湿热之气蕴于带脉之间。而肝不藏血，亦渗于带脉之内，皆由脾气受伤，运化无力，湿热之气随气下陷，同血俱下，所以似血非血之形象，现于其色也。其实血与湿不能两分，世人以赤带属之心火，误矣。治法须清肝火而扶脾气，则庶几可愈。方用清肝止淋汤。

Reddish vaginal discharge looks like blood dripping constantly. The reddish vaginal discharge is also a dampness syndrome. Dampness is the deficient qi corresponding to the spleen/stomach (earth).

The discharge is red due to extreme heat (excess) in the body caused by dampness stagnation. The *dai mai* runs between the waist and the belly button and is located near the place that is the most-yin in the body (kidney), where heat excess cannot exist. However, since the *dai mai* connects with the kidneys, and the kidney qi connects with the liver, the excess heat reaches the liver organ. Stress and negative emotions such as worry and anger hurt both the spleen, making it more deficient, and the liver, making the qi more stagnant, which builds up more heat. The stagnated fire in the liver meridian burns inside and goes downward to restrict spleen qi. The spleen qi fails to transform and transport and makes pathogenic dampness and heat accumulate around the *dai mai*.

Because of the excess heat, the liver fails to store blood, so the blood penetrates the *dai mai*. Because the spleen qi is hurt and is powerless in transformation and transportation, dampness and heat sink and goes downward with blood. That is why

13

the discharge looks like blood. Blood and dampness cannot be divided thoroughly. People are misled by the belief that reddish vaginal discharge belongs to the heart fire.

Treatment: Clearing the liver fire and reinforcing the spleen qi. *Qīng Gān Zhǐ Lín Tāng* (清肝止淋汤, Liver-Clearing and Discharge Stopping Decoction) is recommended.

白芍（一两，醋炒）　　　　当归（一两，酒洗）

生地（五钱，酒炒）　　　　阿胶（三钱，白面炒）

粉丹皮（三钱）　　　　　　黄柏（二钱）

牛膝（二钱）　　　　　　　香附（一钱，酒炒）

红枣（十个）　　　　　　　小黑豆（一两）

bái sháo (white peony root), 1 *liang* (dry-fried with vinegar)

dāng guī (Chinese angelica), 1 *liang* (washed with millet wine)

shēng dì (rehmannia root), 5 *qian* (dry-fried with millet wine)

ē jiāo (donkey-hide gelatin), 3 *qian* (dry-fried with wheat flour)

fěn dān pí (tree peony bark), 3 *qian*

huáng bǎi (amur cork-tree bark), 2 *qian*

niú xī (two-toothed achyranthes root), 2 *qian*

xiāng fù (cyperus), 1 *qian* (dry-fried with millet wine)

hóng zǎo (jujube), 10 pieces

xiǎo hēi dòu (small black soybean), 1 *liang*

水煎服。一剂少止，二剂又少止，四剂全愈，十剂不再发。此方但主补肝之血，全不利脾之湿者，以赤带之为病，火重而湿轻也。夫火之所以旺者，由于血之衰，补血即足以制火。且水与血合而成赤带之症，竟不能辨其是湿非湿，则湿亦尽化而为血矣，所以治血则湿亦除，又何必利湿之多事哉！此方之妙，妙在纯于治血，少加清火之味，故奏功独奇。倘一利其湿，反引火下行，转难遽效矣。或问曰：先生前言助其脾土之气，今但补其肝木之血何也？不知用芍药以平肝，则肝气得舒，肝气舒自不克土，脾不受克则脾土自旺，是平肝正所以扶脾耳，又何必加人参、白术之品，以致累事哉！

The above herbs are decocted in water and taken orally. Minor relief is obtained with one *ji* taken. Further relief is obtained with the second *ji* taken. The condition is dispelled with four *ji* taken, and the patient will not have a relapse with ten *ji* taken.

Functions: Tonify liver blood to restrict fire and clear heat. Nourish liver blood and soothe liver qi.

Indications: Reddish vaginal discharge looks like blood dripping constantly.

This prescription focuses on tonifying liver blood rather than removing dampness because reddish vaginal discharge mainly results from pathogenic heat instead of dampness. As for the excess of fire, it is due to the deficiency of blood. Nourishing blood can restrict the liver fire fully. Moreover, water can integrate with blood and transform into a reddish discharge. It even makes it hard to distinguish whether it is dampness or not. It turns out to be all dampness transforming into blood. So, treating blood is necessary and treating dampness is unnecessary; therefore, there is no need to remove dampness on purpose. The mystery in this prescription lay in the simple treatment of blood and assisted with a few herbs clearing fire. It achieves a magical effect. If applying the method of removing dampness, it will lead the fire to go downward and will not quickly resolve the condition.

Some doctors would ask, previously you said to assist the qi of spleen earth, and why do you simply nourish liver blood now? Because people do not know using *sháo yào* (芍药, peony root) to calm the liver, and the liver qi works well. The soothed liver qi can help the spleen qi. When the liver is calmed, it helps the spleen. So there is no need to use *rén shēn* (人参, ginseng), *bái zhú* (白术, white atractylodes rhizome) or other herbs to stress the spleen.

Volume Two

Uterine Bleeding (Metrorrhagia)

血崩

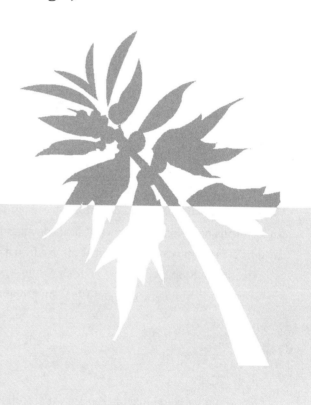

血崩昏暗

妇人有一时血崩，两目黑暗，昏晕在地，不省人事者。人莫不谓火盛动血也。然此火非实火，乃虚火耳。世人一见血崩，往往用止涩之品，虽亦能取效于一时，但不用补阴之药，则虚火易于冲击，恐随止随发，以致经年累月不能全愈者有之。是止崩之药，不可独用，必须于补阴之中行止崩之法。方用固本止崩汤。

When suffering from uterine bleeding, the patient, for a short while, can easily faint and fall, and become unconscious. It is because of the flourishing heat that pushes the blood out. The heat is not an excess condition. It is due to a deficiency of yin. Once seeing uterine bleeding, doctors use hemostats to curb the bleeding. This method works temporarily, but without herbs nourishing yin, deficient heat continues to attack. Bleeding may reoccur at any time. It may last years and cannot be resolved. So the hemostats cannot be used alone.

Treatment: Stop bleeding by nourishing yin. *Gù Běn Zhǐ Bēng Tāng* (固本止崩汤, Constitution Strengthening and Bleeding Stopping Decoction) is recommended.

大熟地（一两，九蒸）　　　　白术（一两，土炒焦）
黄芪（三钱，生用）　　　　　当归（五钱，酒洗）
黑姜（二钱）　　　　　　　　人参（三钱）

shú dì (prepared rehmannia root), 1 *liang* (fully steamed)

bái zhú (white atractylodes rhizome), 1 *liang* (dry-fried with earth until scorched)

huáng qí (astragalus root), 3 *qian* (raw)

dāng guī (Chinese angelica), 5 *qian* (washed with millet wine)

hēi jiāng (charred ginger), 2 *qian*

rén shēn (ginseng), 3 *qian*

水煎服。一剂崩止，十剂不再发。倘畏药味之重而减半，则力薄而不能止。方妙在全不去止血而惟补血，又不止补血而更补气，非惟补气而更补火。盖血崩而至于黑暗昏晕，则血已尽去，仅存一线之气，以为护持。若不急补其气以生血，而先补其血而遗气，则有形之血恐不能隧生，而无形之气必且至尽散，此所以不先补血而先补气也。然单补气则血又不易生，单补血而不补火，则血又必凝滞，而不能随气而速生。况黑姜引血归经，是补中又有收敛之妙，所以同补气补血之药并用之耳。

This formula is decocted in water and taken orally. When one *ji* is taken, the bleeding stops. If ten *ji* is taken, the patient will not relapse. If we are afraid that the dosage is high and cut it by half, the efficacy is weakened, and bleeding cannot be stopped. The formula has no herbs for stopping bleeding. It focuses not only on nourishing blood but also on strengthening qi. It supplements yang as well.

Large amounts of bleeding result in fainting, which means the bulk of the blood has gone, and there is very little qi to sustain life. Suppose we do not strengthen qi quickly to generate blood and only focus on nourishing blood first. In that case, tangible blood cannot be generated quickly enough, and invisible qi will all disappear. That is why we first strengthen qi instead of nourishing blood.

Strengthening qi alone cannot generate blood quickly. We must also supplement yang. If we nourish blood alone but not supplement yang, it will lead to the stagnation of blood. Therefore, the blood cannot be generated with qi quickly. Since prepared charred ginger guides blood to return to the meridians, it has a magical effect of astringency along with the function of strengthening qi. Therefore, it is used along with herbs for nourishing blood and strengthening qi.

若血崩数日，血下数斗，六脉俱无，鼻中微微有息，不可遽服此方，恐气将脱不能受峻补也。有力者用辽人参（去芦）三钱煎成，冲贯众炭末一钱服之，待气息微旺，然后服此方，仍加贯众炭末一钱，无不见效。

If excess bleeding lasts for days, too much blood will be lost. Also, pulses cannot be felt, and there will be only a weak breath through the nose. This decoction, therefore, should not be given to the patient abruptly because qi is at the edge of dispersion and cannot bear powerful tonification.

For the patient who is not too weak, decoct 3 *qian* of *rén shēn* (人参, ginseng) produced in Liaoning province, with the little rhizomes on the top removed. Dissolving *guàn zhòng tàn* (贯众炭, charred cyrtomii rhizome) 1 *qian* with the ginseng decoction and take it orally. The patient may be administered *Gù Běn Zhǐ Bēng Tāng* (固本止崩 汤, Constitution Strengthening and Bleeding Stopping Decoction) when her breathing gets stronger; *guàn zhòng tàn* (贯众炭, charred cyrtomii rhizome) (1 *qian*) is still added to this mixture. An instant effect will be seen.

Chapter Seven

Uterine Bleeding (Metrorrhagia) of Older Women

年老血崩

妇人有年老血崩者，其症亦与前血崩昏暗者同，人以为老妇之虚耳，谁知是不慎房帏之故乎。方用加减当归补血汤。

When an older woman* suffers from uterine bleeding, the patient feels dizzy and has very dim or dark vision. People mistakenly believe that this is due to the older woman's physical weakness, but indeed, it is due to improper sexual intercourse.

Treatment: *Jiā Jiǎn Dāng Guī Bǔ Xuè Tāng* (加减当归补血汤, Chinese Angelica Blood-Supplementing Variant Decoction) is recommended.

当归（一两，酒洗）　　　　黄芪（一两，生用）
三七根末（三钱）　　　　　桑叶（十四片）

dāng guī (Chinese angelica), 1 *liang* (washed with millet wine)

huáng qí (astragalus root), 1 *liang* (raw)

sān qī (pseudo-ginseng), 3 *qian* (root ends powder)

sāng yè, (mulberry leaf), 14 pieces

水煎服。二剂而血少止，四剂不再发。然必须断欲始除根，若再犯色欲，未有不重病者也。夫补血汤乃气血两补之神剂，三七根乃止血之圣药，加入桑叶者，所以滋肾之阴，又有收敛之妙耳。但老妇阴精既亏，用此方以止其暂时之漏，实有奇功，而不可责其永远之绩者，以补精之味尚少也。服此四剂后，再增入：

白术（五钱）　　　　　　　熟地（一两）
山药（四钱）　　　　　　　麦冬（三钱）
北五味（一钱）

服百剂，则崩漏之根可尽除矣。

（亦有孀妇年老血崩者，必系气冲血室，原方加杭芍炭三钱，贯众炭三钱，极效。）

The above herbs are decocted in water and taken orally. If 2 *ji* is taken, the bleeding lessens. After 4 *ji* is taken, the patient should be symptom-free. During treatment, the patient must cease all sexual activity; otherwise, the condition will worsen. This decoction is a magic formula for reinforcing both qi and blood. *Sān qī gēn* (三七根，pseudoginseng root) is an effective medicine for stopping bleeding. *Sang ye* (桑叶，mulberry leaf) is added for nourishing kidney yin and achieving the function of astringency. As the older woman has depletion of yin, although this formula can stop hemorrhage effectively, the effect is only temporary. The lasting function of this formula cannot be expected because there are fewer herbs for nourishing essence. For a more lasting effect, after taking 4 ji *Dāng Guī Bǔ Xuè Tāng* (当归补血汤，Chinese Angelica Blood-Supplementing Decoction), add the following herbs.

bái zhú (white atractylodes rhizome), 5 *qian*

shú dì (prepared rehmannia root), 1 *liang*

shān yào (common yam rhizome), 4 *qian*

mài dōng, (dwarf lilyturf tuber), 3 *qian*

wǔ wèi zǐ, (Chinese magnolivine fruit), 1 *qian*

Taking one hundred *ji* of this formula would allow for a complete recovery.

There is also the example of the aged widow who suffers from uterine bleeding caused by qi invasion of the uterus. In this case, the formula can render a positive effect by adding the following to the above prescription: *háng sháo tàn* (杭芍炭，charred Hangzhou white peony root)* 3 *qian* and *guàn zhòng tàn* (贯众炭，charred cyrtomii rhizome)* 3 *qian*.

*

The term "older women" in this context refers to the book "Yellow Emperor's Canon of Internal Medicine, Suwen (Plain Questions)," where the concept of "menopausal transition," sometimes known as "pre-menopausal" in the west, is discussed. There, women between the ages of 45~55 were regarded as being in menopausal transition and consequently were regarded as older women.

Háng sháo tàn functions to soothe liver qi and stop bleeding and *guàn zhòng tàn* functions to clear heat and stop bleeding.

Chapter Eight

Uterine Bleeding (Metrorrhagia) of Young Married Woman

少妇血崩

有少妇甫娠三月，即便血崩，而胎亦随堕，人以为挫闪受伤而致，谁知是行房不慎之过哉。夫少妇行房，亦事之常尔，何使血崩？盖因其元气衰弱，事难两愿，一经行房泄精，则妊娠无所依养，遂至崩而且堕。凡妇人之气衰，即不耐久战，若贪欢久战，则必泄精太甚，气每不能摄夫血矣。况气弱而又妊娠，再加以久战，内外之气皆动，而血又何能固哉！其崩而堕也，亦无怪其然也。治法自当以补气为主，而少佐以补血乏品，斯为得之。方用固气汤。

Suppose a young married woman who is pregnant for three months or longer suddenly has uterine bleeding, and a consequent miscarriage happens. In that case, doctors mistakenly think it results from being bruised or sprained from a fall or some other physical injury type. It is actually caused by inappropriate* sexual intercourse during pregnancy.

It is quite common for a young married woman to have an active sexual life. How can it cause bleeding? Generally, it is because of the primordial (original) qi weakness that makes it challenging for there to be a balance between the embryo and the ordinary sex life.

Once the patient has sexual intercourse, the kidney essence's emission due to orgasm causes the embryo to lose its nourishment resource, causing bleeding and miscarriage. Commonly, a woman whose qi is declining cannot endure sexual intercourse for a long time. Otherwise, she is bound to have excessive kidney essence emission, and consequently, qi cannot control blood. If qi's declination is coupled with pregnancy, together with excessive sexual intercourse, it destabilizes both internal and external qi. Therefore, it is not surprising to have bleeding and miscarriage.

Treatment: Reinforcing qi complemented by nourishing blood. *Gù Qì Tāng* (固

气汤，Qi Consolidating Decoction) is recommended.

人参（一两）	白术（五钱，土炒）
大熟地（五钱，九蒸）	当归（三钱，酒洗）
白茯苓（二钱）	甘草（一钱）
杜仲（三钱，炒黑）	山萸肉（二钱，蒸）
远志（一钱，去心）	五味子（十粒，炒）

rén shēn (ginseng), 1 *liang*

bái zhú (white atractylodes rhizome), 5 *qian*

shú dì (prepared rehmannia root), 5 *qian* (big ones, fully steamed)

dāng guī (Chinese angelica), 3 *qian*

bái fú líng (poria), 2 *qian*

gān cǎo (licorice root), 1 *qian*

dù zhòng, (eucommia bark), 3 *qian* (charred)

shān yú ròu, (fructus corni), 2 *qian* (steamed)

yuǎn zhì, (thin-leaf milkwort root), 1 *qian* (pitch-removed)

wǔ wèi zǐ, (Chinese magnolivine fruit), 10 pieces (dry-fried)

水煎服。一剂而血止，连服十剂全愈。此方固气而兼补血。已去之血，可以速生，将脱之血，可以尽摄。凡气虚而崩漏者，此方最可通治，非仅治小产之崩。其最妙者，不去止血，而止血之味，含于补气之中也。

（妊娠宜避房事，不避者纵幸不至崩，往往堕胎，即不堕胎，生子亦难养。慎之！戒之！）

This formula is decocted in water and taken orally. When one *ji* is taken, the bleeding may stop, and if ten *ji* is taken, the patient should be symptom-free. The formula can consolidate qi and nourish blood as well.

It will cause blood to be regenerated quickly and therefore control the blood loss. All patients with qi deficiency and bleeding may use this formula besides those who have a miscarriage. The magic in the formula lies in that it is not to stop bleeding; what causes the bleeding to stop lies in reinforcing qi.

(Generally speaking, pregnant women should refrain from sexual intercourse. Otherwise, even though she may not suffer bleeding, the woman can be subject to miscarriage. Moreover, if she does not suffer from miscarriage, the infant's survival rate is meager. Be cautious! Be sure to refrain from it!)

*

The word "inappropriate" here can mean either excessive sexual intercourse or sexual intercourse during pregnancy.

Chapter Nine
Bleeding Due to Sexual Intercourse

交感出血

妇人有一交合则流血不止者，虽不至于血崩之甚，而终年累月不得愈，未免血气两伤，久则恐有血枯经闭之忧。此等之病，成于经水正来之时，贪欢交合，精冲血管也。夫精冲血管，不过一时之伤，精出宜愈，何以久而流红？不知血管最娇嫩，断不可以精伤。凡妇人受孕，必于血管已净之时，方保无虞。倘经水正旺，彼欲涌出而精射之，则欲出之血反退而缩入，既不能受精而成胎，势必至集精而化血。交感之际，淫气触动其旧日之精，则两相感召，旧精欲出，而血亦随之而出。治法须通其胞胎之气，引旧日之集精外出，而益之以补气补精之药，则血管之伤，可以补完矣。方用引精止血汤。

Bleeding due to sexual intercourse may not be as severe as uterine bleeding, although it can injure the qi and blood if it continues for months and years. If it lasts long, amenorrhea due to blood depletion may happen. This kind of disease is due to sexual intercourse during the menstruation period where the semen fluid enters the woman's vessels. The semen fluid entering into the vessels is only a temporary injury, and it may recover with the outflow of the semen fluid.

Why will it result in long term bleeding? Vessels are exceptionally delicate and must not be injured by semen. Fertilization can only be safe when the vessels are clean. Suppose profuse menstruation is about to gush forth at the moment ejaculation of semen occurs. The blood which is about to flow out is forced to retreat and retract. Fertilization is then impossible, and the semen is accumulated and mixed with the blood. At the moment of orgasm, the residual semen in the vessels and the ejaculated semen work in concert. As a result, the residual semen will flow out, along with the blood at the same time.

Treatment: In order to facilitate fertilization, we must drain off the residual accumulated semen. We must also use herbs to reinforce qi and nourish essence in order to resolve the injury to the vessels. Therefore, *Yǐn Jīng Zhǐ Xuè Tāng*(引精止

血汤，Semen Drawing and Bleeding Stopping Decoction) is recommended.

人参（五钱）　　　　　　　白术（一两，土炒）

茯苓（三钱，去皮）　　　　　熟地（一两，九蒸）

山萸肉（五钱，蒸）　　　　　黑姜（一钱）

黄柏（五分）　　　　　　　　芥穗（三钱）

车前子（三钱，酒炒）

rén shēn (ginseng), 5 *qian*

bái zhú (*white atractylodes rhizome*), 1 *liang*（*dry-fried with earth*）

fú líng (poria), 3 *qian* (peeled)

shú dì (prepared rehmannia root), 1 *liang* (fully steamed)

shān yú ròu, (fructus corni), 5 *qian* (steamed)

hēi jiāng (prepared dried ginger), 1 *qian*

huáng bǎi (amur cork-tree bark), 5 *fen*

jiè suì (fineleaf schizonepeta spike), 3 *qian*

chē qián zǐ (plantago seed), 3 *qian* (dry-fried with millet wine)

水煎。连服四剂愈，十剂不再发。此方用参、术以补气，用地、萸以补精，精气既旺，则血管流通。加入茯苓、车前以利水与窍，水利则血管亦利。又加黄柏为引，直入血管之中，而引凤精出于血管之外。芥穗引败血出于血管之内，黑姜以止血管之口。一方之中，实有调停曲折之妙，故能祛旧病而除沉疴。然必须慎房帏三月，破者始不至重伤，而补者始不至重损，否则不过取目前之效耳。其慎之哉，宜寡欲。

This formula is decocted in water and taken orally. When four *ji* is taken in succession, the bleeding may stop, and if ten *ji* is taken, there will not be a relapse. This prescription uses *rén shēn* (人参, ginseng) and *bái zhú* (白术, white atractylodes rhizome) to reinforce qi and *shú dì huáng* (熟地黄, prepared rehmannia root) and *shān yú ròu* to nourish essence. As essence and qi are vigorous, the vessels may have good circulation. *fú líng* (茯苓, poria) and *chē qián zǐ* (车前子, plantago seed) are used to drain water and open orifice. As the water is drained, the vessels may be made smooth. *Huáng bǎi* (黄柏, amur cork-tree bark) is used as a guiding herb to drain the residual semen out of vessels. *Jiè suì* (芥穗, fineleaf schizonepeta spike) guides blood out of the vessels. *Hēi jiāng* (黑姜, prepared dried ginger) can heal the wound of vessels.

So the formula involves herbs for draining water and tonics for tonifying qi.

The patient must keep away from sexual intercourse for three months. Only in this way can the herbs for draining not be so violent to hurt the vessels, and the tonics are unlikely to add new damage to the patient. Otherwise, the prescription cannot be effective. Be cautious! Have less desire.

Chapter Ten

Uterine Bleeding (Metrorrhagia) Due to Melancholia

郁结血崩

妇人有怀抱甚郁，口干舌渴，呕吐吞酸，而血下崩者。人皆以火治之，时而效，时而不效，其故何也？是肝气之郁结也。夫肝主藏血，气结而血亦结，何以反至崩漏？盖肝之性急，气结则其急更甚，更急则血不能藏，故崩不免也。治法宜以开郁为主。若徒开其郁，而不知平肝，则肝气大开，肝火更炽，而血亦不能止矣。方用平肝开郁止血汤。

At times, some women feel desperately depressed, have a parched mouth with a tongue scorched, along with vomiting, acid regurgitation, and uterine bleeding. Interns all treat this as a fire syndrome. Sometimes this method may yield results, while sometimes, it may not. What is the reason? They fail to see it is due to severe stagnation of the liver qi.

The liver stores blood. The liver qi stagnates, and so does the liver blood. How then could this result in uterine bleeding? It is because the liver is impetuous by nature, and qi stagnation makes it more irritable. So it fails to store blood, which makes bleeding unavoidable. The treatment is based on relieving depression. However, if we relieve depression without soothing the liver, the liver qi would be too relaxed, and the hyperactivity of exuberant liver fire would be blazing. Therefore, uterine bleeding could not be stopped.

Treatment: *Píng Gān Kāi Yù Zhǐ Xuè Tāng* (平肝开郁止血汤, Liver Soothing, Depression Relieving, and Blood Stopping Decoction) is recommended.

白芍（一两，醋炒）	白术（一两，土炒）
当归（一两，酒洗）	丹皮（三钱）
三七根（三钱，研末）	生地（三钱，酒炒）
甘草（二钱）	黑芥穗（二钱）

柴胡（一钱）

bái sháo (white peony root), 1 *liang* (dry-fried with vinegar)

bái zhú (white atractylodes rhizome), 1 *liang* (dry-fried with earth)

dāng guī (Chinese angelica), 1 *liang* (washed with millet wine)

dān pí (tree peony bark), 3 *qian*

sān qī gēn (pseudoginseng root), 3 *qian* (ground)

shēng dì (rehmannia root), 3 *qian* (dry-fried with millet wine)

gān cǎo (licorice root), 2 *qian*

hēi jiè suì (charred fineleaf schizonepeta spike), 2 *qian*

chái hú (bupleurum), 1 *qian*

水煎服。一剂呕吐止，二剂干渴除，四剂血崩愈。方中妙在白芍之平肝，柴胡之开郁，白术利腰脐，则血无积住之虞；荆芥通经络，则血有归还之乐。丹皮又清骨髓之热，生地复清脏腑之炎，当归、三七于补血之中以行止血之法，自然郁结散而血崩止矣。

（此方入贯仲炭三钱更妙。）

The formula is decocted in water and taken orally. If one *ji* is taken, vomiting will stop. When two *ji* is taken, the thirsty feeling will disappear, and when four *ji* is taken, the bleeding will be stopped, and the patient will have a full recovery. The imaginative use of *bái sháo* (白芍, white peony root) for calming the liver, *chái hú* (柴胡, bupleurum) for expelling depression, and *bái zhú* (白术, white atractylodes rhizome) for removing stagnation between the waist and navel make blood flow smoothly. *Jīng jiè* (荆芥, fineleaf schizonepeta spike) clears the meridians and collaterals and makes blood go back into the vessels. *Dān pí* (丹皮, cortex moutan) clears away the heat in the bone marrow. *Shēng dì* (生地, rehmannia root) clears up the inflammation in the zang and fu-organs. *Dāng guī* (当归, Chinese angelica) and *sān qī gēn* promote the circulation of the blood because they nourish the blood.

[*Adding guàn zhòng tān* (贯众碳 Charred cyrtomii rhizoma) 3 *qian* makes the formula stronger.]

Chapter Eleven

Uterine Bleeding (Metrorrhagia) Due to Falling and Strain

闪跌血崩

妇人有高坠落，或闪挫受伤，以致恶血下流，有如血崩之状者。若以崩治，非徒无益而又害之也。盖此症之状，必手按之而疼痛，久之则面色萎黄，形容枯搞，乃是瘀血作祟，并非血崩可比。倘不知解瘀而用补涩，则瘀血内攻，疼无止时，反致新血不得生，旧血无由化，死不能悟，岂不可伤哉！治法须行血以去瘀，活血以止疼，则血自止而愈矣。方用逐瘀止血汤。

Injury for falling from high places, and sudden strain or contusion of a muscle, may lead to an outflow of extravasated blood, similar to metrorrhagia. This condition should not be treated as metrorrhagia because it will be made worse. Generally, patients with this syndrome feel pain when pressure is applied with the hands. As time goes on, they show a sallow complexion, emaciation, and have a dried-up appearance, all caused by blood stasis.

If we do not relieve the blood stasis while using tonics and astringent therapy, the inner invasion of blood stasis will produce endless pain. The improper therapy will lead to new blood not being produced and extravasated blood not being removed. What a pity if an inexperienced doctor cannot realize the mistake!

Treatment: Promoting blood circulation, removing blood stasis, and relieving pain. Doing these three things will stop the bleeding naturally. *Zhū Yū Zhǐ Xuè Tāng* (逐瘀止血汤, Blood Stasis Removing and Bleeding Stopping Decoction) is recommended.

生地（一两，酒炒）　　　大黄（三钱）

赤芍（三钱）　　　　　　丹皮（一钱）

当归尾（五钱）　　　　　枳壳（五钱，炒）

龟板（三钱，醋炙）　　　桃仁（十粒，泡，炒，研）

shēng dì (rehmannia root), 1 *liang* (dry-fried with millet wine)

dà huáng (rhubarb root and rhizome), 3 *qian*

chì sháo, (red peony root), 3 *qian*

dān pí (cortex moutan), 1 *qian*

dāng guī wěi (Chinese angelica root), 5 *qian*

zhǐ qiào, (bitter orange), 5 *qian* (dry-fried)

guī bǎn, (tortoise plastron), 3 *qian* (prepared with vinegar)

táo rén, (peach kernel), 10 pieces (soaked, dry-fried and ground)

水煎服。一剂疼轻，二剂疼止，三剂血亦全止，不必再服矣。此方之妙，妙于活血之中，佐以下滞之品，故逐瘀如扫，而止血如神。或疑跌闪升坠，是由外而伤内，虽不比内伤之重，而既已血崩，则内之所伤，亦不为轻，何以只治其瘀而不顾气也？殊不知跌闪升坠，非由内伤以及外伤者可比。盖本实不拨，去其标病可耳。故曰：急则治其标。

Decoct the above medicine in water and take it orally. After one *ji* is taken, the pain will be ameliorated. After two *ji* is taken, the pain may be stopped. When three *ji* is taken, the bleeding stops with no relapse, and there is no need to take it anymore. The prescription's magic effect lies in that purgative drugs are used as an adjuvant along with drugs for removing blood stasis. Therefore, blood stasis can be removed, and the bleeding is stopped magically. When one falls from a high place, the sudden strain or contusion of a muscle leading to bleeding is the internal injury caused by the body's exterior injury. Which means the internal injury is severe. Why don't we care about qi while treating blood stasis? Interns hardly realize that when one falls from high places, the sudden strain or contusion of a muscle is unlike the outside injury caused by inside diseases. Generally speaking, when the disease's root cause is an excess pattern, and it is difficult to remove soon, the treatment should concentrate on symptoms (the manifestations). As it is said to treat acute disease, treat the symptoms first (concentrate on the disease's manifestations first).

（凡跌打损伤致唾血、呕血，皆宜如此治法。若血聚胃中，宜加川厚朴一钱半，姜汁炒。）

[All spitting or vomiting blood caused by injuries from falls, contusions, and strains can be treated this way. If blood accumulates in the stomach, *hòu pò* (厚朴 magnolia bark) (one and a half *qian*, dry-fried with Ginger juice) should be added.]

Chapter Twelve

Uterine Bleeding Due to Excessive Heat in the Sea of Blood

血海太热血崩

妇人有每行人道，经水即来，一如血崩。人以为胞胎有伤，触之以动其血也。谁知是子宫血海因太热而不固乎。夫子宫即在胞胎之下，而血海又在胞胎之上。血海者，冲脉也。冲脉太寒而血即亏，冲脉太热而血即沸。血崩之为病，正冲脉之火热也。然既由冲脉之热，则应常崩而无有止时，何以行人道而始来，果（脾）与肝木无羔耶？夫脾健则能摄血，肝平则能藏血。人未入房之时，君相二火寂然不动，虽冲脉独热，而血亦不至外驰。及有人道之感，则子宫大开，君相火动，以热招热，同气相求，翕然齐动，以鼓其精房，血海泛滥，有不能止遏之势，肝欲藏之而不能，脾欲摄之而不得，故经水随交感而至，若有声应之捷，是惟火之为病也。治法必须滋阴降火，以清血海而和子宫，则终身之病，可半载而除矣。然必绝欲三月而后可。方用清海丸。

Some women start to menstruate the moment they have sexual intercourse, just like metrorrhagia. Some people think this is because the uterus is injured, and blood flows out once sexual intercourse begins, but instead, it is due to the insecurity of the sea of blood caused by excessive heat. The sea of blood is *chong mai*. Extreme cold of *chong mai* leads to depletion of blood, while extreme heat of *chong mai* leads the blood to "boil," which results in uterine bleeding. Why does this happen only when the patient has sexual intercourse and does not happen before and after? It is because the spleen and the liver are in good health. A healthy spleen controls blood, and a soothed liver stores blood.

Immediately preceding sexual intercourse, both heart (monarch) fire and liver (minister) fire are inactive. Although *chong mai* (thoroughfare vessel) has pathogenic heat, blood is unlikely to flow out. When the patient begins to feel excited during intercourse, the uterus opens, both heart (monarch) fire and liver (minister) fire are disturbed. So heat attracts heat, as like attracts like. The heart (monarch) fire and liver (minister) fire are restless and build up in the essence chamber, and the sea of blood (*chong mai*) overflows and seems uncontrollable. At this point, the liver cannot store the blood, and the spleen cannot control blood anymore. So the menstruation comes with the excitement of intercourse. It comes so quickly, just like echo and sound, because the disease is caused by pestilence fire.

Treatment: Enriching yin to reduce fire, clear *chong mai* and uterus. The patient must refrain from sexual intercourse at least for three month.

Qīng Hǎi Wan (清海丸 , Sea of Blood Clearing Bolus) is recommended.

大熟地（一斤，九蒸）　　　　山萸（十两，蒸）
山药（十两，炒）　　　　　　丹皮（十两）
北五味（二两，炒）　　　　　麦冬肉（十两）
白术（一斤，土炒）　　　　　白芍（一斤，酒炒）
龙骨（二两）　　　　　　　　地骨皮（十两）
干桑叶（一斤）　　　　　　　元参（一斤）
沙参（十两）　　　　　　　　石斛（十两）

shú dì (prepared rehmannia root), 1 *jin* (fully steamed)

shān yú, (fructus corni), 10 *liang* (steamed)

shān yào (common yam rhizome), 10 *liang* (dry-fried)

dān pí (cortex moutan),10 *liang*

wǔ wèi zǐ, (Chinese magnolivine fruit), 2 *liang* (dry-fried)

mài dōng, (dwarf lilyturf tuber), 10 *liang*

bái zhú (white atractylodes rhizome), 1 *jin* (dry-fried with earth)

bái sháo (white peony root), 1 *jin* (dry-fried with millet wine)

lóng gǔ, (dinosaur bone), 2 *liang*

dì gǔ pí, (Chinese wolfberry root-bark), 2 *liang*

gān sāng yè, (dried mulberry leaf), 1 *jin*

yuán shēn, (figwort root), 1 *jin*

shā shēn, (radix adenophorae seu glehniae), 10 *liang*

shí hú, dendrobium, 10 *liang*

上十四味，各为细末，合一处，炼蜜丸桐子大。早晚每服五钱，白滚水送下。半载全愈。此方补阴而无浮动之虑，缩血而无寒凉之苦。日计不足，月计有余，潜移默夺，子宫清凉，而血海自固。倘不揣其本而齐其末，徒以发灰、白矾、黄连炭、五倍子等药末，以外治其幽隐之处，则恐愈涩而愈流，终必至于败亡也。

可不慎与！

   Grind the above herbs into a fine powder, and mix the powder with honey to make boluses like semen firmianae. Take 5 *qian* each time with water in the morning and evening, respectively. If the bolus is taken for half a year, the patient will recover. Even if the disease has lasted for the patient's entire life, it may be resolved in half a year. This prescription has the function of nourishing yin and stopping bleeding. There is no need to worry about the side effect of cold herbs. As the days accumulate and the months increase, an invisible, formative influence happens. The uterus regains its cool and refreshing state, and the sea of blood recovers its stability. If we do not find the root of the disease and only use powder of burnt hair, *bái fán* (白矾, alum), *huáng lián tàn* (黄连碳, charred coptis rhizome), and *wǔ bèi zǐ* (五倍子, gallnut of Chinese sumac) to stop bleeding, then the bleeding will become more serious, and finally will lead to death. Be cautious!

Volume Three

Menstruation Regulating

调经

Chapter Thirteen
Earlier Onset of Menstruation (Hypermenorrhea)

经水先期（而多）

　　妇人有先期经来者，其经甚多，人以为血热之极也，谁知是肾中水火太旺乎。夫火太旺则血热，水太旺则血多，此有余之病，非不足之症也。似宜不药，有喜。但过于有余则子宫太热，亦难受孕，更恐有烁干男精之虑，过者损之，谓非既济之道乎！然而火不可任其有余，而水断不可使之不足。治之法但少清其热，不必泄其水也。方用清经散。

Some women suffer from a short menstruation cycle and hypermenorrhea. Interns think it is because of extreme blood heat. In fact, it is caused by excessive exuberance of kidney water and fire. Excessive exuberance of fire may cause blood heat, and excessive exuberance of water can lead to excess blood in the blood vessels, which cannot be held there. So the patient bleeds. This is an excess syndrome and not a deficiency one. It seems that there is no need to use a medicine, and the woman can still conceive a baby. However, the extreme excess heat makes the uterus extremely hot, which may lead to difficulty conceiving and result in the burning of kidney essence. As for the excess, it must be reduced. When reduced, it will balance water and fire. We can neither allow the fire to be in excess nor can the water be in deficiency.

Treatment: Mildly clear heat. There's no need to drain water. *Qīng Jīng Sǎn* (清经散, Meridians Clearing Powder) is recommended.

丹皮（三钱）　　　　　　　地骨皮（五钱）

白芍（三钱，酒炒）　　　　大熟地（三钱，九蒸）

青蒿（二钱）　　　　　　　白茯苓（一钱）

黄柏（五分，盐水浸炒）

dān pí (cortex moutan), 3 *qian*

dì gǔ pí, (Chinese wolfberry root-bark), 5 *qian*

bái sháo (white peony root), 3 *qian* (dry-fried with millet wine)

shú dì (prepared rehmannia root), 3 *qian* (big ones, fully steamed)

qīng hāo, sweet wormwood , 2 *qian*

bái fú líng (poria), 1 *qian*

huáng bǎi (amur cork-tree bark), 5 *fen* (soked in salt water and dry-fried)

水煎服。二剂而火自平。此方虽是清火之品，然仍是滋水之味，火泄而水不与俱泄，损而益也。

This formula is decocted in water and taken orally. If two *ji* is taken, the heat can be reduced. Although this formula is for clearing fire, it still has some ingredients for nourishing water. The fire will be cleared while the water will not be affected. By clearing fire, we achieve the purpose of nourishing water.

经水先期（而少）
Earlier onset of menstruation (hypomenorrhea)

又有先期经来只一二点者，人以为血热之极也，谁知肾中火旺而阴水亏乎！夫同是先期之来，何以分虚实之异？盖妇人之经最难调，苟不分别细微，用药鲜克有效。

Some other patients also have a short menstruation cycle, while the amount of menstrual blood is small. Interns think it is because of a high level of blood heat. In fact, it is the result of the excess fire and the inadequacy of yin (water) in the kidney. With the same symptoms of a short menstruation cycle, they belong to different syndromes: deficiency and excess. Menstruation regulating is not easy. If we do not make a cautious syndrome differentiation, the medicine will not be beneficial.

先期者火气之冲，多寡者水气之验。故先期而来多者，火热而水有余也；先期而来少者，火热而水不足也。倘一见先期之来，俱以为有余之热，但泄火而不补水，或水火两泄之，有不更增其病者乎！ 治之法不必泄火，只专补水，水既足而火自消矣，亦既济之道也。方用两地汤。

The short menstruation cycle results from the heat of fire, while the amount of bleeding shows whether the water is deficient or not. When the menstruation period is short and the amount of bleeding is heavy, it is due to fire and a surplus of water. If the period is short and the quantity is little, it is because of the fire's heat while the water is insufficient. If we think that all short menstrual cycles are caused by excess fire and only clear and discharge fire while not nourishing water or discharge both fire and water, the patient's condition is bound to worsen.

To treat it, we do not need to discharge fire. What we should do is focus on replenishing water. When there is enough water, the fire would be put out naturally. This is the coordination between water and fire. In this case, *Liǎng Dì Tāng* (两地汤, Rehmannia Root and Chinese Wolfberry Root-Bark Decoction) is recommended.

大生地（一两，酒炒）　　　　元参（一两）

白芍药（五钱，酒炒）　　　　麦冬肉（五钱）

地骨皮（三钱）　　　　　　　阿胶（三钱）

shēng dì (rehmannia root), 1 *liang* (big ones, dry-fried with millet wine)

yuán shēn, figwort root, 1 *liang*

bái sháo (white peony root), 5 *qian* (dry-fried with millet wine)

mài dōng, dwarf lilyturf tuber, 5 *qian*

dì gǔ pí, (Chinese wolfberry root-bark), 3 *qian*

ē jiāo (donkey-hide gelatin), 3 *qian*

水煎服。四剂而经调矣。此方之用地骨、生地，能清骨中之热。骨中之热，由于肾经之热，清其骨髓，则肾气自清，而又不损伤胃气，此治之巧也。况所用诸药，又纯是补水之味，水盛而火自平理也。此条与上条参观，断无误治先期之病矣。

This formula is decocted in water and taken orally. After four *ji* is taken, the menstruation will become regular. *Dì gǔ pí* (地骨皮, Chinese wolfberry root-bark) and *shēng dì* (生地, rehmannia root) may clear the heat in the bone. The heat in the bone comes from the heat in the kidney meridian. The kidney will be clean to clear the bone marrow heat, and it does not harm the stomach qi. That is the subtlety of this formula. Besides, all medicine used here has the function of replenishing water. Sufficient water will surely cool down the fire. If one compares this formula with the above formula, misdiagnosis and mistreatment will not happen.

Chapter Fourteen
Menstruation Behind Schedule

经水后期

　　妇人有经水后期而来多者，人以为血虚之病也，谁知非血虚乎。盖后期之多少，实有不同，不可执一而论。盖后期而来少，血寒而不足；后期而来多，血寒而有余。夫经本于肾，而其流五脏六腑之血皆归之。故经来而诸经之血尽来附益，以经水行而门启不遑迅阖，诸经之血乘其隙而皆出也。但血既出矣，则成不足。治法宜于补中温散之，不得曰：后期者俱不足也。方用温经摄血汤。

Some women have menstruation behind schedule (or delayed menstrual flow) in great amounts. Interns think it is a syndrome of blood deficiency. It is indeed not. A different diagnosis depend on the blood amount in a late period. We should not stick to only one judgement (treating all late periods without further classification). Late periods with a small amount of flow indicate cold, insufficient blood (blood deficiency). While late periods with a great quantity of flow means cold, superabundant blood (blood excess). The menstrual flow originates in the kidneys, and the blood of the five *zang* and six *fu* organs all infuse it. Therefore, when the menstruation blood comes, blood from all the meridians come and infuse it. When the menstruation blood flows, the door opens and it is so abrupt that there's not enough time to close the door. Blood from all meridians seizes the opportunity and flows out, while the blood loss will lead to deficiency.

Treatment: Dissipate cold and warm the meridians and replenish blood. We cannot say all patients with delayed menstruation have a deficiency syndrome. *Wēn Jīng Shè Xuě Tang* (温经摄血汤, Meridians Warming and Blood Controlling Decoction) is recommended.

大熟地（一两，九蒸）　　　　　白芍（一两，酒炒）

川芎（五钱，酒洗）　　　　　　白术（五钱，土炒）

柴胡（五分）　　　　　　　　　五味子（三分）

续断（一钱）　　　　　　　　　肉桂（五分，去粗，研）

shú dì (prepared rehmannia root), 1 *liang* (big ones, fully steamed)

bái sháo (white peony root), 1 *liang* (dry-fried with millet wine)

chuān xiōng, (Sichuan lovage root), 5 *qian* (washed with millet wine)

bái zhú (white atractylodes rhizome), 5 *qian* (dry-fried with earth)

chái hú (bupleurum), 5 *fen*

wǔ wèi zǐ, (Chinese magnolivine fruit), 3 *fen*

xù duàn, (himalayan teasel root), 1 *qian*

ròu guì, (cinnamon bark), 5 *fen* (ground)

水煎服。三剂而经调矣。此方大补肝、肾、脾之精与血。加肉桂以祛其寒，柴胡以解其郁，是补中有散，而散不耗气；补中有泄，而泄不损阴，所以补之有益，而温之收功。此调经之妙药也，而摄血之仙丹也。凡经来后期者，俱可用。倘元气不足，加人参一二钱亦可。

This formula is decocted in water and taken orally. After three *ji* is taken, the menstruation will be regulated. The formula may greatly tonify the essence and blood of the liver, kidney, and spleen. Add *ròu guì*, (肉桂，cinnamon bark) to expel cold, and *chái hú* (柴胡，bupleurum) to dispel melancholy. There is dispelling in tonification, and the dispelling will not consume qi. There is discharging in replenishment, and the discharging will not cause the impairment of yin. Both tonifying and warming can get a corresponding result. This is a magic formula for regulating menstruation and controlling blood. All patients with delayed menstruation may use it. If the patient has an insufficiency of primordial qi, *rén shēn*(人参，Ginseng 1 or 2 *liang*) may be added.

Chapter Fifteen
Irregular Menstruation

经水先后无定期

妇人有经来断续，或前或后无定期。人以为气血之虚也，谁知是肝气之郁结乎。夫经水出诸肾，而肝为肾之子，肝郁则肾亦郁矣。肾郁而气必不宣，前后之或断或续，正肾之或通或闭耳。或曰：肝气郁而肾气不应，未必至于如此。殊不知子母关切，子病而母必有顾复之情，肝郁而肾不无缱绻之谊，肝气之或开或闭，即肾气之或去或留，相因而致，又何疑焉。治法宜舒肝之郁，即开肾之郁也。肝肾之郁既开，而经水自有一定之期矣。方用定经汤。

Some women menstruate intermittently. Sometimes it comes earlier, and sometimes it is delayed. Interns think it is because of the deficiency of qi and blood. Actually, it is from the stagnation of liver qi. Menstruation comes from the kidneys, and the liver is the son organ of the kidneys. The stagnation of the liver qi will lead to the stagnation of the kidneys. The stagnation of kidneys will lead to the failure of qi to diffuse. The cause of the irregular menstruation (intermittently, short period, or long period) is that the kidneys are sometimes obstructed and sometimes are not. Some say it is because the liver qi is stagnated, and the kidneys do not cooperate with it.

When the son organ is sick, the mother organ must keep an eye on the son. When the liver qi is stagnated, the kidneys will indeed have mutual sympathy. The opening or closing of the liver qi is just the flowing or stagnation of the kidney qi.

Treatment: Disperse the stagnated liver qi, and expel the obstructed kidney qi. When the stagnation of the liver and kidneys is expelled, the menstruation will be regular. *Dìng Jīng Tāng* (定经汤, Menstruation Regulating Decoction) is recommended.

菟丝子（一两，酒炒）　　　　白芍（一两，酒炒）
当归（一两，酒洗）　　　　　大熟地（五钱，九蒸）

山药（五钱，炒）　　　　　　白茯苓（三钱）

芥穗（二钱，炒黑）　　　　　　柴胡（五分）

tù sī zǐ, (dodder seed), 1 *liang* (dry-fried with millet wine)

bái sháo (white peony root), 1 *liang* (dry-fried with millet wine)

dāng guī (Chinese angelica), 1 *liang* (washed with millet wine)

shú dì (prepared rehmannia root), 5 *qian* (big ones, fully steamed)

bái fú líng (poria), 3 *qian*

shān yào (common yam rhizome), 5 *qian* (dry-fried)

jiè suì (charred schizonepeta), 3 *qian*

chái hú (bupleurum), 5 *fen*

水煎服。二剂而经水净，四剂而经期定矣。此方舒肝肾之气，非通经之药也；补肝肾之精，非利水之品也。肝肾之气舒而精通，肝肾之精旺而水利。不治之治，正妙于治也。

The medicine is decocted with water and taken orally. If 2 *ji* is taken, the menstruation stops, and if 4 *ji* is taken, it turns regular. This formula may soothe the liver qi and kidney qi. It is not a medicine for inducing menstruation. It is for supplementing the liver and kidney essence and not for alleviating water retention. When the liver qi and kidney qi are unobstructed, the liver and kidney essence are flourishing, and the water metabolism is normal. It looks like this medicine is not for treating irregular menstruation, but it has quite a magical effect in regulating menstruation.

［以上调经三条，辨论明晰，立方微妙，但恐临时或有外感、内伤不能见效。有外感者宜加苏叶一钱，有内伤者宜加神曲二钱（炒），有因肉食积滞者再加东山楂肉二钱（炒），临症须酌用之。若肝气郁抑又当以逍遥散为主，有热加栀炭、丹皮，即加味逍遥散。］

[The above three chapters are for regulating menstruation and have a precise treatment plan according to syndrome differentiation. The formulas contain a delicate way of treatment. However, if a temporary occurrence of the disease is caused by an exogenous pathogenic factor or internal injury, it cannot produce the desired result. For diseases caused by exogenous pathogenic factors, add *sū yè* (苏叶, perilla leaf) 1 *qian*. For diseases caused by internal injury, add *shén qū* (神曲, medicated leaven) 2 *qian*. As for the patient with retention of meat food, add *shān zhā ròu* (山楂肉, Chinese hawthorn fruit) 2 *qian*. If the patient suffers from liver qi stagnation, we should use *Xiāo Yáo Sǎn* (逍遥散，Free Wanderer Powder) as the main ingredient. For the patient with heat, add *zhī tàn* (栀炭，charred gardenia) and *dān pí* (丹皮，tree peony bark) , that is, *Jiā Wèi Xiāo Yáo Sǎn* (加味逍遥散，Supplemented Free Wanderer Powder).]

Chapter Sixteen

Intermittent or Irregular Menstruation

经水数月一行

妇人有数月一行经者，每以为常，亦无或先或后之异，亦无或多或少之殊。人莫不以为异，而不知非异也。盖无病之人，气血两不亏损耳。夫气血既不亏损，何以数月而一行经也？妇人之中，亦有天生仙骨者，经水必一季一行。盖以季为数，而不以月为盈虚也。真气内藏，则坎中之真阳不损，倘加以炼形之法，一年之内，便易飞腾。无如世人不知，见经水不应月来，误认为病，妄用药饵，本无病而治之成病，是治反不如其不治也。山闻异人之教，特为阐扬，使世人见此等行经，不必妄行治疗，万勿疑为气血之不足，而轻一试也。虽然天生仙骨之妇人，世固不少。而嗜欲损夭之人，亦复甚多，又不可不立一疗救之方以辅之，方名助仙丹。

Some women have menstruation that only happens once every several months, neither earlier nor later, and with a constant flow. Interns all consider such cases abnormal. There is nothing abnormal. It may be seen in healthy persons without any deficiency of qi and blood. If there is no depletion or damage of qi and blood, why does it come only once every several months? For some healthy women, menstruation happens once every season. It is not related to the wax and wane of the moon. They have genuine qi and genuine yang maintained inside. Interns mistake it for a disease of some kind and use medicine in vain, resulting in more difficulties. Employing medicine cannot do better than no medicine. While some women damage their qi and blood by over-indulgence in sexual intercourse, it is necessary to design a formula to rescue them. The formula is called *Zhù Xiān Dan* (助仙丹, Immortal Assisting Pill).

白茯苓（五钱）	陈皮（五钱）
白术（三钱，土炒）	白芍（三钱，酒炒）
山药（三钱，炒）	菟丝子（二钱，酒炒）

杜仲（一钱，炒黑）　　　　　　甘草（一钱）

bái fú líng (poria), 5 *qian*

chén pí (aged tangerine peel), 5 *qian*

bái zhú (white atractylodes rhizome), 3 *qian* (dry-fried with earth)

bái sháo (white peony root), 3 *qian* (dry-fried with millet wine)

shān yào (common yam rhizome), 3 *qian* (dry-fried)

tù sī zǐ, (dodder seed), 2 *qian* (dry-fried with millet wine)

dù zhòng, (eucommia bark), 1 *qian* (charred)

gān cǎo (licorice root), 1 *qian*

河水煎服。四剂而仍如其旧，不可再服也。此方平补之中，实有妙理。健脾益肾而不滞，解郁清痰而不泄，不损天然之气血，便是调经之大法，何得用他药以冀通经哉！

This formula is decocted in water and taken orally. If the condition remains the same as before after four *ji* is taken, no more should be administered. This formula has a subtle mechanism in mild supplements indeed. It invigorates the spleen and benefits the kidney without bringing about stagnation. Resolving depression and clearing phlegm without resulting in drainage, not damaging natural qi and blood, it is an excellent method of regulating menstruation. No other medicine is needed to stimulate menstrual flow.

Chapter Seventeen

Recommencement of Menstruation in Older Women

年老经水复行

妇人有年五十外，或六、七十岁忽然行经者，或下紫血块、或如红血淋。人或谓老妇行经，是还少之象，谁知是血崩之渐乎。夫妇人至七七之外，天癸已竭，又不服济阴补阳之药，如何能精满化经，一如少妇。然经不宜行而行者，乃肝不藏、脾不统之故也。非精过泄而动命门之火，即气郁甚而发龙雷之炎，二火交发，而血乃奔矣，有似行经而实非经也。此等之症，非大补肝脾之气血，而血安能骤止。方用安老汤。

Some older women over 50 or even 60 to 70 years old can suddenly start menstruating again. Some may have a dark blood clot; others may have fresh blood dripping. Interns say older women having menstruation is the renewing of their youth. To our surprise, it is a sign of metrorrhagia. For women above 49 years of age, their tiangui (reproduction-stimulating essence) is exhausted. Without taking medicine to nourish yin and tonify yang, how can their essence be full enough to transform into menses the way a young woman does?

That the menstruation appears when it should not results from the liver failing to store blood and the spleen failing to contain it. It is caused either by the undue drainage of the essence, and the stirring of *mìng mén* fire (命门, gate of vitality) or the severe stagnation of qi transforms into inflammation. The two fires break out by turn so that blood runs frantically. It seems to be the flowing of menstruation, but it is not.

Treatment: In order to stop bleeding immediately, there is no other choice but to drastically tonify qi and blood of the liver and the spleen. The formula to use is *Ān Lǎo Tāng* (安老汤, The Decoction for Calming the Aged).

人参（一两）　　　　　　　黄芪（一两，生用）

大熟地（一两，九蒸）　　　白术（五钱，土炒）

当归（五钱，酒洗）　　　　山萸（五钱，蒸）

阿胶（一两，蛤粉炒）　　　黑芥穗（一钱）

甘草（一钱）　　　　　　　香附（五分，酒炒）

木耳炭（一钱）

rén shēn (ginseng), 1 *liang*

huáng qí (astragalus root), 1 *liang* (raw)

shú dì (prepared rehmannia root), 1 *liang* (big ones, fully steamed)

bái zhú (white atractylodes rhizome), 5 *qian* (dry-fried with earth)

dāng guī (Chinese angelica), 5 *qian* (washed with millet wine)

shān yú, (fructus corni), 5 *qian* (steamed)

ē jiāo (donkey-hide gelatin), 1 *liang* (dry-fried with clam shell powder)

hēi jiè suì, (charred fineleaf schizonepeta spike), 1 *qian*

gān cǎo (licorice root), 1 *qian*

xiāng fù (cyperus), 5 *fen* (dry-fried with millet wine)

mù ěr tān, (charred wood ear), 1 *qian*

水煎服。一剂减，二剂尤减，四剂全减，十剂愈。此方补益肝脾之气，气足自能生血而摄血。尤妙大补肾水，水足而肝气自舒，肝舒而脾自得养，肝藏之而脾统之，又安有泄漏者，又何虑其血崩哉！

This formula is decocted in water and taken orally. When one *ji* is taken, the bleeding is relieved; when the second *ji* is taken, the bleeding will have a more marked reduction; when the fourth *ji* is taken, the bleeding will stop; If ten *ji* is taken, the patient will have a full recovery. This formula supplements the qi of the liver and the spleen. Once qi is abundant, blood is naturally generated and contained. What is magic is its great supplementation of kidney water. Once water is abundant, liver qi is naturally soothed, and once the liver qi is soothed, the spleen naturally is nurtured. Since the liver plays the role of storing blood, and the spleen contains it, leakage cannot occur, and there is no need to worry about bleeding.

（加贯众炭一钱，研细末，以药冲服尤妙。）

[It is better to take the formula with 1 *qian* of finely ground *guàn zhòng tàn* (贯众炭, charred cyrtomii rhizome), brewed in it.]

Chapter Eighteen
Menstruation Comes Intermittently with Intermittent Pain

经水忽来忽断时疼时止

妇人有经水忽来忽断，时疼时止，寒热往来者。人以为血之凝也，谁知是肝气不舒乎。夫肝属木而藏血，最恶风寒。妇人当行经之际，腠理大开，适逢风之吹寒之袭，则肝气为之闭塞，而经水之道路亦随之而俱闭。由是腠理经络，各皆不宣，而寒热之作，由是而起。其气行于阳分则生热，其气行于阴分则生寒，然此犹感之轻者也。倘外感之风寒更甚，则内应之热气益深，往往有热入血室，而变为如狂之症。若但往来寒热，是风寒未甚而热未深耳。

For some women, their menstruation comes suddenly and ceases suddenly. Alternate attacks of chills and fever accompany it. People suppose that it is because of the coagulation of blood. It is actually due to the discomfort of the liver qi indeed. The liver belongs to the wood element and stores blood and is averse to wind and cold. During the period of menstruation, women's *cǒu lǐ* (striae and interstices of skin) are wide open. If the wind and cold happen to attack, the liver qi may be blocked, and thereupon the passageways of menstrual flow will be blocked. As a result, *cǒu lǐ* (striae and interstices of skin) and the meridians and collaterals all fail to diffuse. And then chills and fever arise. When the qi travels in the yang phase, heat is engendered. When it travels in the yin phase, cold is engendered. However, this is only a slight case of invasion. The more serious the external invasion of wind-cold is, the deeper the responding internal hot qi penetrates. Sometimes, the hot qi syndrome enters into the blood chamber and causes mania-like diseases. If there are only alternate chills and fever appearing, that means the wind-cold is not too serious, and heat has not penetrated deep.

治法宜补肝中之血，通其郁而散其风，则病随手而效。所谓治风先治血，血和风自灭。此其一也。方用加味四物汤。

Treatment: supplement blood in the liver, relieve depression, and disperse wind. In this way, the patient can recover soon. This is what is said "to treat wind, blood should be treated first, then the wind dies down of itself once blood is harmonized". *Jiā Wèi Sì Wù Tāng* (加味四物汤, Supplemented Four Substances Decoction) is recommended.

大熟地（一两，九蒸）　　　　白芍（五钱，酒炒）
当归（五钱，酒洗）　　　　　川芎（三钱，酒洗）
白术（五钱，土炒）　　　　　粉丹皮（三钱）
元胡（一钱，酒炒）　　　　　甘草（一钱）
柴胡（一钱）

shú dì (prepared rehmannia root), 1 *liang* (big ones, fully steamed)

bái sháo (white peony root), 5 *qian* (dry-fried with millet wine)

dāng guī (Chinese angelica), 5 *qian* (washed with millet wine)

chuān xiōng, (Sichuan lovage root), 3 *qian* (washed with millet wine)

bái zhú (white atractylodes rhizome), 5 *qian* (dry-fried with earth)

fěn dān pí (cortex moutan), 3 *qian*

yuán hú, (corydalis tuber), 1 *qian* (stir-fired with millet wine)

gān cǎo (licorice root), 1 *qian*

chái hú (thotowax root), 1 *qian*

水煎服。此方用四物以滋脾胃之阴血；用柴胡、白芍、丹皮以宣肝经之风郁；用甘草、白术、元胡以利腰脐而和腹疼，入于表里之间，通乎经络之内。用之得宜，自奏功如响也。

The formula is decocted in water and taken orally. This formula uses the Four ingredients: *dāng guī* (当归, Chinese angelica), *bái sháo* (白芍, white peony root), *Shú dì* (熟地, prepared rehmania root), *chuān xiōng* (川芎, Sichuan lovage root), to nourish the spleen and stomach's yin-blood. *Chái hú* (柴胡, bupleurum), *bái sháo* (白芍, white peony root), *dān pí* (丹皮, tree peony bark) are used to disperse the wind in the liver meridian. *Gān cǎo* (甘草, licorice root), *bái zhú* (白术, white atractylodes rhizome), *yuán hú*, (元胡, corydalis tuber) to strengthen the waist and the spine and relieve abdominal pain. This formula's efficacy works in both the exterior and interior and finds its way into both meridians and collaterals. If it is used appropriately, its effect will appear as quickly as an echo follows a sound.

【加荆芥穗（炒黑）一钱，尤妙。】

[Add *jīng jiè suì* (荆芥穗, fineleaf schizonepeta spike, slightly charred, 1 *qian* for a better effect.]

经水未来腹先疼

妇人有经前腹疼数日，而后经水行者，其经来多是紫黑块。人以为寒极而然也，谁知是热极而火不化乎。夫肝属木，其中有火，舒则通畅，郁则不扬。经欲行而肝不应，则抑拂其气而疼生。然经满则不能内藏，而肝中之郁火焚烧，内逼经出，则其火亦因之而怒泄。其紫黑者，水火两战之象也；其成块者，火煎成形之状也。经失其为经者，正郁火内夺其权耳。治法似宜大泄肝中之火。然泄肝之火，而不解肝之郁，则热之标可去，而热之本未除也，其何能益！方用宣郁通经汤。

Some women have abdominal pain several days ahead of menstruation, and then, the menstruation comes with many purple or black blood clots. Interns think it is due to extreme cold. In fact, it is because of the extreme heat, which leads to fire failing to be transmitted. The liver belongs to the wood element and gives birth to fire. So long as it is soothed, it will be unobstructed. When it is stagnated, the function of the liver qi becomes inactive. So it fails to respond when menstruation flow is about to start. Since the liver qi is burdened and inactive, pain is the result.

Jammed-up menstruation cannot be stored in the interior while stagnated fire in the liver is burning and forcing the menstruation to flow out. With the discharge of the menses, the fire drains out furiously. The dark purple color is a sign of the battle between water and fire. The forming of blood clots is due to the work of the scorching of fire. The abnormal menstruation is due to the stagnated fire struggling in the interior.

It seems that the treatment should be discharging fire in the liver meridian drastically. While if we solely discharge the fire in the liver and do not soothe the liver's stagnation, the heat manifestation can be removed, but the root cause of the heat cannot. So, in this case, the formula to use is *Xuān Yù Tōng Jīng Tāng* (宣郁通经汤, Depression Relieving and Menstruation Promoting Decoction).

白芍（五钱，酒炒）　　　　当归（五钱，酒洗）

丹皮（五钱）　　　　　　　山栀子（三钱，炒）

白芥子（二钱，炒，研）　　柴胡（一钱）

香附（一钱，酒炒）　　　　川郁金（一钱，醋炒）

黄芩（一钱，酒炒）　　　　生甘草（一钱）

bái sháo (white peony root), 5 *qian* (dry-fried with millet wine)

dāng guī (Chinese angelica), 5 *qian* (washed with millet wine)

dān pí (tree peony bark), 5 *qian*

shān zhī (gardenia), 3 *qian* (dry-fried)

bái jiè zǐ, white mustard seed, 2 *qian* (dry-fried and ground)

chái hú (bupleurum), 1 *qian*

xiāng fù (cyperus), 1 *qian* (dry-fried with millet wine)

yù jīn, turmeric root tuber, 1*qian* (dry-fried with vinegar)

huáng qín, scutellaria root, 1*qian* (dry-fried with millet wine)

shēng gān cǎo (fresh licorice root), 1 *qian* (raw)

水煎。连服四剂，下月断不先腹疼而后行经矣。此方补肝之血而解肝之郁，利肝之气而降肝之火，所以奏功之速。

The formula is decocted in water. If four *ji* is taken in succession, there will be no abdominal pain before the coming of menses. This formula supplements the liver blood, soothes the liver qi, and calms down the liver fire. It works swiftly.

Chapter Twenty

Menstruation Followed by Lower Abdominal Pain

行经后少腹疼痛

妇人有少腹疼于行经之后者，人以为气血之虚也，谁知是肾气之涸乎。夫经水者，乃天之真水也，满则溢而虚则闭，亦其常耳。何以虚能作疼哉？盖肾水一虚，则水不能生木，而肝木必克脾土，木土相争，则气必逆，故尔作疼。治法必须以舒肝气为主，而益之以补肾之味，则水足而肝气益安，肝气安而逆气自顺，又何疼痛之有哉！方用调肝汤。

Some women have lower abdominal pain after menstruation. Interns consider this to be a deficiency of qi and blood. In fact, it is due to the exhaustion of kidney qi. Menstruation flow is the genuine water that is a natural base of life. When it is full, it is always the case that it overflows outwardly, and when it is deficient, it stops (amenorrhea). So why would a deficient syndrome result in pain? The reason is that once the kidney (water) is insufficient, the water cannot generate wood. Then the liver (wood) is bound to restrain the spleen (earth). The struggle between wood and earth results in the counter-flow of qi. Thus, pain is produced.

The treatment should be to soothe liver qi as the basic idea and add some medicine to strengthen the kidneys. When water is made abundant, liver qi is boosted and becomes calm. As long as the liver qi is calm, the counter-flow of qi is automatically normalized. *Tiáo Gān Tāng* (调肝汤, Liver Regulating Decoction) is recommended.

山药（五钱，炒）	阿胶（三钱，白面炒）
当归（三钱，酒洗）	白芍（三钱，酒炒）
山萸肉（三钱，蒸熟）	巴戟（一钱，盐水浸）
甘草（一钱）	

shān yào (common yam rhizome), 5 *qian* (dry-fried)

ē jiāo (donkey-hide gelatin), 3 *qian* (dry-fried with wheat flour)

dāng guī (Chinese angelica), 3 *qian* (washed with millet wine)

bái sháo (white peony root), 3 *qian* (dry-fried with millet wine)

shān yú ròu, (fructus corni), 3 *qian* (steamed)

bā jǐ, (morinda root), 1 *qian* (soaked in salt water)

gān cǎo (licorice root), 1 *qian*

水煎服。此方平调肝气，既能转逆气，又善止郁疼。经后之症，以此方调理最佳。不特治经后腹疼之症也。

The formula is decocted in water and taken orally. This formula levels and regulates the liver qi in a tempered way. It can reverse qi counter-flow, and it is also good at relieving pain due to qi stagnation. It is an ideal formula to regulate post menstruation disorders, not a specific formula merely to treat post-menstrual pain.

（经前、经后腹痛二方极妙，不可加减。若有别症，亦宜此方为主，另加药味治之。原方不可减去一味。）

[This formula, along with *Xuān Yù Tōng Jīng Tāng* (宣郁通经汤, *Depression Relieving and Menstruation Promoting Decoction*) from chapter 19 for abdominal pain before and after menstruation, respectively, are quite miraculous and should not be modified. In case there are complications, these formulas should be used as a foundation, and then they can be supplemented with certain medicines. However, not one ingredient is allowed to be deleted from them.]

Chapter Twenty-one

Abdominal Pain and Vomiting of Blood Before Menstruation

经前腹疼吐血

妇人有经未行之前一二日忽然腹疼而吐血。人以为火热之极也，谁知是肝气之逆乎。夫肝之性最急，宜顺而不宜逆。顺则气安，逆则气动。血随气为行止，气安则血安，气动则血动，亦勿怪其然也。

Some women have sudden abdominal pain and vomit blood one or two days before menstruation. Interns consider it an extreme heat condition. Actually, it is due to the counter-flow of the liver qi. The liver is the most impetuous of all organs by nature. The flow of liver qi should be guided to its normal and should never be in counter-flow. When its flow is normal, qi is calm. If it counter-flows, qi is stirred up. Blood always acts in response to qi. When qi is calm, blood is calm. When qi is stirred up, so is blood. There is nothing strange about this correspondence.

或谓经逆在肾不在肝，何以随血妄行，竟至从口上出也，是肝不藏血之故乎？抑肾不纳气而然乎？殊不知少阴之火急如奔马，得肝火直冲而上，其势最捷，反经而为血，亦至便也，正不必肝不藏血，始成吐血之症，但此等吐血与各经之吐血有不同者。盖各经之吐血，由内伤而成；经逆而吐血，乃内溢而激之使然也。其症有绝异，而其气逆则一也。

Some interns ascribe the counter-flow of menses to the kidney rather than the liver. How can it flow with blood in such a reckless way that it eventually comes out from the mouth? Is it because the liver fails to store blood? Or, is it because the kidneys fail to control respiring qi? It is hardly imaginable that the pestilence fire in the *shaoyin* meridian is impetuous like a galloping horse. It can surge straight up once aided by liver fire. It moves so forcefully that it is relatively easy for it to reverse the flow of menses and cause blood vomiting. The liver does not need to fail in storing blood to cause the symptom of vomiting blood. However, this type of vomiting blood is different from that of other meridians due to internal injury. Vomiting of blood is caused by menstrual counter-flow results from the provocation of internal spillage. Their syndromes may differ significantly, while their symptom of qi counter-flow is the same.

治法似宜平肝以顺气，而不必益精以补肾矣。虽然经逆而吐血，虽不大损夫血，而反复颠倒，未免太伤肾气，必须于补肾之中，用顺气之法，始为得当。方用顺经汤。

Treatment: Calm and sooth liver qi. Move qi downward.

It is not necessary to nourish yin to strengthen kidneys. Blood vomiting caused by menstrual blood counter-flow, although it does not incur blood loss in large amounts, would probably cause severe damage to the kidneys due to repeated reversion of the menses. The only appropriate method is to guide the flow of qi downward during the process of strengthening kidneys. The formula to use is *Shùn Jīng Tāng* (顺经汤, Menses Normalizing Decoction).

当归（五钱，酒洗）　　　大熟地（五钱，九蒸）
白芍（二钱，酒炒）　　　丹皮（五钱）
白茯苓（三钱）　　　　　沙参（三钱）
黑芥穗（三钱）

dāng guī (Chinese angelica), 5 *qian* (washed with millet wine)

shú dì (prepared rehmannia root), 5 *qian* (fully steamed)

bái sháo (white peony root), 2 *qian* (dry-fried with millet wine)

dān pí (tree peony bark), 5 *qian*

bái fú líng (poria), 3 *qian*

shā shēn, (radix adenophorae seu glehniae), 3 *qian*

hēi jiè suì (charred schizonepeta), 3 *qian*

水煎服。一剂而吐血止，二剂而经顺，十剂不再发。此方于补肾调经之中，而用引血归经之品，是和血之法，实寓顺气之法也。肝不逆而肾气自顺，肾气既顺，又何经逆之有哉！

The formula is decocted in water and taken orally. When one *ji* is taken, vomiting of blood ceases; if the second *ji* is taken, the menses is normalized. After 10 *ji* is taken, relapse will not happen. In this formula for strengthening kidney and regulation menses, medicines for inducing blood to return to meridians are used. The method of guiding qi is contained in the method of regulating blood. When the liver (qi) is not counter-flowing, the kidney qi would naturally be smooth.

（妇人年壮吐血往往有之，不可作劳症治。若认为劳症，必至肝气愈逆，非劳反成劳矣。方加茜草一钱，怀牛膝八分尤妙。）

[Vomiting of blood is often seen in women in the prime of life. It should not be treated as a consumption syndrome. Otherwise, the counter-flow of liver qi will be bound to get worse, and, consequently, what began not as a consumption syndrome will become one. It is better if 1 *qian* of *qiàn cǎo* (茜草 , india madder root) and 8 *fen* of *huái niú xī* (怀牛膝 , two-toothed achyranthes root) are added to this formula.]

Chapter Twenty-two

Aching and Pain Below the Navel Before the Period Is About to Come

经水将来脐下先疼痛

　　妇人有经水将来三五日前而脐下作疼，状如刀刺者，或寒热交作，所下如黑豆汁，人莫不以为血热之极，谁知是下焦寒湿相争之故乎。夫寒湿乃邪气也。妇人有冲任之脉，居于下焦。冲为血海，任主胞胎，为血室，均喜正气相通，最恶邪气相犯。经水由二经而外出，而寒湿满二经而内乱，两相争而作疼痛，邪愈盛而正气日衰。寒气生浊，而下如豆汁之黑者，见北方寒水之象也。治法利其湿而温其寒，使冲任无邪气之乱，脐下自无疼痛之疚矣。方用温脐化湿汤。

　　Some women have aching below their navel 3~5 days before their period is about to come. The pain feels like a puncture wound, or there may be alternating fever and chills with the menstrual flow, which looks like black soybean juice. Interns suppose this is due to extreme blood heat. In fact, this is due to the struggle between cold and dampness in the lower *jiao*. Cold and dampness are both evil qi (pathogenic qi). Women have *chong mai* and *ren mai* in the lower *jiao*. *Chong mai* is the sea of blood, while *ren mai*, which governs *baotai* (fetus), and it is *xueshi* (blood chamber). These two vessels both like or desire the free flow of healthy qi but hate the invasion of evil qi. Menstruation blood comes from the two vessels. If cold and dampness fill them and cause an internal disorder, the struggle between these two evils provokes pain. As the evils become more and more vigorous, the healthy qi becomes feebler day by day. Cold qi engenders turbidity. Like black soybean juice, the black discharge is a sign of cold water in the north (it refers to the kidneys).

　　Treatment: remove the dampness and warm the cold to eliminate the disturbing evil qi from *chong mai* and *ren mai*. In this way, the aching and pain below the navel is relieved. The formula to use is *Wēn Qì Huà Shī Tāng* (温脐化湿汤，Navel Warming and Dampness Dispelling Decoction).

白术（一两，土炒）　　　白茯苓（三钱）

山药（五钱，炒）　　　　巴戟肉（五钱，盐水浸）

扁豆（炒，捣，三钱）　　　白果（十枚，捣碎）

建莲子（三十枚，不去心）

bái zhú (white atractylodes rhizome), 1 *liang* (stirred with earth)

bái fú líng (poria), 3 *qian*

shān yào (common yam rhizome), 5 *qian* (dry-fried)

bā jǐ ròu, (morinda root), 5 *qian* (soaked in salt water)

biǎn dòu, (hyacinth bean), 3 *qian* (dry-fried, pounded)

bái guǒ (ginkgo nut), 10 pieces (pounded)

lián zǐ, (lotus seed), 30 pieces (plumules preserved, produced in Fujian Province)

水煎服。然必须经未来前十日服之。四剂而邪气去，经水调，兼可种子。此方君白术以利腰脐之气，用巴戟、白果以通任脉；扁豆、山药、莲子以卫冲脉，所以寒湿扫除而经水自调，可受妊矣。倘疑腹疼为热疾，妄用寒凉，则冲任虚冷，血海变为冰海，血室反成冰室，无论难于生育，而疼痛之止，又安有日哉！

（冲任之气宜通不宜降，故化湿不用苍术、薏仁。余宜类参。）

The formula is decocted in water and taken orally. It should be administered ten days before menstruation. When four *ji* is taken, the evil qi will be dispelled, the menses will be regulated, and conception will become possible. This formula uses *bái zhú* (白术, white atractylodes rhizome) as the ruler to disinhibit the qi of the waist and navel. It uses *bā jǐ ròu*, (巴戟肉, morinda root) and *bái guǒ* (白果, ginkgo nut) to free the flow of *ren mai*. It uses *biǎn dòu*, (扁豆, hyacinth bean), *shān yào* (山药, common yam rhizome), and *lián zǐ*, (莲子, lotus seed) to protect *chong mai*. Thus, cold and dampness are dispelled, and menstruation is automatically regulated to make conception possible. If this abdominal pain is mistaken for a heat syndrome and cool and cold medicines are utilized in haste, then *chong mai* and *ren mai* will be deficient and cold. The blood sea turns into an icy sea, and the blood chamber becomes an icy chamber. Pregnancy would be hardly possible, and the relieving of the pain would be far away.

[As for the qi of *chong mai* and *ren mai*, it is proper to use flow-freeing but not down bearing medicines. Therefore, *cāng zhú* (苍术, atractylodes rhizome) and *yì rén* (薏仁, coix seed) are not used to transform dampness. This should also be taken into consideration in similar cases.]

经水过多

　　妇人有经水过多，行后复行，面色萎黄，身体倦怠，而困乏愈甚者。人以为血热有余之故，谁知是血虚而不归经乎。夫血旺始经多，血虚当经缩，今日血虚而反多经，是何言与？

Some women have a menstrual flow that is excessive in amount, which has one period following in the wake of another, with a sallow yellow facial complexion, generalized fatigue, and deep languor. Interns suppose this is due to heat and the surplus of blood. In fact, it is due to blood deficiency and blood failing to return to the meridians. Only when blood is abundant should the menses come in large quantity, and when blood is deficient, the menses should dwindle. While here, on the contrary, menstrual flow is said to be abundant due to blood deficiency. How can this be?

　　殊不知血归于经，虽旺而经亦不多；血不归经，虽衰而经亦不少。世之人见经水过多，谓是血之旺也，此治之所以多错耳。倘经多果是血旺，自是健壮之体，须当一行即止，精力如常，何至一行后而再行，而困乏无力耶？惟经多是血之虚，故再行而不胜其困乏，血损精散，骨中髓空，所以不能色华于面也。治法宜大补血而引之归经，又安有行后复行之病哉！方用加减四物汤。

As we all know, if blood returns to the meridians, even if it is abundant, the menses does not increase. However, if the blood fails to circulate in the vessels, even if it is feeble, menses does not decrease. Interns nowadays attribute excessive menstrual flow to abundant blood. This results in a failed treatment. If the excessive menstrual flow is due to blood effulgence, the constitution should undoubtedly be healthy, and the menstrual flow would come to an apparent stop in due course. Subsequently, the energy would be usual. What makes one period follow in the wake of another, and what results in the fatigue and languor? The only explanation is that excessive menstrual flow is due to blood deficiency. Therefore, menstruation occurs time and again, and the patient becomes weak and feels exceptionally fatigued. As large amounts of blood are lost, the essence is dispersed, marrow becomes vacuous in the bones, and luster cannot appear on the face.

Treatment: supplement blood greatly and guide it back to the meridians. This treatment will resolve the problem of one period persistently following another. The formula to use is *Jiā Jiǎn Sì Wù Tāng* (加减四物汤, Four Substances Variant Decoction).

大熟地（一两，九蒸）　　　白芍（三钱，酒炒）

当归（五钱，酒洗）　　　　川芎（二钱，酒洗）

白术（五钱，土炒）　　　　黑芥穗（三钱）

山萸（三钱，蒸）　　　　　续断（一钱）

甘草（一钱）

shú dì (prepared rehmannia root), 1 *liang* (big ones, fully steamed)

bái sháo (white peony root), 3 *qian* (dry-fried with millet wine)

dāng guī (Chinese angelica), 5 *qian* (washed with millet wine)

chuān xiōng, (Sichuan lovage root), 2 *qian* (washed with millet wine)

bái zhú (white atractylodes rhizome), 5 *qian* (dry-fried with earth)

hēi jiè suì (charred fineleaf schizonepeta spike), 3 *qian*

shān yú, (fructus corni), 3 *qian* (streamed)

xù duàn, (himalayan teasel root), 1 *qian*

gān cǎo (licorice root), 1 *qian*

水煎服。四剂而血归经矣。十剂之后，加人参三钱，再服十剂，下月行经，适可而止矣。夫四物汤乃补血之神品。加白术、荆芥，补中有利；加山萸、续断，止中有行；加甘草以调和诸品，使之各得其宜。所以血足而归经，归经而血自静矣。

This formula is decocted in water and taken orally. If four *ji* is taken, the blood will return to the vessels. After ten *ji* is taken, add *rén shēn* (人参, ginseng) 3 *qian* and administer ten more *ji*. Then the next menstruation flow will stop in due time. *Sì Wù Tāng* (Four Substances Decoction) is the medicine for nourishing blood and has a magic effect. Add *bái zhú* (白术, white atractylodes rhizome) and *jīng jiè* (荆芥, schizonepeta), and the formula will have the function of soothing and nourishment. Add *shān yú*, (山萸, fructus corni) and *xù duàn*, (续断, himalayan teasel root), and it will have the function of promoting circulation and stopping the menstrual flow. Add *gān cǎo* (甘草, licorice root) to harmonize all herbs and help them play their roles. Thus, blood is made abundant and returns to the vessels, and when it returns to the vessels, it will be at peace.

（荆芥穗炭能引血归经。方妙极，不可轻易加减。）

[*Jīng jiè suì tàn* (荆芥穗炭, charred fineleaf schizonepeta spike) has the function of guiding blood to the vessels. This formula is quite marvelous and should not be modified without careful consideration.]

Chapter Twenty-four

Watery Discharge Prior to Menstruation

经前泄水

妇人有经未来之前，泄水三日，而后行经者。人以为血旺之故，谁知是脾气之虚乎。夫脾统血，脾虚则不能摄血矣。且脾属湿土，脾虚则土不实，土不实而湿更甚，所以经水将动，而脾先不固。脾经所统之血，欲流注于血海，而湿气乘之，所以先泄水而后行经也。调经之法，不在先治其水，而在先治其血。抑不在先治其血，而在先补其气。盖气旺而血自能生，抑气旺而湿自能除，且气旺而经自能调矣。方用健固汤。

Some women have three days of watery discharge preceding their menstrual flow. Interns consider it effulgent blood. In fact, it is spleen qi deficiency. The spleen governs the blood. When it is deficient, it is no longer able to contain the blood.

Furthermore, as the spleen belongs to the Earth element, when it becomes deficient, the earth becomes not secure (not solid). Conversely, when earth is not secure, dampness becomes more serious. Suppose spleen becomes insecure before the menstrual flow starts. In that case, blood, which is governed by spleen meridian and is about to pour into the sea of blood, is overwhelmed by dampness and, therefore, the menstrual flow is preceded by a watery discharge.

Treatment: The method of regulating menstruation does not give priority to the treatment of water but to that of blood. Alternatively, it does not give priority to the treatment of blood but to the supplement of qi. It is because when qi is effulgent, blood will be naturally be engendered. On the other hand, when qi is effulgent, dampness will be naturally eliminated. Furthermore, when qi is effulgent, the menses will be restored to normal by itself. The formula to use is *Jiàn Gù Tāng* (健固汤，Strengthening and Consolidating Decoction).

人参（五钱）　　　　　　白茯苓（三钱）
白术（一两，土炒）　　　巴戟（五钱，盐水浸）

薏苡仁（三钱，炒）

rén shēn (ginseng), 5 *qian*

bái fú líng (poria), 3 *qian*

bái zhú (white atractylodes rhizome), 1 *liang*(dry-fried with earth)

bā jǐ, (morinda root), 5 *qian* (soaked in salt water)

yì yǐ rén, (coix seed), 3 *qian* (dry-fried)

水煎。连服十剂，经前不泄水矣。此方补脾气以固脾血，则血摄于气之中，脾气日盛，自能运化其湿，湿既化为乌有，自然经水调和，又何至经前泄水哉。

This formula is decocted in water. After 10 *ji* is taken in succession, water will no longer be discharged before menstruation. This formula supplements the spleen qi to secure the spleen blood. The blood is contained within qi, and spleen qi gradually becomes exuberant; it regains its ability to transport and transform dampness. When dampness is reduced to naught, menstruation will naturally be regulated and harmonized.

经前大便下血

　　妇人有行经之前一日大便先出血者。人以为血崩之症，谁知是经流于大肠乎。夫大肠与行经之路，各有分别，何以能入乎其中？不知胞胎之系，上通心而下通肾，心肾不交，则胞胎之血两无所归，而心肾二经之气不来照摄，听其自便，所以血不走小肠而走大肠也。治法若单止大肠之血，则愈止而愈多。若击动三焦之气，则更拂乱而不可止。盖经水之妄行，原因心肾之不交，今不使水火之既济，而徒治其胞胎，则胞胎之气无所归，而血安有归经之日？故必大补其心与肾，使心肾之气交，而胞胎之气自不散，则大肠之血自不妄行，而经自顺矣。方用顺经两安汤。

　　Some women have blood in their stool one day before menstruation. Interns suppose that is metrorrhagia. In fact, it is the menses flowing into the large intestine. Since the menstrual flow takes a different route from that of the stool, how can it enter the large intestine? The uterus communicates with the heart above and the kidneys below. If there is disharmony between the heart and the kidney, the blood in the *bāo tāi* (uterus) can return to neither of them, and the qi of the heart and kidney meridians stop warming and controlling the blood and letting it flow free. Consequently, blood runs into the large intestine instead of the small intestine.

　　If the treatment were to stop the bleeding in the large intestine solely, then the more that is done to stop bleeding, the more bleeding would be seen. If the qi of *sanjiao* is hit and stirred, blood will be more seriously disturbed and impossible to stop. This reckless wandering of the menstrual flow results from the disharmony between the heart and kidneys. If no effort is made to coordinate water (kidneys) and fire (heart) but merely treat the *bāo tāi* (uterus), which makes the qi of the *bāo tāi* (uterus) have no place to stay, how can blood return to the menses?

　　So, the heart and kidneys should be significantly supplemented to restore the harmony between the heart and kidneys' qi. When this is done, the *bāo taī* (uterus) qi will no longer disperse, and the blood in the large intestine will not move recklessly. Menstruation will be restored to normal naturally. The formula to use is *Shùn Jīng liǎng ān Tang* (顺经两安汤 Menstruation Normalizing and Heart and Kidneys Calming Decoction).

当归（五钱，酒洗）　　　　　白芍（五钱，酒炒）
大熟地（五钱，九蒸）　　　　山萸肉（二钱，蒸）
人参（三钱）　　　　　　　　白术（五钱，土炒）
麦冬（五钱，去心）　　　　　黑芥穗（二钱）
巴戟肉（一钱，盐水浸）　　　升麻（四分）

dāng guī (Chinese angelica), 5 *qian* (washed with millet wine)

bái sháo (white peony root), 5 *qian* (dry-fried with millet wine)

shú dì (prepared rehmannia root), 5 *qian* (big ones, fully steamed)

shān yú ròu, (fructus corni), 2 *qian* (steamed)

rén shēn (ginseng), 3 *qian*

bái zhú (white atractylodes rhizome), 5 *qian* (dry-fried with earth)

mài dōng, (dwarf lilyturf tuber), 5 *qian* (pith discarded)

hēi jiè suì (charred fineleaf schizonepeta spike), 2 *qian*

bā jǐ ròu, (morinda root), 1 *qian* (soaked in salt water)

shēng má, (black cohosh rhizome), 4 *fen*

水煎服。二剂大肠血止，而经从前阴出矣；三剂经止，而兼可受妊矣。此方乃大补心、肝、肾三经之药，全不去顾胞胎，而胞胎有所归者，以心肾之气交也。盖心肾虚则其气两分，心肾足则其气两合。心与肾不离，而胞胎之气听命于二经之摄，又安有妄动之形哉。然则心肾不交，补心肾可也，又何兼补夫肝木耶？不知肝乃肾之子、心之母也，补肝则肝气往来于心肾之间，自然上引心而下入于肾，下引肾而上入于心，不啻介绍之助也。此便心肾相交之一大法门，不特调经而然也，学者其深思诸。

Decoct in water and take orally. When two *ji* is taken, the large intestine bleeding is stopped, and the menstrual flow is led out from the external genitalia. After three *ji* is taken, the menstrual flow is stopped, and conception is possible. This formula dramatically supplements the three meridians of the heart, liver and kidneys with no care for the *bāo taī* (uterus). The *bāo taī* now finds somewhere to return the menses because the heart and kidneys regain harmony. When the heart and kidneys are deficient, their qi separates. When they are healthy, their qi unites with each other. The heart and kidneys are closely linked, and these two meridians govern the qi of *bāo taī*.

How can it behave recklessly? It is understandable to supplement the heart and kidneys in case of disharmony between the heart and kidneys. However, why is it necessary to simultaneously supplement the liver (wood)? The liver is the child organ of the kidney and the mother organ of the heart as well. When the liver is supplemented, its qi travels to and from between the heart and kidneys. It naturally goes up to conduct the heart qi down to the kidneys and goes down to guide kidney qi up to the heart. It serves as an intermediary. This is an essential method for restoring the coordination between the heart and kidneys. It is not limited to the regulation of menstruation. Students should have a serious reflection on it.

【若大便下血过多，精神短少，人愈消瘦，必系肝气不舒，久郁伤脾，脾伤不能统血又当分别治之。方用补血汤，嫩黄芪二两（生熟各半），归身四钱（酒洗，炒黑），杭芍炭二钱，焦白术五钱（土炒），杜仲二钱（炒断丝），荆芥炭二钱，姜炭二钱，引用贯仲炭一钱冲入服之，四剂必获愈，愈后减半再服二剂。经入大肠，必当行经之际而大便下血也，初病血虽错行，精神必照常，若脾不统血，精神即不能照常矣。用者辨之。】

[If there is excessive blood in the stool, and the patient feels slouchy and looks emaciated day by day, it must be due to stagnation of hepatic (liver) qi. Long time stagnation, in turn, damages the spleen, and the damaged spleen fails to govern blood. This requires a different treatment. *Bǔ Xuè Tāng* (补血汤, Blood Supplementing Decoction) is recommended.

huáng qí (astragalus root), 2 *liang* (half raw and half prepared)

dāng guī (Chinese angelica), 4 *qian* (washed with millet wine, charred)

bái sháo tàn (charred white peony root), 2 *qian*

bái zhú (white atractylodes rhizome), 5 *qian* (dry-fried with earth)

dù zhòng, (eucommia bark), 2 *qian* (dry-fried till the fibers break off)

jīng jiè tàn, (charred schizonepeta), 2 *qian*

Jiāng tàn, (prepared dried ginger), 2 *qian*

The formula is taken with *guàn zhòng tàn*, (贯仲炭, charred cyrtomii rhizoma) 1 *qian* as a guider. When four *ji* is taken, the patient will surely recover. After recovery, reduce the amount to half and administer two more *ji*. Trespassing of blood into the large intestine invariably happens during the menstrual period. At the initial stage, the patient's essence-spirit remains normal. However, failure of the spleen to govern blood must result in abnormal essence-spirit. This should be distinguished.]

年未老经水断

经云：女子七七而天癸绝。有年未至七七而经水先断者。人以为血枯经闭也，谁知是心肝脾之气郁乎。使其血枯，安能久延于人世。医见其经水不行，妄谓之血枯耳。其实费血之枯，乃经之闭也。且经原非血也，乃天一之水，出自肾中，是至阴之精而有至阳之气，故其色赤红似血，而实非血，所以谓之天癸。世人以经为血，此千古之误，牢不可破。倘果是血，何不名之曰血水，而曰经水乎！经水之名者，原以水出于肾，乃癸干之化，故以名之。无如世人沿袭而不深思其旨，皆以血视之。

Huáng Dì Nèi Jīng (黄帝内经, *The Yellow Emperor's Inner Classic*) states: "Females, at the age around 49 (7 times 7), the *tiān guǐ* (reproduction-stimulating essence) is exhausted." However, there are cases of menopause under the age of 49.

People suppose this is amenorrhea due to blood exhaustion. Actually, it is the qi stagnation of the heart, liver, and spleen. How could life be sustained for a long time in the case of blood exhaustion? Some interns diagnose it arbitrarily as blood exhaustion whenever they encounter menopause. In fact, it is menopause rather than the exhaustion of blood.

What is more, the menstruation is not blood but heavenly water or the *tiān guǐ* (reproduction-stimulating essence). Originated in the kidneys, it is the essence of extreme yin that contains the qi of extreme yang. Therefore, it is red like blood but not blood at all. It is called *tiān guǐ* (reproduction-stimulating essence). Interns mistakenly take it as blood. This is an incorrect assumption for one thousand years. If it were blood, it would be named *Xuè Shuǐ* (blood flow) rather than *Jīng Shuǐ* (menstrual flow). The name for *Jīng Shuǐ* (menstrual flow), is derived from the belief that it comes from the kidneys and is transformed by one of the ten heavenly stems called *guǐ*. It is nothing more than the fact that people accept conventional ideas without considering the profound implications and look upon menstruation as blood.

然则经水早断，似乎肾水衰涸，吾以为心肝脾气之郁者。盖以肾水之生，原不由于心肝脾；而肾水之化，实有关于心肝脾。使水位之下无土气以承之，则水滥灭火，肾气不能化；火位之下无水气以承之，则火炎铄金，肾气无所生；木位之下无金气以承之，则木妄破土，肾气无以成。倘心肝脾有一经之郁，则其气不能入于肾中，肾之气即郁而不宣矣。况心肝脾俱郁，即肾气真足而无亏，尚有茹而难吐之势。矧肾气本虚，又何能盈满而化经水外泄耶！

While it seems that premature menopause is due to the debilitation and exhaustion of kidney (water), I believe that is because of the qi stagnation of the heart, liver, and kidneys. Kidney (water) is not generated from the heart, liver, and kidneys, while kidney (water) transformation is of importance with these three organs. If there is no earth qi to control water from beneath, water will flood over to extinguish fire, and kidney qi will be unable to transform. If there is no water qi to control fire from beneath, flaming Fire will burn and melt metal, and kidney qi will have no place to be generated. If there is no metal qi to control wood from beneath, wood will become wild to break earth, and kidney qi cannot be generated. If there is stagnation of any one of the meridians in the heart, liver, and spleen, their qi cannot enter the kidneys, and the kidney qi will be stagnated and fail to diffuse. If qi stagnation happens in all the heart, liver, and spleen meridians, even if the kidney qi is sufficient, it would be in a predicament similar to a lump stuck in the throat (in which case, it is difficult to spit out what is taken in). Moreover, if kidney qi is deficient, how can it be brimful and transformed into menstrual flow and discharge?

经曰：亢则害。此之谓也。此经之所以闭塞，有似乎血枯，而实非血枯耳。治法必须散心肝脾之郁，而大补其肾水，仍大补其心肝脾之气，则精溢而经水自通矣。方用益经汤。

This is what is implied in *Huáng Dì Nèi Jīng* (黄帝内经, *The Yellow Emperor's Inner Classic*), that "hyperactivity is harmful." This is why amenorrhea seems due to blood exhaustion, but, practically speaking, it is not.

Treatment: Dissipate depression of the heart, liver, and spleen and greatly supplement kidney (water). To supplement kidney (water) significantly is to supplement the heart, liver, and spleen qi. As a result, the essence will be full enough to spill, and the menses will recover its free flow naturally. *Yì Jīng Tāng* (益经汤, Menses Nourishing Decoction) is recommended.

大熟地（一两，九蒸）　　　白术（一两，土炒）

山药（五钱，炒）　　　　　当归（五钱，酒洗）

白芍（三钱，酒炒）　　　　生枣仁（三钱，捣碎）

丹皮（二钱）　　　　　　　沙参（三钱）

柴胡（一钱）　　　　　　　杜仲（一钱，炒黑）

人参（二钱）

shú dì (prepared rehmannia root), 1 *liang* (big ones, fully steamed)

bái zhú (white atractylodes rhizome), 1 *liang* (dry-fried with earth)

dāng guī (Chinese angelica), 5 *qian* (washed with millet wine)

bái sháo (white peony root), 3 *qian* (dry-fried with millet wine)

zǎo rén, (spiney date seed), 3 *qian* (raw, pounded)

dān pí (tree peony bark), 2 *qian*

shā shēn, (radix adenophorae seu glehniae), 3*qian*

chái hú (bupleurum), 1 *qian*

dù zhòng, (eucommia bark), 1 *qian* (charred)

rén shēn (ginseng), 2 *qian*

水煎。连服八剂而经通矣，服三十剂而经不再闭，兼可受孕。此方心肝脾肾四经同治药也。妙在补以通之，散以开之。倘徒补则郁不开而生火，徒散则气益衰而耗精。设或用攻坚之剂，辛热之品，则非徒无益而又害之矣。

This formula is decocted in water and taken orally. When 8 *ji* is taken in succession, the menstruation will recover its free flow. After thirty *ji* is taken, the menstrual block will disappear, making conception possible as well. This formula treats the meridians of the heart, liver, spleen and kidneys simultaneously. Its subtlety lies in freeing the flow of supplementation and opening (stagnation) through dissipation. If only supplementation were applied, stagnation would not be removed but instead would engender fire. If only dissipating were employed, qi would become more debilitated and essence more consumed. Medicines for attacking hardness or herbs pungent in taste and heat in nature would bring no good but harm.

Volume Four

Promoting Conception

种子

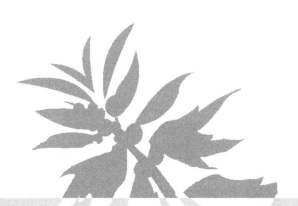

Chapter Twenty-seven
Infertility Due to Emaciation

身瘦不孕

妇人有瘦怯身躯，久不孕育，一交男子，即卧病终朝。人以为气虚之故，谁知是血虚之故乎。或谓血藏于肝，精涵于肾，交感乃泄肾之精，与血虚何与？殊不知肝气不开，则精不能泄，肾精既泄，则肝气亦不能舒。以肾为肝之母，母既泄精，不能分润以养其子，则木燥乏水，而火且暗动以铄精，则肾愈虚矣。况瘦人多火，而又泄其精，则水益少而火益炽，水虽制火，而肾精空乏，无力以济，成火在水上之卦，所以倦怠而卧也。此等之妇，偏易动火。然此火因贪欲而出于肝木之中，又是偏燥之火，绝非真火也。且不交合则已，交合又偏易走泄，此阴虚火旺不能受孕。即偶尔受孕，必致逼干男子之精，随种而随消者有之。治法必须大补肾水而平肝木，水旺则血旺，血旺则火消，便成水在火上之卦。方用养精种玉汤。

Some women, who are extremely thin and unable to conceive a child for a long time, will be ill in bed for a long time once they have sexual intercourse. Interns consider it due to qi deficiency. Actually, it is a result of blood deficiency. Some interns would ask: "Blood is stored in the liver. The essence is stored in the kidneys. Sexual intercourse is the emission of kidney essence. Is there any relationship between infertility and blood deficiency?" If the liver qi is not soothed, the essence can not be emitted. However, if the kidney essence has been emitted, the liver qi is still not soothed. As the kidney is the mother organ of the liver, the mother organ has already emitted its essence and cannot nourish its child organ. This leads to Wood's dryness, and then the essence is condensed by fire, and is stirred quietly.

Moreover, the kidney would be more deficient. Also, thin people are more likely to have an exuberance of fire. In this case, when the essence has been emitted, it leads to less water and more flaming of fire. Although water may restrain fire, the kidney essence has been destitute and cannot assist in restraining. The hexagram image* of fire above water is formed. So the patient feels lassitude and stays in bed.

If they have sexual intercourse, it causes fire from liver wood to be stirred up easily. It belongs to the dryness of fire and is by no means genuine fire. If there is no sexual intercourse, it could stay normal. Once having intercourse, the fire would tend to leak out. This would also lead to infertility caused by blazing fire due to yin deficiency. Even if the woman has a chance of pregnancy, the sperm would be condensed and dried, and the amphicytula cannot survive.

Treatment: supplement the kidney water greatly, and calm the liver wood. When the water is abundant, the blood will be exuberant. When the blood is exuberant, the fire would burn itself out. It will turn into the hexagram image* of water being above fire. The formula to use is *Yǎng Jīng zhòng yù Tāng* (养精种玉汤, Essence Nourishing and Fertilization Improving Decoction).

大熟地（一两，九蒸）　　　　当归（五钱，酒洗）
白芍（五钱，酒洗）　　　　　山萸肉（五钱，蒸熟）

shú dì (prepared rehmannia root), 1 *liang* (big ones, fully steamed)

dāng guī (Chinese angelica), 5 *qian* (washed with millet wine)

bái sháo (white peony root), 5 *qian* (washed with millet wine)

shān yú ròu, (fructus corni), 5 *qian* (steamed)

水煎服。三月便可身健受孕，断可种子。此方之用，不特补血而纯于填精，精满则子宫易于摄精，血足则子宫易于容物，皆有子之道也。惟是贪欲者多，节欲者少，往往不验。服此者果能节欲三月，心静神清，自无不孕之理。否则不过身体健壮而已，勿咎方之不灵也。

The formula is decocted in water and taken orally. If it is taken for three months, the woman will be in good condition and get pregnant. This formula aims to nourishing essence instead of supplementing blood. When the essence is full, the uterus is capable of controlling essence. Furthermore, when the blood is abundant, the uterus will be able to contain an embryo. These are the principles of pregnancy. Unfortunately, more people are addicted to sexual intercourse, and fewer people consider abstinence, which often makes this formula not efficacious. If people who take this formula can stay abstinent for three months, keep a calm and quiet mind, there is no possibility for infertility. If they cannot, they can only try to build a healthy body but cannot say that the formula does not work.

服药三月后不受孕，仍照原方加杜仲二钱（炒断丝），续断二钱，白术五钱

（土炒焦），云苓三钱，服数剂后必受孕。

If the patient can not get pregnant after taking this formula for three months, add the following herbs to the original formula: *dù zhòng*, (杜仲, eucommia bark), 2 *qian* (dry-fried to have the hair off); *xù duàn*, (续断, himalayan teasel root), 2 *qian*; *bái zhú* (白术, white atractylodes rhizome), 5 *qian* (dry-fried with earth until scorched); *yún líng* (云苓; poria), 3 *qian*.

Taking it for a few days, the patient can get pregnant without failure.

*

Hexagram image, recorded in, *Yì Jīng* (易经, *The Book of Changes*), which is also called divinatory symbols, or the eight diagrams (eight combinations of three whole or broken lines formerly used in divination).

Chapter Twenty-eight

Infertility with Chest Fullness and No Appetite

胸满不思食不孕

妇人有饮食少思，胸膈满闷，终日倦怠思睡．一经房事，呻吟不已。人以为脾胃之气虚也，谁知是肾气不足乎。夫气宜升腾，不宜消降。升腾于上焦则脾胃易于分运，降陷于下焦则脾胃难于运化。人乏水谷之养，则精神自尔倦怠，脾胃之气可升而不可降也明甚。然则脾胃之气虽充于脾胃之中，实生于两肾之内。无肾中之水气，则胃之气不能腾；无肾中之火气，则脾之气不能化。惟有肾之水火二气，而脾胃之气始能升腾而不降也。然则补脾胃之气，可不急补肾中水火之气乎？治法必以补肾气为主，但补肾而不兼补脾胃之品，则肾之水火二气不能提于至阳之上也。方用并提汤。

Some women have no appetite and feel fatigued and drowsy. There is fullness and oppression in the chest and diaphragm. Once having sexual intercourse, they groan (in pain) continuously. Interns think that is due to the deficiency of the spleen qi. They never think the deficiency of kidney qi causes it. qi is supposed to rise rather than being dispersed and dropped-down. When qi rises to the upper *jiao*, the spleen and stomach can transport and transform. When qi is stuck in the lower *jiao*, the spleen and stomach will not transport and transform. Then the patient has no nourishing of water and food, so she feels fatigued. The qi of the spleen and stomach should be raised rather than being lowered. Although the qi of the spleen and stomach stays in the spleen and stomach, it is originated from the two kidneys. If there is no water-qi from the kidneys, the stomach-qi cannot rise.

Moreover, without fire-qi from the kidneys, the spleen-qi cannot be transformed. Depending on both the water-qi and fire-qi from the kidneys, the spleen and stomach qi may rise and not dropdown. To supplement the qi of spleen and stomach, we must strengthen water-qi and fire-qi in kidneys first.

Treatment should focus on tonifying kidney qi. Tonifying kidney qi without bringing together medicines for tonifying spleen and stomach will result in the water-qi and fire-qi in kidneys failing to rise to the extreme yang. *Bìng tí Tāng* (并提汤, Double Lifting Decoction) is recommended.

大熟地（一两，九蒸）　　　巴戟（一两，盐水浸）

白术（一两，土炒）　　　　人参（五钱）

黄芪（五钱，生用）　　　　山萸肉（三钱，蒸）

枸杞（二钱）　　　　　　　柴胡（五分）

shú dì (prepared rehmannia root), 1 *liang* (big ones, fully steamed)

bā jǐ, (morinda root), 1 *liang* (soaked in salt water)

bái zhú (white atractylodes rhizome), 1 *liang* (dry-fried with earth)

rén shēn (ginseng), 5 *qian*

huáng qí (astragalus root), 5 *qian* (raw)

shān yú ròu, (Fructus Corni), 3 *qian* (steamed)

gǒu qǐ, (Chinese wolfberry fruit), 2 *qian*

chái hú (bupleurum), 5 *fen*

水煎服。三月而肾气大旺。再服一月，未有不能受孕者。此方补气之药多于补精，似乎以补脾胃为主矣。孰知脾胃健而生精自易，是脾胃之气与血，正所以补肾之精与水也。又益以补精之味，则阴气自足，阳气易升，自尔腾越于上焦矣。阳气不下陷，则无非大地阳春，随遇皆是化生之机，安有不受孕之理与！

This formula is decocted in water and taken orally. If patients take the decoction for three months, the kidney qi will be significantly strengthened. If taken one more month, all patients can get pregnant. In this formula, there are more medicines for supplementing qi than that for supplementing kidney essence. It seems tonifying the spleen and stomach is the main task. When the spleen and stomach are strong, the production of essence will be much easier. The qi and blood in the spleen and kidneys are for tonifying the essence and water of kidneys. Added with the medicines for supplementing essence, the yin qi becomes sufficient, and yang qi can rise to the upper *jiao*. When yang-qi does not sink, it is like the warm spring on earth. There are chances for the transformation and growth of all things, and there is no reason for sterility.

（胸满不孕。人每误为脾胃虚寒，不能克食。用扶脾消导之药。肾气愈虚，何能受孕。妙在立方不峻补肾火，所以不用桂附等药，但专补肾气，使脾胃之气不复下陷，则带脉气充，胞胎气暖，自然受孕无难矣。）

[For infertility with chest fullness, interns always mistake it for spleen and stomach's deficiency cold, resulting in indigestion. Medicines for strengthening spleen and promoting digestion to remove retained food make the kidney qi weaker. How can fertilization be possible? This formula's subtlety is that it does not supplement kidney fire drastically with *ròu guì* (肉桂, cinnamon bark) or *fù zǐ* (附子, prepared aconite root), for example. However, it concentrates on kidney qi's supplementing, making the spleen and stomach qi not sink any more. Therefore, the *dai mai* has enough qi, and the uterus is warm, and conception is not a difficult thing.]

下部冰冷不孕

妇人有下身冰冷，非火不暖，交感之际，阴中绝无温热之气。人以为天分之薄也，谁知是胞胎寒之极乎！夫寒冰之地，不生草木；重阴之渊，不长鱼龙。今胞胎既寒，何能受孕。虽男子鼓勇力战，其精甚热，直射于子宫之内，而寒冰之气相逼，亦不过茹之于暂而不能不吐之于久也。夫犹是人也，此妇之胞胎，何以寒凉至此，岂非天分之薄乎？非也。盖胞胎居于心肾之间，上系于心而下系于肾。胞胎之寒凉，乃心肾二火之衰微也。故治胞胎者，必须补心肾二火而后可。方用温胞饮。

Some women feel ice-cold at lower abdomen. When having sexual intercourse, there's not any warm feeling in their vaginas. Interns think it is because they are born thin and weak. Actually, it is because their uterus's are extremely cold. Just like in the natural world, there's no grass and plants that grow in ice-cold places, and there's no fish that will stay in an extreme yin abyss. When pathogenic cold settles in the uterus, how can fertilization happen? Even if the man's seminal fluid is warm, when it arrives at the uterus, the pathogenically cold uterus cannot accept it. Why is this woman's cold uterus so distinct from other women? Isn't it because they are congenitally deficient? No. It is because the uterus is located between the heart and the kidneys. It connects with the heart upward and links with the kidneys downward. The coldness of the uterus is caused by the wane of the fire in the heart and the kidneys. Thus, to treat the disease of the uterus, we must first supplement the fire in the heart and the kidneys. *Wēn Bāo Yǐn* (温胞饮，Uterus Warming Decoction) is recommended.

白术（一两，土炒）	巴戟（一两，盐水浸）
人参（三钱）	杜仲（三钱，炒黑）
菟丝子（三钱，酒浸炒）	山药（三钱，炒）

芡实（三钱，炒）　　　　　肉桂（三钱，去粗，研）

附子（二分，制）　　　　　补骨脂（二钱，盐水炒）

bái zhú (white atractylodes rhizome), 1 *liang* (dry-fried with earth)

bā jǐ, (morinda root), 1 *liang* (soaked in salt water)

rén shēn (ginseng), 2 *qian*

dù zhòng, (eucommia bark), 3 *qian* (slightly charred)

tù sī zǐ, (dodder Seed), 3 *qian* (soaked in millet wine and dry-fried)

shān yào (common yam rhizome), 3 *qian* (dry-fried)

qiàn shí (euryale seed), 3 *qian* (dry-fried)

ròu guì, (cinnamon bark), 3 *qian* (ground)

fù zǐ, (processed aconite root), 3 *fen* (processed)

bǔ gǔ zhī, (psoralea fruit), 2 *qian* (dry-fried with salt water)

水煎服。一月而胞胎热。此方之妙，补心而即补肾，温肾而即温心。心肾之气旺，则心肾之火自生。心肾之火生，则胞胎之寒自散。原因胞胎之寒，以至茹而即吐，而今胞胎既热矣，尚有施而不受者乎？若改汤为丸，朝夕吞服，尤能摄精，断不至有伯道无儿之叹也。

Decoct the formula in water and take the decoction orally. When the decoction is taken for one month, the uterus will be warm. The subtlety of this formula lies in that tonifying the heart is strengthening the kidneys. When the qi of the heart and kidneys is vigorous, the fire in the heart and the kidneys will grow naturally. And then, the pathogenic cold in the uterus would be dispersed. Now that the uterus is warm, fertilization is not a difficult thing. If the decoction is changed into bolus and taken every morning and night, it would be specially good at reinforcing and holding the essence.

今之种子者多喜服热药，不知此方特为胞胎寒者设，若胞胎有热则不宜服。审之。

Nowadays, most people who want to get pregnant take medicine with a warm property. They don't know this formula is for women who have pathogenic cold in the uterus. It is not suitable for women who have pathogenic heat in their uterus. Doctors must differentiate carefully.

Chapter Thirty
Infertility with Chest Fullness and Poor Appetite

胸满少食不孕

妇人有素性恬淡，饮食少则平和，多则难受，或作呕泄，胸膈胀满，久不受孕。人以为赋禀之薄也，谁知是脾胃虚寒乎。夫脾胃之虚寒，原因心肾之虚寒耳。盖胃土非心火不能生，脾土非肾火不能化。心肾之火衰，则脾胃失生化之权，即不能消水谷以化精微矣。既不能化水谷之精微，自无津液以灌溉于胞胎之中。欲胞胎有温暖之气以养胚胎，必不可得。纵然受胎，而带脉无力，亦必堕落。此脾胃虚寒之咎，故无玉麟之毓也。治法可不急温补其脾胃乎？然脾之母原在肾之命门，胃之母原在心之包络。欲温脾胃，必须补二经之火。盖母旺子必不弱，母热子必不寒，此子病治母之义也。方用温土毓麟汤。

Some women are always quiet. They may be placid when eating less. However, when eating more, they feel unwell, having fullness of the chest and the diaphragm, and sometimes have vomiting or diarrhea. They cannot get pregnant for a long time. Interns think it is because they are thin and weak constitutionally.

In contrast, the root lies in the deficiency cold of the spleen and stomach. Moreover, the spleen and stomach's deficiency cold results from the heart and kidneys' deficiency cold. Because the stomach-earth cannot grow without the heart-fire, and the spleen-earth cannot transform without the kidney-fire. When the heart and kidney-fire is weak, the spleen and stomach may lose production and transformation power. That is, they cannot digest the nutrients of food and water and transform them into essence. So, naturally, there is no body fluid to irrigate the uterus.

Furthermore, there is no warm qi in the uterus to nourish the embryo. Fertilization is impossible. Even if the conceiving happens, *dai mai* lacks strength, and spontaneous miscarriage is inevitable. This problem is due to the spleen and stomach's deficiency cold, which makes the uterus unable to get its nutrition.

To treat it, is it right not to warm and tonify the spleen and stomach? The spleen's mother originates in the life gate of the kidney, and the mother of the stomach originates in the collateral of the pericardium. To warm the spleen and stomach, we must first supplement the fire in these two meridians. When the mother is strong, the son will not be weak. When the mother is warm, the son will not be cold. This is the principle of treating the mother when the son is sick. The formula *Wēn Tǔ Yù Lín Tā-ng* (温土毓麟汤, Spleen-Earth Warming and Uterus Nourishing Decoction) is recommended.

巴戟（一两，去心，酒浸）　　　覆盆子（一两，酒浸，蒸）
白术（五钱，土炒）　　　　　　人参（三钱）
怀山药（五钱，炒）　　　　　　神曲（一钱，炒）

bā jǐ, (morinda root), 1 *liang* (core removed, soaked in millet wine)

fù pén zǐ, (Chinese raspberry), 1 *liang* (soaked in millet wine, steamed)

bái zhú (white atractylodes rhizome), 5 *qian* (dry-fried in earth)

rén shēn (ginseng), 3 *qian*

huái shān yào, (common yam rhizome), 5 *qian* (dry-fried, produced in Huaiqing)

shén qū, (medicated leaven), 1 *qian* (dry-fried)

水煎服。一月可以种子矣。此方之妙，温补脾胃而又兼补命门与心包络之火。药味不多，而四经并治。命门心包之火旺，则脾与胃无寒冷之虞。子母相顾，一家和合，自然饮食多而善化，气血旺而能任。带脉有力，不虞落胎，安有不玉麟之育哉！

If the formula is decocted in water and taken orally for one month, the patient may get pregnant. This prescription's subtlety lies in that it can warm and tonify the spleen and stomach; meanwhile, it supplements the fire in the life gate and the pericardium. With a few medicines, the four meridians are treated. When the fire in the life gate and pericardium is exuberant, the spleen and stomach will not be cold. The son and the mother can take care of each other and be a harmonious family. Naturally, food and drink could be digested and transformed. Therefore, qi and blood are also exuberant and can nourish the embryo. *Dai mai* is strengthened to keep the fetus intact. There is no need to worry about a miscarriage.

（少食不孕与胸满不思饮食有间，一补肾中之气，一补命门与心包络之火。药味不多，其君臣佐使之妙，宜细参之。）

(There are differences between infertility with poor appetite and infertility with chest fullness and no appetite. One is to strengthen the kidney qi; the other is to supplement the fire in the life gate and pericardium. Only a few medicines are included in the formula, and doctors need to reflect on the subtlety of the combination of the monarch, minister, assistant, and guide in the formula.)

Chapter Thirty-one

Sterility with Tense Feeling at the Lower Abdomen

少腹急迫不孕

妇人有少腹之间自觉有紧迫之状，急而不舒，不能生育。此人人之所不识也，谁知是带脉之拘急乎。夫带脉系于腰脐之间，宜弛而不宜急。今带脉之急者，由于腰脐之气不利也。而腰脐之气不利者，由于脾胃之气不足也。脾胃气虚，则腰脐之气闭，腰脐之气闭，则带脉拘急。遂致牵动胞胎，精即直射于胞胎，胞胎亦暂能茹纳，而力难负载，必不能免小产之虞。况人多不能节欲，安得保其不坠乎？此带脉之急，所以不能生子也。治法宜宽其带脉之急。而带脉之急，不能遽宽也，宜利其腰脐之气。而腰脐之气，不能遽利也，必须大补其脾胃之气与血，而腰脐可利，带脉可宽，自不难于孕育矣。方用宽带汤。

Some women have a tense and tight feeling in the lower abdomen. In fact it is very tight and uncomfortable, accompanied by infertility. Interns do not understand what is happening. In fact, it is *dai mai*'s spasm. As *dai mai* connects with the waist, it is supposed to be relaxed and should not be tight. *Dai mai* contracture is caused by the inhibition (stagnation) of the qi of the waist and umbilicus. The inhibition results from weakness of qi of the spleen and stomach. The spleen and stomach's qi deficiency leads to qi stagnation in the waist and umbilicus, which causes *dai mai*'s spasm. It then affects the uterus. Even if sperm is shot into the uterus, and the uterus can contain them temporarily, amblosis is inevitable.

The treatment should be to release the tension of *dai mai*. In order to relieve the tension of *dai mai*, the qi of the waist and the umbilicus should be soothed first. In order to soothe the qi of the waist and the umbilicus, the qi and blood of the spleen and stomach should be tonified first. Thus, the waist and umbilicus are soothed, and *dai mai* is relieved, and pregnancy is not a difficult thing. *Kuān Dài Tāng* (宽带汤, *Dai mai* Releasing Decoction) is recommended.

白术（一两，土炒） 巴戟（五钱，酒浸）

补骨脂（一钱，盐水炒） 人参（三钱）

麦冬（三钱，去心） 杜仲（三钱，炒黑）

大熟地（五钱，九蒸） 肉苁蓉（三钱，洗净）

白芍（三钱，酒炒） 当归（二钱，酒洗）

五味（三分，炒） 建莲子（二十粒，不去心）

bái zhú (white atractylodes rhizome), 1 *liang* (dry-fried with earth)

bā jǐ, (morinda root), 5 *qian* (soaked in millet wine)

bǔ gǔ zhī, (psoralea fruit), 1 qian (dry-fried with salt water)

rén shēn (ginseng), 3 *qian*

mài dōng, (dwarf lilyturf tuber), 3 *qian* (pitch-discarded)

dù zhòng, (eucommia bark), 3 *qian* (slightly charred)

shú dì (prepared rehmannia root), 5 *qian* (big ones, fully steamed)

ròu cōng róng, (desert cistanche), 3 *qian*

bái sháo (white peony root), 3 *qian* (dry-fried with millet wine)

dāng guī (Chinese angelica), 2 *qian* (washed with millet wine)

wǔ wèi zǐ, (Chinese magnolivine fruit), 3 *fen* (dry-fried)

lián zǐ, (lotus seed), 20 pieces (plumula preserved, produced in Fujian)

水煎服。四剂少腹无紧迫之状，服一月即受胎。此方之妙，脾胃两补，而又利其腰脐之气，自然带脉宽舒，可以载物而胜任矣。或疑方中用五味、白芍之酸收，不增带脉之急，而反得带脉之宽，殊不可解。岂知带脉之急，由于气血之虚，盖血虚则缩而不伸，气虚则挛而不达。用芍药之酸以平肝木，则肝不克脾。用五味之酸以生肾水，则肾能益带。似相妨而实相济也，何疑之有。

Decoct the formula in water and take orally. When four *ji* is taken, the feeling of tension at the lower abdomen is relieved. If it is taken for one month, the patient may get pregnant. The subtlety in this formula lies in that it may tonify both the spleen and stomach and also, it may release the qi of the waist and umbilicus. Naturally, *dai mai* would be soothed and could contain an embryo. Some interns will worry that *wǔ wèi zǐ* (五味子, Chinese magnolivine fruit) and *bái sháo* (白芍, white peony root), with their sour flavor and having the effect of astringency, may aggravate the tension. How can they relieve *dai mai*? The tension of *dai mai* is due to the deficiency of the qi and blood. The blood deficiency will cause contraction and preventing it from being stretched, and the qi deficiency may cause spasm and not be smooth. *Sháo yào* (芍药, white peony root) is used to calm the liver wood so that it does not restrict

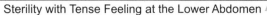

the spleen. *wǔ wèi zǐ* (五味子, Chinese magnolivine fruit)'s sour tastes are used here to generate kidney water, and therefore the kidney will nourish *dai mai*. That is its mutual promotion, and so there is no need to worry.

（凡种子治法，不出带脉胞胎二经。数言已泄造化之秘矣。）

(As for the secret of getting pregnant, it's nothing else but the recovery of the uterus and *dai mai*. God's design is leaked in a few words.)

Chapter Thirty-two
Infertility due to Depression

嫉妒不孕

妇人有怀抱素恶不能生子者，人以为天心厌之也，谁知是肝气郁结乎。夫妇人之有子也，必然心脉流利而滑，脾脉舒徐而和，肾脉旺大而鼓指，始称喜脉。未有三部脉郁而能生子者也。若三部脉郁，肝气必因之而更郁，肝气郁则心肾之脉必致郁之极而莫解。盖子母相依，郁必不喜，喜必不郁也。其郁而不能成胎者，以肝木不舒，必下克脾土而致塞。脾土之气塞，则腰脐之气必不利。腰脐之气不利，必不能通任脉而达带脉，则带脉之气亦塞矣。带脉之气既塞，则胞胎之门必闭，精即到门，亦不得其门而入矣。其奈之何哉？治法必解四经之郁，以开胞胎之门，则几矣。方用开郁种玉汤。

Women who are always depressed and pessimistic cannot get pregnant. The stagnation of the liver qi causes the inability to get pregnant! If a woman has got pregnant, she must have a smooth and slippery heart pulse, a gentle and peaceful spleen pulse, and a full and large kidney pulse, named "happy event pulse" (pregnant pulse). No woman can give birth to a baby while her liver, spleen, and kidney pulse are all stagnated. If the three pulses are all stagnated, the liver qi must be more stagnated. Therefore, the heart and kidney pulse must be stagnated and cannot be relieved, as the son and mother are dependent on each other. Depression makes her unhappy. That depression results in infertility because the liver wood is not soothed, which then restricts the spleen earth and makes it stagnated. The stagnation of spleen earth qi will make the qi of the waist and umbilicus unsmooth, and so the qi of the waist and umbilicus cannot go through *ren mai* and reach *dai mai*. Thus, the qi of *dai mai* will be blocked. When the qi of *dai mai* is blocked, the gate of the uterus will be closed. Even if sperm arrives, it cannot enter the gate. How helpless!

To treat it, we must relieve the stagnation in the four meridians and open the uterus gate. *Kaī Yù Zhòng Yù Tāng* (开郁种玉汤, Stagnation Relieving and Fertilization Improving Decoction) is recommended.

白芍（一两，酒炒）　　香附（三钱，酒炒）

当归（五钱，酒洗）　　白术（五钱，土炒）

丹皮（三钱，酒洗）　　茯苓（三钱，去皮）

花粉（二钱）

bái sháo (white peony root), 1 *liang* (dry-fried with millet wine)

xiāng fù (cyperus), 3 *qian* (dry-fried with millet wine)

dāng guī (Chinese angelica), 5 *qian* (washed with millet wine)

bái zhú (white atractylodes rhizome), 5 *qian* (dry-fried with earth)

dān pí (tree peony bark), 3 *qian* (washed with millet wine)

fú líng (poria), 3 *qian* (peel removed)

tiān huā fěn, (snakegourd root), 2 *qian*

水煎服。一月则郁结之气开，郁开则无非喜气之盈腹，而嫉妒之心亦可以一易，自然两相合好，结胎于顷刻之间矣。此方之妙。解肝气之郁，宣脾气之困，而心肾之气亦因之俱舒，所以腰脐利而任带通达，不必启胞胎之门，而胞胎自启。不特治嫉妒者也。

The formula is decocted in water and taken orally. When it has been taken for one month, the stagnated qi is relieved. Then, there is a full pleasant mood inside, and depression is removed. Getting pregnant is a natural thing. The subtlety of this formula lies in that it can relieve the liver qi's stagnation, dredge and disperse the encumbered spleen, and the qi of the heart and the kidney can be soothed too. Thus, the waist and the umbilicus are soothed, and *ren mai* and *dai mai* are smooth. The gate of the uterus will open naturally. It is not a formula to be used only for the treatment of envy.

Chapter Thirty-three

Infertility Due to Obesity

肥胖不孕

妇人有身体肥胖，痰涎甚多，不能受孕者。人以为气虚之故，谁知是湿盛之故乎。夫湿从下受，乃言外邪之湿也。而肥胖之湿，实非外邪，乃脾土之内病也。然脾土既病，不能分化水谷以养四肢，宜其身躯瘦弱，何以能肥胖乎？不知湿盛者多肥胖，肥胖者多气虚，气虚者多痰涎，外似健壮而内实虚损也。内虚则气必衰，气衰则不能行水，而湿停于肠胃之间，不能化精而化涎矣。夫脾本湿土，又因痰多，愈加其湿。脾不能受，必浸润于胞胎，日积月累，则胞胎竟变为汪洋之水窟矣。且肥胖之妇，内肉必满，遮隔子宫，不能受精，此必然之势也。况又加以水湿之盛，即男子甚健，阳精直达子宫，而其水势滔滔，泛滥可畏，亦遂化精成水矣，又何能成妊哉。治法必须以泄水化痰为主。然徒泄水化痰，而不急补脾胃之气，则阳气不旺，湿痰不去，人先病矣。乌望其茹而不吐乎！方用加味补中益气汤。

Suffering from obesity, some women have an exuberance of phlegm and saliva, and have difficulty in becoming pregnant. Qi deficiency is assumed to be the cause, but the exuberance of dampness is to blame. It is said that the lower part of the body tends to be attacked by pathogenic dampness. It is talking about external pathogenic dampness. However, the dampness of obesity is not the external pathogenic factor. It is an internal disease from the spleen-earth. If the spleen-earth is sick and cannot transform water and food to nourish limbs, the body is apt to be thin and weak. So how could they be overweight? One who has an exuberance of dampness usually suffers from obesity. One who suffers from obesity commonly has qi deficiency.

Moreover, the one who has qi deficiency generally has an exuberance of phlegm and saliva. They look strong externally and feel deficient and asthenic internally. When one is internally deficient, qi debilitation is a certainty. Qi debilitation makes it challenging to move water; thus, the dampness stays in the stomach and intestine and is transformed into phlegm instead of essence. As the spleen is damp in itself, excessive phlegm makes the dampness more serious. It is an unaffordable burden to the spleen. The dampness will certainly invade the uterus. As days accumulate and months increase, the uterus turns into a cave full of water.

Furthermore, those women who suffer from obesity must have more fat in their inner organs. The uterus, therefore, may be barred from fertilization. Added with the excessive water dampness, even if the man is strong enough, the semen may arrive at the uterus, and the water dampness will dissolve the semen into water. How can they get pregnant?

The treatment should be draining water and resolving phlegm instead of urgently supplementing the qi of spleen and stomach, which will make the yang-qi weak, the phlegm not transported, and the patient sick. *Jiā Wèi Bǔ Zhōng Yì Qì Tāng* (加味补中益气汤，Supplemented Middle Tonifying and Qi Benefiting Decoction) is recommended.

人参（三钱）　　　　黄芪（三钱，生用）

柴胡（一钱）　　　　当归（三钱，酒洗）

白术（一两，土炒）　升麻（四分）

陈皮（五分）　　　　茯苓（五钱）

半夏（三钱，制）

rén shēn (ginseng), 3 *qian*

huáng qí (astragalus root), 3 *qian* (raw)

chái hú (bupleurum), 1 *qian*

dāng guī (Chinese angelica), 3 *qian* (washed with millet wine)

bái zhú (white atractylodes rhizome), 1 *liang* (dry-fried with earth)

shēng má, (black cohosh rhizome), 4 *fen*

chén pí (aged tangerine peel), 5 *fen*

fú líng (poria), 5 *qian*

bàn xià, (pinellia rhizome), 3 *qian* (processed)

水煎服。八剂痰涎尽消，再十剂水湿利，子宫涸出，易于受精而成孕矣。其在于昔，则如望洋观海；而在于今，则是马到成功也。快哉！此方之妙，妙在提脾气而升于上，作云作雨，则水湿反利于下行。助胃气而消于下，为津为液，则痰涎转易于上化。不必用消化之品以损其肥，而肥自无碍；不必用浚决之味以开其窍，而窍自能通。阳气充足，自能摄精，湿邪散除，自可受种。何肥胖不孕之足虑乎！

【再十剂，后方加杜仲一钱半（炒断丝），续断钱半（炒），必受孕矣。】

Decoct the formula with water and take it orally. When 8 *ji* is taken, there is no sputum. If ten more *ji* is taken, water dampness will be removed. The uterus will then not be in water dampness, and it is relatively easy to conceive a baby. This formula's subtlety is to raise the spleen-qi to upper *jiao* so that the water dampness goes downward to aid the stomach-qi in resolving it in the lower *jiao*, where it is turned into body fluid. Sputum is also resolved. There is no need to use digestive medicine to relieve obesity because it cannot affect the situation. Also, there is no need to use drastic medicines for opening the orifice because orifices can now be opened naturally. With abundant yang-qi, the semen is controlled, the dampness is removed, and the fertilized eggs can be implanted. Obesity is no longer a worry.

[After 10 *ji* is taken, add *dù zhòng* (杜仲, eucommia bark, dry-fried till the fibers are broken) one and a half *qian*, *xù duàn* (续断, himalayan teasel root, dry-fried) one and a half *qian* so that the woman will get pregnant without fail.]

Chapter Thirty-four

Infertility Due to Bone Steaming and Fever at Night

骨蒸夜热不孕

妇人有骨蒸夜热，遍体火焦，口干舌燥，咳嗽吐沫，难于生子者。人以为阴虚火动也，谁知是骨髓内热乎。夫寒阴之地固不生物，而干旱之田岂能长养？然而骨髓与胞胎何相关切，而骨髓之热，即能使人不嗣，此前贤之所未言者也。山一旦创言之，不几为世俗所骇乎。而要知不必骇也，此中实有其理焉。盖胞胎为五脏外之一脏耳，以其不阴不阳，所以不列于五脏之中。所谓不阴不阳者，以胞胎上系于心包，下系于命门。系心包者通于心，心者阳也；系命门者通于肾，肾者阴也。是阴之中有阳，阳之中有阴，所以通于变化。或生男或生女，俱从此出。然必阴阳协和，不偏不枯，始能变化生人，否则否矣。况胞胎既通于肾，而骨髓亦肾之所化也。骨髓热由于肾之热，肾热而胞胎亦不能不热。且胞胎非骨髓之养，则婴儿无以生骨。骨髓过热，则骨中空虚，惟存火烈之气，又何能成胎？治法必须清骨中之热。然骨热由于水亏，必补肾之阴，则骨热除，珠露有滴濡之喜矣。壮水之主，以制阳光，此之谓也。方用清骨滋肾汤。

Some women suffer from bone steaming and have a fever at night. They feel the whole body is hot and burning. Their throat is parched with thirst, and have coughing and foaming at the mouth. It is difficult for them to conceive a baby. Yin deficiency stirring fire is assumed to be the reason, but actually, bone marrow's interior heat should be blamed. Indeed, a cold and shady place can not grow things. Furthermore, how can drought soil moisten a plant? So what is the relationship between the bone marrow and the uterus?

Pathogenic heat in the bone marrow may lead to sterility, which scholars never mentioned previously. This theory is as follows. The uterus is an organ that is beside the five *zang* organs. Because it belongs to neither yin nor yang, it is not listed in the five *zang* organs. Neither yin nor yang means that the uterus connects up with the pericardium and down with the life gate. The thing which connects with the pericardium communicates with the heart, and the heart is the most yang of all yin organs. The thing connected with the life gate communicates with the kidneys, and the kidneys belong to yin. Thus, there is yin in yang and yang in yin. They communicate with each other and change mutually. So, no matter male or female, both are born from the uterus.

Nevertheless, the yin and yang must be in harmony, not scorched, and then, they can transform sperm and egg into life. Otherwise, it will not work. Moreover, the uterus connects with the kidneys, and the bone marrow is also transformed from the kidneys. So the heat in the bone marrow is originated from the heat in the kidneys. The kidney heat makes the uterus unable to cool down. Without the nourishing of the bone marrow, the bones of the fetus cannot grow. The excessive heat will lead to the emptiness of the bone, and there is only flaming left. How can an embryo come into being in these circumstances?

The treatment should be clearing away the heat in the bone. The heat in the bone is caused by lack of water, so the kidney yin must be supplemented, and then the heat of the bone may be cleared away. This method is also called invigorating the water source to inhibit exuberant yang. *Qīng Gǔ Zī Shèn Tāng* (清骨滋肾汤, Bone Clearing and Kidney Nourishing Decoction) is recommended.

地骨皮（一两，酒洗）　　　　丹皮（五钱）

沙参（五钱）　　　　　　　　麦冬（五钱，去心）

元参（五钱，酒洗）　　　　　五味子（五分，炒，研）

白术（三钱，土炒）　　　　　石斛（二钱）

水煎。连服三十剂而骨热解，再服六十剂自受孕。此方之妙，补肾中之精，凉骨中之热，不清胞胎而胞胎自无太热之患。然阴虚内热之人，原易受妊，今因骨髓过热，所以受精而变燥，以致难于育子，本非胞胎之不能受精。所以稍补其肾，以杀其火之有余，而益其水之不足，便易种子耳。

dì gǔ pí, (Chinese wolfberry root-bark), 1 *liang* (washed with millet wine)

dān pí (tree peony bark), 5 *qian*

shā shēn, (radix adenophorae seu glehniae), 5 *qian*

mài dōng, (dwarf lilyturf tuber), 5 *qian* (pith discarded)

yuán shēn, (figwort root), 5 *qian* (washed with millet wine)

wǔ wèi zǐ, (Chinese magnolivine fruit), 5 *fen* (dry-fried, ground)

bái zhú (white atractylodes rhizome), 3 *qian* (dry-fried with earth)

shí hú, (dendrobium), 2 *qian*

The formula is decocted in water and taken orally. If the patient takes this medicine continually for 30 days, the bone steaming will be relieved. If taking it for 60 days, the patient may get pregnant naturally. The subtlety in this formula lies in that it supplements the kidneys' essence and cools down the bone's heat. Then the uterus no longer suffers from the effects of excessive heat. The woman who has interior heat due to yin deficiency should be able to get pregnant quickly. Without treatment, the bone marrow's excessive heat causes the uterus to be too dry to nourish a baby. It is not because the uterus cannot be fertilized. Therefore, nourishing the kidney, clearing away the excess fire, and supplementing the water deficiency, makes fertilization an easy thing.

· Chapter Thirty-five ·
Infertility with Aching Lumbus and Abdominal Distention

腰酸腹胀不孕

妇人有腰酸背楚，胸满腹胀，倦怠欲卧，百计求嗣不能如愿。人以为腰肾之虚也，谁知是任督之困乎。夫任脉行于前，督脉行于后，然皆从带脉之上下而行也。故任脉虚则带脉坠于前，督脉虚则带脉坠于后，虽胞胎受精亦必小产。况任督之脉既虚，而疝瘕之症必起。疝瘕碍胞胎而外障，则胞胎缩于疝瘕之内，往往精施而不能受。虽饵以玉燕，亦何益哉！治法必须先去其疝瘕之病，而补其任督之脉，则提挈天地，把握阴阳，呼吸精气，包裹成形，力足以胜任而无虞矣。外无所障，内有所容，安有不能生育之理！方用升带汤。

Some women feel an aching in the waist and back, fullness in the chest, abdominal distention, and fatigue to the point of not wanting to get out of bed. They try everything possible to get pregnant but fail. People believe it is the waist and kidneys that should be blamed, while actually, it is due to *ren mai* deficiency or *du mai* deficiency. As we know, *ren mai* runs at the abdominal-anterior, while *du mai* runs at the back. They both run up and down and cross *dai mai*. Therefore, *ren mai*'s deficiency will lead to the anterior abdominal prolapse of *dai mai*. Alternatively, a deficiency of *du mai* will lead to a posterior prolapse of *dai mai*. So even if the egg is fertilized, miscarriage is unavoidable.

Furthermore, *ren mai* deficiency or *du mai* deficiency will indeed cause hernias and movable abdominal masses (such as congestive sclerosis, myomas, and other tumors). The hernias and movable abdominal masses cover the uterus, and the uterus retracts inside. Thus, sperm can arrive at it but cannot be accepted.

To treat it, the hernias and masses must be removed first, and then *ren mai* and *du mai* should be supplemented. Yin and yang can then achieve harmony. When there are no obstacles outside, but there is essence inside, is there any reason for sterility? *Shēng dài Tāng* (升带汤, *Dai mai* Raising Decoction) is recommended.

白术（一两，土炒）　　　　　人参（三钱）

沙参（五钱）　　　　　　　　肉桂（一钱，去粗，研）

荸荠粉（三钱）　　　　　　　鳖甲（三钱，炒）

茯苓（三钱）　　　　　　　　半夏（一钱，制）

神曲（一钱，炒）

bái zhú (white atractylodes rhizome), 1 *liang* (dry-fried with earth)

rén shēn (ginseng), 3 *qian*

shā shēn, (radix adenophorae seu glehniae), 5 *qian*

ròu guì, (cinnamon bark), 1 *qian* (ground into powder)

bí qí fěn, (Chinese water-chestnut), 3 *qian* (ground into powder)

biē jiǎ, (turtle carapace), 3 *qian* (dry-fried)

fú líng (poria), 3 *qian*

bàn xià, (pinellia rhizome), 1 *qian* (prepared)

shén qū, (medicated leaven), 1 *qian* (dry-fried)

水煎。连服三十剂，而任督之气旺。再服三十剂，而疝瘕之症除。此方利腰脐之气，正升补任督之气也。任督之气升，而疝瘕自有难容之势。况方中有肉桂以散寒，荸荠以祛积，鳖甲之攻坚，茯苓之利湿，有形自化于无形，满腹皆升腾之气矣。何至受精而再坠乎哉！

If the formula is decocted in water and taken orally for 30 days, the qi in both *ren mai* and *du mai* will be vigorous. Take it for another 30 days, and the hernias and masses will be removed. This prescription may soothe the qi between the waist and umbilicus while raising and supplementing *ren mai*'s and *du mai*'s qi. When *ren mai*'s and *du mai*'s qi is raised, the hernias and masses will disappear. Moreover, *ròu guì* (肉桂, cinnamon bark) is used to dispel cold, *bí qí fěn* (荸荠粉, Chinese water-chestnut) to eliminate accumulation, *biē jiǎ* (鳖甲 turtle carapace) to attack hernias, *fú líng* (茯苓, poria) to drain dampness. So in sum, the hernias and masses will melt away. The abdomen is full of rising qi. There will be no miscarriage.

【此方为有疝瘕而设，故用沙参、荸荠粉、鳖甲以破坚理气。若无疝瘕，去此三味加杜仲一钱半（炒黑）、泽泻一钱半（炒），甘枸杞二钱，三味服之，腰酸腹胀自除矣。鳖甲破气，不可误服。】

[This formula is designed for patients with hernias and masses; *shā shēn* (沙参, radix adenophorae seu glehniae), *bí qí fěn* (荸荠粉, Chinese water-chestnut), *biē jiǎ* (鳖甲 turtle carapace) are used to break up hernias and soothe qi. If there are no hernias and masses, the three medicines may be taken out, and *dù zhòng* (杜仲, eucommia bark)1 *qian* and 5 *fen* (charred) added, along with *zé xiè* (泽泻, water plantain rhizome), 1 *qian* and 5 *fen* (dry-fried), and *gǒu qǐ zǐ* (枸杞子, Chinese Wolfberry Fruit) 2 *qian*. Soreness of the waist and abdominal distention may disappear. *biē jiǎ* (鳖甲 turtle carapace) has the function of breaking up (dispersing) qi. It should not be administered mistakenly.]

Chapter Thirty-six

Infertility with Difficult Urination, Abdominal Distention, and Dropsy (Edema) of Feet

便涩腹胀足浮肿不孕

妇人有小水艰涩，腹胀脚肿，不能受孕者。人以为小肠之热也，谁知是膀胱之气不化乎。夫膀胱原与胞胎相近，膀胱病而胞胎亦病矣。然水湿之气必走膀胱，而膀胱不能自化，必得肾气相通，始能化水，以出阴器。倘膀胱无肾气之通，则膀胱之气化不行，水湿之气必且渗入胞胎之中，而成汪洋之势矣。汪洋之田，又何能生物也哉？

Some women have infertility, accompanied by difficult urination, abdominal distention, and dropsy (edema) of feet. Interns believe it is because of the small intestine's heat, while actually, it is due to qi transformation failure in the bladder. The urinary bladder is located near the uterus. When the bladder is suffering from some disorder, so is the uterus. Undoubtedly, the water dampness needs to pass through the urinary bladder. While the bladder cannot transform water dampness by itself, it is interrelated with the kidney qi to transform water and discharge it. If the bladder is not interrelated with kidney qi, it will fail in qi transformation. Therefore, water dampness will seep into the uterus. The uterus will become waterlogged. How can a piece of a waterlogged field grow things?

治法必须壮肾气以分消胞胎之湿，益肾火以达化膀胱之水。使先天之本壮，则膀胱之气化；胞胎之湿除，而汪洋之田化成雨露之壤矣。水化则膀胱利，火旺则胞胎暖，安有布种而不发生者哉！方用化水种子汤。

To treat it, we must reinforce the kidney qi to help transform the uterus' dampness and benefit the kidney fire to warm and transform water in the bladder. The dampness in the uterus can be eliminated, and the waterlogged field will change into rich soil. When water can be transformed, the bladder will be soothed. When the fire is exuberant, it will warm the uterus. *Huà Shuǐ zhòng zǐ Tāng* (化水种子汤,

Water Transforming and Conception Promoting Decoction) is recommended.

巴戟（一两，盐水浸）　　白术（一两，土炒）
茯苓（五钱）　　　　　　人参（三钱）
菟丝子（五钱，酒炒）　　芡实（五钱，炒）
车前（二钱，酒炒）　　　肉桂（一钱，去粗，研）

bā jǐ, (morinda root), 1 *liang* (salt water soaked)

bái zhú (white atractylodes rhizome), 1 *liang* (dry-fried with earth)

fú líng (poria), 5 *qian*

rén shēn (ginseng), 3 *qian*

tù sī zǐ, (dodder seed), 5 *qian* (dry-fried with millet wine)

qiàn shí (euryale seed), 5 *qian* (dry-fried)

chē qián zǐ (plantago seed), 2 *qian,* (dry-fried with millet wine)

ròu guì, (cinnamon bark), 1 *qian* (ground)

水煎服。二剂膀胱之气化，四剂难涩之症除，又十剂虚胀脚肿之病形消。再服六十剂，肾气大旺，胞胎温暖易于受胎而生育矣。此方利膀胱之水，全在补肾中之气。暖胞胎之气，全在壮肾中之火。至于补肾之药，多是濡润之品，不以湿而益助其湿乎？然方中之药，妙于补肾之火，而非补肾之水，尤妙于补火而无燥烈之虞，利水而非荡涤之猛。所以膀胱气化，胞胎不湿，而发荣长养无穷与。

Decoct the formula with water and take it orally. When it is taken for two days, qi in the bladder can be transformed. When it is taken for four days, difficult urination will disappear. After it is taken for another ten days, the symptoms like abdominal distention and dropsy (edema) of feet will disappear. Take it for another 60 days, and the kidney qi will be significantly reinforced; also, the uterus will be warmed and easy for fertilization. This formula is for draining water in the bladder, which depends on reinforcing the kidney qi. It is also for warming qi in the uterus, which lies in the kidneys' strengthening. Most of the herbs for tonifying kidneys are nourishing and moist in their property. So will it not make the dampness more serious? The herbs here are for reinforcing the fire in kidneys, not for nourishing kidney water. It is lovely because it supplements fire while not causing dryness; it drains water and does not cause flushing damage. Consequently, qi is transformed in the bladder, and the uterus is nourished forever and not interfered with by dampness.

【便涩、腹胀、足浮肿，此病极多。不惟不能受孕，抑且渐添杂症，久而不愈，甚有成劳瘵不治者。此方补水而不助湿，补火而使归原，善极，不可加减一味。若无好肉桂，以破故纸一钱（炒）代之。用核桃仁二个，（连皮烧黑去皮，用仁）作引。若用好肉桂，即可不用核桃引。】

[Inhibited urination, abdominal distention, and dropsy (edema) of feet are commonly seen in this disease. It not only causes sterility but also adds other problems that last a long time. Some cases even turn into incurable consumption diseases. This formula has the function of supplementing water while not assisting dampness, reinforcing fire, and bringing it back to its origin. No addition and subtraction of any medicines are needed. If there is no good *ròu guì*, (肉桂, cinnamon bark), use *pò gù zhǐ* (破故纸, oroxylum seed) 1 *qian* (dry-fried) instead. 2 walnuts, charred and peeled, may be used as guiding herb. If there is good *ròu guì*, (肉桂, cinnamon bark), the walnuts will not be used.]

Volume Five

Pregnancy

妊娠

Chapter Thirty-seven

Malign Obstruction in Pregnancy (Morning Sickness)

妊娠恶阻

妇人怀娠之后，恶心呕吐，思酸解渴，见食憎恶，困倦欲卧，人皆曰妊娠恶阻也，谁知肝血太燥乎。夫妇人受妊，本于肾气之旺也，肾旺是以摄精，然肾一受精而成娠，则肾水生胎，不暇化润于五脏。而肝为肾之子，日食母气以舒，一日无津液之养，则肝气迫索，而肾水不能应，则肝益急，肝急则火动而逆也。肝气既逆，是以呕吐恶心之症生焉。

Some women suffer from nausea, retching, vomiting, with a desire for sour food to quench thirst, apocleisis (anorexia), fatigue, and somnolence. It is called malign obstruction in pregnancy (morning sickness). The extreme dryness of liver blood causes it. When the kidney qi is exuberant, it can contain essence, which is the foundation of fertilization. While once the kidneys have received essence (sperm) (from the male) and engendered pregnancy, kidney water begins to nourish the fetus and neglect the five *zang* organs' nourishment. In five-element theory, the liver is the son organ of the kidneys and has to be fed by the qi of its mother organ every day to soothe itself. Once there is no nourishing from fluid, the liver qi will demand it more from the kidneys. When the kidney Water can not meet the need, the liver becomes more upset, which may stir up liver fire and result in qi's counter-flow. The counter-flow of the liver qi will consequently cause syndromes like retching, vomiting and nausea.

呕吐纵不至太甚，而其伤气则一也。气既受伤，则肝血愈耗。世人用四物汤治胎前诸症者，正以其能生肝之血也。然补肝以生血，未为不佳，但生血而不知生气，则脾胃衰微，不胜频呕，犹恐气虚则血不易生也。故于平肝补血之中，加以健脾开胃之品，以生阳气，则气能生血，尤益胎气耳。

The syndromes such as retching, vomiting, and nausea may not be too severe, but qi will be damaged all the same inevitably. Now that qi is damaged, liver blood will be more consumed. Doctors use *Sì Wù Tā* (四物汤, Four Substances Decoction) to treat various disorders in pregnancy because this formula can generate liver blood. Although it may not be wrong to supplement the liver to generate its blood, if blood is engendered without making efforts to engender qi, debilitation of the spleen and stomach is unavoidable. The weak spleen and stomach cannot bear frequent retching. As long as the qi is deficient, blood will not be easy to engender. Therefore, the ingredients for soothing the liver and supplementing blood to strengthen spleen and stimulate appetite should be used to engender yang qi. Qi can engender blood, and this is quite helpful for the fetal qi.

或疑气逆而用补气之药，不益助其逆乎？不知妊娠恶阻，其逆不甚，且逆是因虚而逆，非因邪而逆也。因邪而逆者，助其气则逆增；因虚而逆者，补其气则逆转。况补气于补血之中，则阴足以制阳，又何虑其增逆乎。宜用顺肝益气汤。

People may also ask that in using qi supplementing ingredients for the syndrome of counter-flow of qi, will this not promote the counter-flow of qi? Interns should understand that, in terms of morning sickness, the qi counter-flow is not severe. Moreover, the qi counter-flow is caused by deficiency rather than pathogenic factors. If pathogenic factors cause it, assisting qi will make the counter-flow more serious. However, when it is caused by deficiency, supplementing qi will rectify it.

Furthermore, qi supplementation is incorporated into the nourishing of blood, so Yin is then made abundant to restrain Yang. Why should we then worry about the qi counter-flow? It is appropriate to use *Shùn Gān Yì Qì Tāng* (顺肝益气汤, Liver Soothing and Qi Benefiting Decoction).

（亦有肝郁气滞，胸膈膨闷，见食不恶，不能多食，虽系妊娠而非恶阻，宜分别治之。后另有方。）

(Some patients also have the symptoms like liver depression with qi stagnation, depression in the chest, poor appetite. Although it belongs to pregnancy, it is not morning sickness. The treatment is different. There is another formula for it.)

人参（一两）　　　　　　当归（一两，酒洗）

苏子（一两，炒，研）　　白术（三钱，土炒）

茯苓（二钱）　　　　　　熟地（五钱，九蒸）

白芍（三钱，酒炒）　　　麦冬（三钱，去心）

陈皮（三分）　　　　　　砂仁（一粒，炒，研）

神曲（一钱，炒）

rén shēn (ginseng), 1 *liang*

dāng guī (Chinese angelica), 1 *liang* (washed with millet wine)

sū zǐ, (perilla fruit), 1 *liang* (dry-fried, ground)

bái zhú (white atractylodes rhizome), 3 *qian*

fú líng (poria), 2 *qian*

shú dì (prepared rehmannia root), 5 *qian* (big ones, fully steamed)

bái sháo (white peony root), 3 *qian* (dry-fried with millet wine)

mài dōng, (dwarf lilyturf tuber), 3 *qian* (pitch-removed)

chén pí (aged tangerine peel), 3 *fen*

shā rén, (villous amomum fruit), 1 piece (dry-fried and ground)

shén qū, (medicated leaven), 1 *qian*, (dry-fried)

水煎服。一剂轻，二剂平，三剂全愈。此方平肝则肝逆除，补肾则肝燥息，补气则血易生。凡胎病而少带恶阻者，俱以此方投之无不安，最有益于胎妇，其功更胜于四物焉。

Decoct the formula in water. When one *ji* is taken, it will mitigate the symptoms. If a second *ji* is taken, more improvement is effected. After the third *ji* is taken, complete recovery is effected. This formula soothes the liver, and the counterflow of liver qi is eliminated. It supplements the kidneys, and the liver dryness is put to an end. It supplements qi, making it easy to engender blood. This formula can be used for any fetal disorder with slight morning sickness and be effective without fail. It is beneficial for pregnant women, being even more effective than *Sì Wù Tāng* (四物汤, Four Substances Decoction).

（方极效。但苏子一两，疑是一钱之误。）

[This formula is quite useful. It is suspected that *sū zǐ*, (苏子, perilla fruit) 1 *liang* is mistaken for 1 *qian*.]

疏肝化滞汤：

全当归（酒洗，六钱）	杭芍（酒炒，三钱）
党参（去芦，三钱）	白扁豆（去皮，四钱）
云苓（二钱）	香附（炒焦，二钱）
砂仁（炒、研，钱半）	条芩（炒焦，八钱）

神曲（炒焦，钱半）　　　　广皮（八分）

薄荷（六分）　　　　　　　甘草（五分）

Shū Gān Huà Zhì Tāng（疏肝化滞汤，Liver Soothing and Stagnation Transforming Decoction）：

quán dāng guī (Chinese angelica), 6 *qian* (whole, washed with millet wine)

háng sháo (Hangzhou white peony root), 3 *qian* (dry-fried with millet wine)

dǎng shēn, (codonopsis root), 3 *qian* (the little rhizomes on the top are removed)

bái biǎn dòu (white hyacinth bean), 4 *qian* (peel-removed)

yún líng (poria), 2 *qian*

xiāng fù (cyperus), 1 *qian* and 5 *fen* (dry-fried until scorched)

shā rén, (villous amomum fruit), 1 qian and 5 fen (dry-fried, ground)

tiáo qín, (scutellaria root), 8 *fen* (charred)

shén qū, (medicated leaven), 1 *qian* and 5 *fen* (charred)

guǎng pí, (pericarpium citri reticulatae chachiensis) 8 *fen*,

bò he, (field mint), 6 *fen*

gān cǎo (licorice root), 5 *fen*

Chapter Thirty-eight
Edema during pregnancy

妊娠浮肿

妊妇有至五个月，肢体倦怠，饮食无味，先两足肿，渐至遍身头面俱肿。人以为湿气使然也，谁知是脾肺气虚乎。夫妊娠虽有按月养胎之分，其实不可拘于月数，总以健脾补肺为大纲。盖脾统血，肺主气，胎非血不荫，非气不生，脾健则血旺而荫胎，肺清则气旺而生子。苟肺衰则气馁，气馁则不能运气于皮肤矣；脾虚则血少，血少则不能运血于肢体矣。气与血两虚，脾与肺失职，所以饮食难消，精微不化，势必至气血下陷，不能升举，而湿邪即乘其所虚之处，积而成浮肿症，非由脾肺之气血虚而然耶。治法当补其脾之血与肺之气，不必祛湿，而湿自无不去之理。方用加减补中益气汤。

In the fifth month of pregnancy, some women suffer from fatigue, poor appetite, and edema that gradually spreads from the feet to the whole body, including the head and face. Interns think this is due to dampness. Actually, it is due to the deficiency of the lungs. Although the fetus is nourished during pregnancy according to a monthly regularity, in practice, treatment should not be limited to the number of months. Spleen strengthening and lung tonifying should be used as a general principle. The reason is that the spleen controls blood, the lungs govern qi, the fetus cannot sprout without the nourishment of blood and cannot grow without(the exuberance) of qi. When the spleen is fortified, the blood would be effulgent to nourish the fetus. When the lungs are made clear, qi would be effulgent to give birth to a baby. If the lungs are weakened, qi will be deficient and cannot transport itself to the skin. If the spleen is deficient, there would be no enough blood to reach the limbs. Now that both qi and blood are deficient, the spleen and lungs will fail to do their duty. Food is difficult to be digested, and refined essence is no longer transformed. Consequently, qi and blood will collapse and cannot uplift. The dampness will take advantage of the deficiency to accumulate and develop into edema.

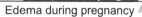
The treatment should be to nourish blood in the spleen and to supplement qi in the lungs instead of dispelling dampness. The dampness will depart without retention. The formula to use is *Jiā Jiǎn Bǔ Zhōng Yì Qì Tāng* (加减补中益气汤，Middle Tonifying and qi Benefiting Variant Decoction)

人参（五钱）　　　　黄芪（三钱，生用）

柴胡（一钱）　　　　甘草（一分）

当归（三钱，酒洗）　白术（五钱，土炒）

茯苓（一两）　　　　升麻（三分）

陈皮（三分）

rén shēn (ginseng), 5 *qian*

huáng qí (astragalus root) 3 *qian* (raw)

chái hú (bupleurum), 1 *qian*

gān cǎo (licorice root), 1 *fen*

dāng guī (Chinese angelica), 3 *qian* (washed with millet wine)

bái zhú (white atractylodes rhizome), 5 *qian*

fú líng (poria), 1 *liang*

shēng má, black cohosh rhizome, 3 *fen*

chén pí (aged tangerine peel), 3 *fen*

水煎服。四剂即愈，十剂不再犯。夫补中益气汤之立法也，原是升提脾肺之气似乎益气而不补血，然而血非气不生，是补气即所以生血。观当归补血汤用黄芪为君，则较著彰明矣。况湿气乘脾肺之虚而相犯，未便大补其血，恐阴太盛而招阴也。

Decoct the formula in water. When four *ji* is taken, the edema disappears. Taking 10 *ji* may prevent a relapse. *Bǔ Zhōng Yì Qì Tāng* (补中益气汤，Center-Supplementing and Qi-Boosting Decoction) is designed initially to uplift the qi of the spleen and lungs. It seems to boost the qi without supplementing the blood. Blood cannot be engendered without qi. Supplementing qi is precisely what engenders blood. This issue becomes apparent when this formula is compared with *Dāng Guī Bǔ Xuè Tāng* (当归补血汤，Chinese Angelica Blood Supplementing Decoction), in which, *huáng qí* (黄芪，asastragalus root) is used as the monarch herb. Moreover, dampness takes advantage of the deficiency of the spleen and lungs to invade; therefore, it is not proper to supplement blood greatly for fear that too exuberant yin may bring in pathogenic yin.

只补气而助以利湿之品，则气升而水尤易散，血亦随之而生矣。然则何以重用茯苓而至一两，不凡以利湿为君乎？磋！磋！湿症而不以此药为君，将以何者为君乎？况重用茯苓于补气之中，虽曰渗湿，而仍是健脾清肺之意。且凡利水之品，多是耗气之药，而茯苓与参术合，实补多于利，所以重用之以分湿邪，即以补气血耳。

To supplement qi and add herbs for draining dampness, the qi then may go up, and water will be dispersed quickly. Blood will then be engendered soon. However, why is *fú líng* (茯苓, poria) used heavily (as much as 1 *liang*)? Surely it means that we are using ingredients for draining dampness as the monarch herb. What is more, using large amounts of *fú líng* (茯苓, poria), together with ingredients to supplement qi, is for reinforcing the spleen and for clearing the lungs, although it is said that it is used for removing dampness. Generally speaking, herbs used for draining water are qi-consuming. However, considerable amounts of *fú líng* (茯苓, poria), together with *rén shēn* (人参, ginseng) and *bái zhú* (白术, white atractylodes rhizome), are much more tonifying and less water draining. Therefore we use considerable amounts of *fú líng* (茯苓, poria) to disperse dampness, which, in turn, results in supplementing qi and blood.

Chapter Thirty-nine

Lower Abdominal Pain During Pregnancy

妊娠少腹疼

妊娠少腹作疼，胎动不安，如有下堕之状，人只知带脉无力也，谁知是脾肾之亏乎。夫胞胎虽系于带脉，而带脉实关于脾肾。脾肾亏损，则带脉无力，胞胎即无以胜任矣。况人之脾肾亏损者，非饮食之过伤，即色欲之太甚。脾肾亏则带脉急，胞胎所以有下坠之状也。然则胞胎之系，通于心与肾，而不通于脾，补肾可也，何故补脾？然脾为后天，肾为先天，脾非先天之气不能化，肾非后天之气不能生，补肾而不补脾，则肾之精何以遽生也？是补后天之脾，正所以补先天之肾也；补先后二天之脾与肾，正所以固胞胎之气与血，脾肾可不均补乎！方用安奠二天汤。

Interns think lower abdominal pain during pregnancy, and excessive movement of the fetus threatening abortion, are merely due to *dai mai* atony. However, it is caused by the deficiency of the spleen and kidneys. The fetus is linked with *dai mai*, which is closely related to the spleen and kidneys. When the spleen and kidneys are depleted and damaged, *dai mai* will have atony, and the uterus would be incompetent. Furthermore, deficiency of the spleen and kidneys are caused either by the damage of overeating or indulging in sexual pleasure. When the spleen and kidneys are depleted, *dai mai* becomes spasmodic, and the uterus shows signs of sagging. Since the uterus communicates with the heart and kidneys rather than the spleen, it is reasonable to supplement the kidneys.

Nevertheless, why is it necessary to supplement the spleen? As the spleen is the postnatal base of life and the kidneys are the innate base of life, the spleen cannot perform its transforming function without the innate qi of life, while the kidneys cannot engender essence without the innate qi of life. To supplement the kidneys without reinforcing the spleen, how can the kidneys' essence be engendered quickly?

Treatment: supplementing the postnatal spleen is equal to reinforcing the innate essence of the kidneys. Therefore, both the innate and the postnatal spleen and kidneys are supplemented, and qi and blood of the uterus are strengthened. *Ān Diàn Èr Tiān Tāng* (安奠二天汤, Innate and Postnatal Tocolysis Decoction).

人参（一两，去芦）　　　　熟地（一两，九蒸）

白术（一两，土炒）　　　　山药（五钱，炒）

炙草（一钱）　　　　　　　山萸（五钱，蒸，去核）

杜仲（三钱，炒黑）　　　　枸杞（二钱）

扁豆（五钱，炒，去皮）

rén shēn (ginseng), 1 *liang* (with the little rhizomes on the top removed)

shú dì (prepared rehmannia root), 1 *liang* (big ones, fully steamed)

bái zhú (white atractylodes rhizome), 1 *liang* (dry-fried with earth)

shān yào (common yam rhizome), 5 *qian* (dry-fried)

zhì gān cǎo (prepared licorice root), 1 *qian*

shān yú ròu, fructus corni, 5 *qian* (steamed and decored)

dù zhòng, eucommia bark, 3 *qian* (charred)

gǒu qǐ , Chinese wolfberry fruit, 2 *qian*

biǎn dòu, hyacinth bean, 5 *qian* (dry-fried and peeled)

水煎服。一剂而疼止，二剂而胎安矣。夫胎动乃脾肾双亏之症，非大用参、术、熟地补阴补阳之品，断不能挽回于顷刻。世人往往畏用参、术，或少用，以冀建功，所以寡效。此方正妙在多用也。

The formula is decocted in water and taken orally. When one *ji* is taken, the pain is relieved. When the second *ji* is taken, the fetus becomes quiet. As threatened abortion belongs to the syndrome of deficiency of the spleen and kidneys, it can be saved quickly when only the herbs for supplementing yin and yang such as *rén shēn* (人参, ginseng), *bái zhú* (白术, white atractylodes rhizome), *shú dì* (熟地, are extensively used. Interns usually dare not use or only use a little *rén shēn* (人参, ginseng) and *bái zhú* (白术, white atractylodes rhizome). Therefore, they rarely achieve any effect. The subtlety of this formula lies in using them in large amounts.

（人参一两，或以党参代之，无上党参者，以嫩黄芪代之。）

[*Rén shēn* (人参, ginseng), 1 *liang*, could be substituted by *dǎng shēn* (党参, codonopsis root). If there is no good *dǎng shēn* (党参, codonopsis root), use young *huáng qí* (黄芪, asastragalus root).]

Chapter Forty
Dry Mouth and Sore Throat During Pregnancy

妊娠口干咽疼

妊娠三四个月，自觉口干舌燥，咽喉微痛，无津以润，以至胎动不安，甚则血流如经水，人以为火动之极也，谁知是水亏之甚乎；夫胎也者，本精与血之相结而成。逐月养胎，古人每分经络，其实均不离肾水之养，故肾水足而胎安，肾水亏而胎动。虽然肾水亏又何能动胎，必肾经之火动，而胎始不安耳。然而火之有余，仍是水之不足，所以火炎而胎必动，补水则胎自安，亦既济之义也。惟是肾水不能遽生，必须滋补肺金，金润则能生水，而水有逢源之乐矣。水既有本，则源泉混混矣，而火又何难制乎？再少加以清热之品，则胎自无不安矣。方用润燥安胎汤。

Some women in the third or fourth month of pregnancy experience dryness in the mouth, parched tongue, slight sore throat accompanied by an absence of fluid to moisten it, a restlessness of the fetus, and may even suffer from bleeding like menstrual flow. Interns would suspect this is because of a powerfully stirred fire. In fact, it is due to the severe depletion of water. The fetus is originally the combination of essence and blood and is nourished by a monthly natural law. The ancients used to assign the meridians to each month's nourishment or development. Kidney water is indispensable in nourishing the fetus all the time. When the kidney water is abundant, the fetus is healthy. When the kidney water is depleted, the fetus will be restless (showing symptoms of an impending abortion). How can the depletion of kidney water result in threatened abortion? It must be caused by agitated kidney fire. At the same time, the excessive fire is still the result of the deficiency of water. The flaming of fire will lead to the restlessness of the fetus (impeding abortion). Supplementing water will make the fetus peaceful, which is adding (kidney water) to balance fire and water. However, kidney water cannot be produced soon if lung metal is not nourished. When the metal is nourished, the water can be produced naturally. When water has its abundant resource, it can easily overwhelm fire. If a small amount of heat-clearing medicine is added, the fetus will be calm. The formula to use is *Rùn Zào Ān Tāi Tāng* (润燥安胎汤, Dryness Moistening and Fetus Calming Decoction).

熟地（一两，九蒸）　　　　生地（三钱，酒炒）

山萸肉（五钱，蒸）　　　　麦冬（五钱，去心）

五味子（一钱，炒）　　　　阿胶（二钱，蛤粉炒）

黄芩（二钱，酒炒）　　　　益母（二钱）

shú dì (prepared rehmannia root), 1 *liang* (fully steamed)

shēng dì (rehmannia root), 3 *qian* (dry-fried with millet wine)

shān yú ròu, (fructus corni), 5 *qian* (steamed)

mài dōng, dwarf lilyturf tuber, 5 *qian* (pith discarded)

wǔ wèi zǐ, Chinese magnoliavine fruit, 1 *qian* (dry-fried)

ē jiāo (donkey-hide gelatin), 2 *qian* (dry-fried with gecko powder)

huáng qín, scutellaria root, 2 *qian* (dry-fried with millet wine)

yì mǔ, motherwort, 2 *qian*

水煎服。二剂而燥息，再二剂而胎安。连服十剂，而胎不再动矣。此方专填肾中之精，而兼补肺。然补肺仍是补肾之意，故肾经不干燥，则火不能灼，胎焉有不安之理乎。

The formula is decocted in water. When two *ji* is taken, dryness is ended; When two more *ji* is taken, the fetus is calm. This formula is specially designed to supplement the essence in the kidneys, and at the same time, it can supplement the lungs. Supplementing the lungs still serves the purpose of supplementing the kidneys. Therefore, the kidney meridian is free from dryness, and fire can no longer burn. How can the fetus be restless?

Chapter Forty-one
Vomiting, Diarrhea, and Abdominal Pain During Pregnancy

妊娠吐泻腹疼

妊妇上吐下泻，胎动欲堕，腹疼难忍，急不可缓，此脾胃虚极而然也。夫脾胃之气虚，则胞胎无力，必有崩坠之虞。况又上吐下泻，则脾与胃之气，因吐泻而愈虚，欲胞胎之无恙也得乎。然胞胎疼痛而究不至下坠者，何也？全赖肾气之固也。胞胎系于肾而连于心，肾气固则交于心，其气通于胞胎，此胞胎之所以欲坠而不得也。且肾气能固，则阴火必来生脾；心气能通，则心火必来援胃，脾胃虽虚而未绝，则胞胎虽动而不堕，可不急救其脾胃乎！然脾胃当将绝而未绝之时，只救脾胃而难遽生，更宜补其心肾之火，使之生土，则两相接续，胎自固而安矣。方用援土固胎汤。

Some pregnant women suffer from vomiting, diarrhea, excessive fetus movement threatening abortion, unbearable acute abdominal pain too severe to be relieved. It is due to extreme deficiency and weakness of the spleen and stomach. When the spleen and stomach qi are deficient, the uterus will become weak, and there will undoubtedly exist the danger of bleeding and miscarriage. The spleen and stomach qi are made even more deficient and weak in combination with vomiting and diarrhea. How can the fetus be expected to be safe under these circumstances?

So, what is the reason why, despite the pain of the uterus, abortion does not occur? It depends on the security of the kidney qi. The uterus connects with the kidneys and links with the heart. When the kidney qi is secure, it will communicate with the heart and flow to the fetus. That is why the fetus threatens but does not miscarry.

Moreover, when the kidney qi is secure, the yin fire will surely come to engender the spleen. When the heart qi can flow freely, the heart fire will surely assist the stomach. The spleen and stomach are weak but not exhausted. Therefore, the fetus is restless but not aborted yet. So, is there any choice but to save the spleen and stomach?

The spleen and stomach, though not yet exhausted, are already on the edge of exhaustion. It is consequently difficult to engender them quickly if they alone are rescued. Therefore, it is proper to supplement the heart and kidneys' fire in order for them to engender earth. That way, the two are brought into contact, and the fetus will become secure and calm. The formula to use is *Yuán Tǔ Gù Tāi Tāng* (援土固胎汤, Earth Supporting and Fetus Securing Decoction).

人参（一两）	白术（二两，土炒）
山药（一两，炒）	肉桂（二钱，去粗，研）
制附子（五分）	续断（三钱）
杜仲（三钱，炒黑）	山萸（一两，蒸，去核）
枸杞（三钱）	菟丝子（三钱，酒炒）
砂仁（三粒，炒，研）	炙草（一钱）

rén shēn (ginseng), 1 *liang*

bái zhú (white atractylodes rhizome), 2 *liang* (dry-fried with earth)

shān yào (common yam rhizome), 1 *liang* (dry-fried)

ròu guì, (cinnamon bark), 2 *qian* (ground)

zhì fù zǐ (prepared aconite root), 5 fen

xù duàn, himalayan teasel root, 3 qian

dù zhòng, eucommia bark, 3 qian (charred)

shān yú fructus corni, 1 liang (steamed, stoned)

gǒu qǐ, Chinese wolfberry fruit, 3 qian

tù sī zǐ dodder seed, 3 qian (dry-fried with millet wine)

shārén, villous amomum fruit, 3 pieces (dry-fried, ground)

zhì cǎo (prepared licorice root), 1 *qian*

水煎服。一剂而泄止，二剂而诸病尽愈矣。此方救脾胃之土十之八，救心肾之火十之二也。救火轻于救土者，岂以土欲绝而火未甚衰乎？非也。盖土崩非重剂不能援，火衰虽小剂而可助，热药多用，必有太燥之虞，不比温甘之品也。况胎动系土衰而非火弱，何用太热。妊娠忌桂附，是恐伤胎，岂可多用。小热之品计之以钱，大热之品计之以分者，不过用以引火，而非用以壮火也。其深思哉！

Decoct the formula in water and take it. When one *ji* is taken, diarrhea is stopped. After the second *ji* is taken, all other problems are solved. Eight-tenths of the functions and effects of this formula are allotted to saving the spleen and stomach earth, while two-tenths are allotted to the saving of the fire of the heart and kidneys. Is saving fire given less priority to saving earth because the earth borders on exhaustion while the fire is not yet so debilitated? No. When earth is about to collapse, it cannot be saved unless a large dose is used. At the same time, debilitated fire can be assisted by a small dose. The large number of hot ingredients, which are unlike warm, sweet ingredients, is sure to incur the danger of over-dryness.

What is more, excessive fetus movement is due to the debilitated earth rather than to weak fire. What is the point of using hot herbs? Women in pregnancy should avoid *fù zǐ* (附子, prepared aconite root) and *ròu guì* (肉桂, cinnamon bark), because they may hurt the fetus. How can they be used in large amounts? Slightly hot herbs may be used only by *qian* (3.125 *gram*), while herbs that are extremely hot in nature only by *fen* (0.3125 *gram*). They are used to guide fire rather than to invigorate fire. It deserves deep thought.

妊娠子悬肋疼

妊妇有怀抱忧郁，以致胎动不安，两胁闷而疼痛，如弓上弦，人止知是子悬之病也，谁知是肝气不通乎。夫养胎半系于肾水，然非肝血相助，肾水实有独力难支之势。故保胎必滋肾水，而肝血断不可不顾，使肝气不郁，则肝之气不闭，而肝之血必旺，自然灌溉胞胎，合肾水而并协养胎之力。

Some pregnant women are overwhelmed by depression that they have a threatened abortion, hypochondriac fullness, and pain like a fully drawn bow-string. Interns know that is "zixuan"*. Actually, it is liver qi stagnation. The fetus growing relies half on kidney water for nourishment, but if there is no liver blood assistance, kidney water finds it challenging to persist. Therefore, to secure the fetus, kidney water must be enriched, and the liver blood also must be taken into account. Thus the liver qi is free from depression and being blocked. Liver blood would then undoubtedly become effulgent and be able to irrigate the uterus. Moreover, it will join kidney water to nourish the fetus.

今肝气因忧郁而闭塞，则胎无血荫，肾难独任，而胎安得不上升以觅食，此乃郁气使然也。莫认为子之欲自悬，而妄用泄子之品则得矣。治法宜开肝气之郁结，补肝血之燥干，则子悬自定矣。方用解郁汤。

When the liver qi is blocked due to depression, the fetus loses nourishment from the blood, and the kidneys find it challenging to fulfill their duty single-handed. How can the fetus not go upward to search for food? Of course, it is due to qi's depression. Please do not believe that it will be all right when medicines to drain the fetus are employed to assume that the fetus can suspend itself by its own will.

Treatment: Relieve the depression of the liver qi and nourish dried liver blood. Then the suspended fetus will settle back into place. *Jiě yù Tāng* (解郁汤，Depression Relieving Decoction) is recommended.

人参（一钱）　　　　　　白术（五钱，土炒）

白茯苓（三钱）　　　　　当归（一两，酒洗）

白芍（一两，酒炒）　　　枳壳（五分，炒）

砂仁（三粒，炒，研）　　山栀子（三钱，炒）

薄荷（二钱）

rén shēn (ginseng), 1 *qian*

bái zhú (white atractylodes rhizome), 5 *qian* (dry-fried with earth)

bái fú líng (poria), 3 *qian*

dāng guī (Chinese angelica), 1 *liang* (washed with millet wine)

bái sháo (white peony root), 1 *liang* (dry-fried with millet wine)

zhǐ qiào (bitter orange), 5 *fen* (dry-fried)

shā rén (villous amomum fruit), 3 pieces (dry-fried, ground)

shān zhī zǐ (gardenia), 3 *qian* (dry-fried)

bò he, (field mint), 2 *qian*

水煎服。一剂而闷痛除，二剂而子悬定，至三剂而全安。去栀子，再多服数剂不复发。此乃平肝解郁之圣药，郁开则木不克土，肝平则火不妄动。方中又有健脾开胃之品，自然水精四布，而肝与肾有润泽之机，则胞胎自无干燥之患，又何虑上悬之不愈哉。

（方加薏仁三四钱尤妙。）

Decoct the formula in water. When one *ji* is taken, the depression and pain are relieved. When the second *ji* is taken, the fetal suspension is settled. When the third *ji* is taken, a complete recovery will be achieved. Then, if several more *ji* with *zhī zǐ* (栀子，gardenia) removed is taken, relapse will be prevented. It is an effective formula for soothing the liver and relieving depression. When the depression is relieved, wood will no longer restrain earth. Once the liver is soothed, the fire will no longer be stirred recklessly. This formula also includes medicines for strengthening spleen and promoting appetite. Water essence will be distributed all through the body. The liver and kidneys may have the chance of getting moisture, and the fetus will naturally exist without the affliction of dryness. No need to worry that fetal suspension will not be cured.

[It is even better if 3~4 *qian* of *yì rén* (薏仁 coix seed) is added.]

*

Zixuan, its literal translation is "fetal suspension" which implies that the fetus has moved up too far under the ribs. It is not being carried down low enough in the abdomen. In fact, it is the distention feeling in chest during pregnancy.

Chapter Forty-three
Impact Injury During Pregnancy

妊娠跌损

妊妇有失足跌损，致伤胎元，腹中疼痛，势如将堕者，人只知是外伤之为病也，谁知有内伤之故乎。凡人内无他症，胎元坚固，即或跌扑闪挫，依然无恙。惟内之气血素亏，故略有闪挫，胎便不安。

Some pregnant women experience impact injury from falling and suffer from damage of the embryo, have abdominal pain, and impending abortion. Interns believe this is a disease resulting from external injury. Actually, it is caused by existing internal damage. So long as the patient has no other interior disease, the fetal origin (embryo) is strong and secure. Even in case of falling, wrenching, or contusion, they are safe and sound. Only if the internal qi and blood have been frequently depleted can the fetus be disturbed by contusion or wrenching, however slight it be.

若止作闪挫外伤治，断难奏功，且恐有因治而反堕者，可不慎欤！必须大补气血，而少加以行瘀之品，则瘀散胎安矣。但大补气血之中，又宜补血之品多于补气之药，则无不得之。方用救损安胎汤。

If this is treated simply as an external injury due to contusion or wrenching, the cure is nearly impossible, and there are cases where abortion is induced by therapeutic error. How can we not be cautious? It is necessary to supplement qi and blood significantly and use a small number of medicines to remove stasis. Then stasis will be dispersed, and the fetus will become normal. Blood-supplementing medicines should be used more than qi-supplementing ones. An almost magic effect will be the result without fail. *Jiù Sǔn Ān Tāi Tāng* (救损安胎汤, Injury Rescuing and Fetus Calming Decoction) is recommended.

当归（一两，酒洗）　　　　　　白芍（三钱，酒炒）

生地（一两，酒炒）　　白术（五钱，土炒）

炙草（一钱）　　　　　人参（一钱）

苏木（三钱，捣碎）　　乳香（一钱，去油）

没药（一钱，去油）

dāng guī (Chinese angelica), 1 *liang* (washed with millet wine)

bái sháo (white peony root), 3 *qian* (dry-fried with millet wine)

shēng dì (rehmannia root), 1 *liang* (dry-fried with millet wine)

bái zhú (white atractylodes rhizome), 5 *qian* (dry-fried with earth)

zhì cǎo (prepared licorice root), 1 *qian*

rén shēn (ginseng), 1 *qian*

sū mù, (sappan wood), 3 *qian* (pound to pieces)

rǔ xiāng (frankincense), 1 *qian* (deoil)

mò yào (myrrh), 1 *qian* (deoil)

水煎服。一剂而疼痛止，二剂而势不下坠矣，不必三剂也。此方之妙，妙在既能祛瘀而不伤胎，又能补气补血而不凝滞，固无通利之害，亦痊跌闪之伤。有益无损，大建奇功，即此方与。然不特治怀孕之闪挫也，即无娠闪挫，亦可用之。

The formula is decocted in water. After one *ji* is taken, the pain is relieved. When the second *ji* is taken, the likelihood of abortion is thwarted. Taking the third *ji* is unnecessary. This formula's subtlety lies in its ability to remove stasis without injury to the fetus and to supplement qi and blood without causing congealing and stagnation. There is no risk caused by smoothing and unblocking. However, it can treat the impact injury, being beneficial without causing any harm. It is a formula with magic power. What is more, it is a formula specifically effective for contusion and wrenching during pregnancy and efficacious for injures of patients who are not pregnant.

Chapter Forty-four

Vaginal Bleeding During Pregnancy

妊娠胎漏

妊妇有胎不动腹不疼，而小便中时常有血流出者，人以为血虚胎漏也，谁知气虚不能摄血乎。夫血只能荫胎，而胎中之荫血，必赖气以卫之，气虚下陷，则荫胎之血亦随气而陷矣。然则气虚下陷，而血未尝虚，似不应与气同陷也。不知气乃血之卫，血赖气以固，气虚则血无凭依，无凭依必燥急，燥急必生邪热；血寒则静，血热则动，动则外出而莫能遏，又安得不下流乎。倘气不虚而血热，则必大崩，而不止些微之漏矣。治法宜补其气之不足，而泄其火之有余，则血不必止而自无不止矣。方用助气补漏汤。

Some pregnant women frequently have blood in the urine (vaginal bleeding) with no fetal stirring (excessive fetal movement) and no abdominal pain. Interns believe it is due to blood deficiency. Actually, it results from deficient qi failing to control blood as blood nourishes the fetus, while blood (yin) in the fetus depends on qi for its defense.

Deficient qi will lead to the collapse of blood in the fetus. Moreover, deficient qi fall does not necessarily mean blood deficiency. The blood seems like it should not collapse with qi. However, the fact is that qi provides the defense of blood, and blood depends on qi to consolidate itself. When qi is deficient, blood will have nothing to depend on to defend it, which will lead to dryness and impetuosity of blood. This dryness and impetuosity then engender pathogenic heat.

In a cold circumstance, blood is tranquil, but it is agitated and stirred in a hot circumstance. Once stirred, it must go out and cannot be stopped. How can it not flow downward? If qi is not deficient and blood is hot, this will undoubtedly lead to blood flooding. It is not a small amount of leakage.

Treatment: supplement insufficient qi and drain superabundant fire. In this way, bleeding is stopped automatically without using a hemorrhage stopping medicine. The prescription to use is *Zhù Qì Bǔ Lòu Tāng* (助气补漏汤，Qi Assisting and

Bleeding Stopping Decoction).

人参（一两）　　　　　白芍（五钱，酒炒）

黄芩（三钱，酒炒黑）　　生地（三钱，酒炒黑）

益母草（一钱）　　　　　续断（二钱）

甘草（一钱）

rén shēn (ginseng), 1 *liang*

bái sháo (white peony root), 5 *qian* (dry-fried with millet wine)

huáng qín (scutellaria root), 3 *qian* (charred with millet wine)

shēng dì (rehmannia root), 3 *qian* (charred with millet wine)

yì mǔ cǎo (motherwort) , 1 *qian*

xù duàn (himalayan teasel root), 2 *qian*

gān cǎo (licorice root), 1 *qian*

水煎服。一剂而血止，二剂再不漏矣。此方用人参以补阳气，用黄芩以泄阴火。火泄则血不热而无欲动之机，气旺则血有依而无可漏之窍，气血俱旺而和协，自然归经而各安其所矣，又安有漏泄之患哉！

Decoct the formula in water. When one *ji* is taken, flooding is stopped. After the second *ji* is taken, metrostaxis is stopped. *Rén shēn* (人参, ginseng) is used to reinforce yang qi, and *huáng qín* (黄芩, scutellaria root) is used to drain yin fire. When fire is drained, blood will be no longer hot and has no chance to agitate. When qi is made effulgent, blood can depend on it and has no chance to leak out. When qi and blood are both effulgent and in harmony, they naturally return to the channels and become calm in their abodes.

Chapter Forty-five

Fetal Crying in Pregnancy

妊娠子鸣

妊妇怀胎至七八个月，忽然儿啼腹中，腰间隐隐作痛，人以为胎热之过也，谁知是气虚之故乎。治宜大补其气，方用扶气止啼汤。

In the seventh or eighth month of pregnancy, some women suddenly experience the fetus crying from within the abdomen accompanied by a dull pain in the lumbar region. People suppose this is due to fetal heat. Who would suspect that it is caused by qi deficiency?

Treatment: supplement qi greatly. The formula to use is *Fú Qì Zhǐ Tí Tā-ng* (扶气止啼汤, Qi Supporting and Cry Stopping Decoction).

人参（一两）　　　　　　黄芪（一两，生用）
麦冬（一两，去心）　　　当归（五钱）
橘红（五分）　　　　　　甘草（一钱）
花粉（一钱）

rén shēn (ginseng), 1 *liang*

huáng qí (astragalus root), 1 *liang* (raw)

mài dōng, (dwarf lilyturf tuber), 1 *liang* (pitch discarded)

dāng guī (Chinese angelica), 5 *qian*

jú hóng, (red tangerine peel), 5 *fen*

gān cǎo (licorice root), 1 *qian*

huā fěn (snakegourd root), 1 *qian*

水煎服。一剂而啼即止，二剂不再啼。此方用人参、黄芪、麦冬以补肺气，使肺气旺则胞胎之气亦旺，胞胎之气旺，则胞中之子气有不随母之气以为呼吸者，未之有也。

Decoct the formula in water. After one *ji* is taken, crying is brought to a pause.

After the second *ji* is taken, the crying stops. *Rén shēn* (人参, ginseng), *huáng qí* (黄芪, astragalus root) and mài dōng (麦冬, dwarf lilyturf tuber) are used to supplement the lung qi. When the lung qi is effulgent, the qi of the uterus also becomes effulgent. Then, how can the fetal qi in the uterus not breathe in pace with its mother's qi? It is impossible.

Chapter Forty-six

Lumber and Abdominal Pain, Thirst, Sweating, and Mania During Pregnancy

妊娠腰腹疼渴汗躁狂

妇人怀妊有口渴汗出，大饮冷水，而烦躁发狂，腰腹疼痛，以致胎欲堕者。人莫不谓火盛之极也，抑知是何经之火盛乎。此乃胃火炎炽，熬煎胞胎之水，以致胞胎之水涸，胎失所养，故动而不安耳。夫胃为水谷之海，多气多血之经，所以养五脏六腑者。盖万物皆生于土，土气厚而物始生，土气薄而物必死。

Some women become thirsty, sweat spontaneously, drink cold water in significant quantities, and then suffer from vesania, agitation, mania, lumber, and abdominal pain, which eventually induces abortion. Interns all say it is due to extreme fire exuberance, but do they know in which channel the fire is so effulgent? It is fire in the stomach that is flaming intensely and boils water in the uterus. As a result, water in the uterus is dried up, and the fetus loses what nourishes it. Therefore, the fetus stirs and becomes restless. The stomach is the sea of water and grain, and a channel abundant in qi and blood. It nourishes the five zang-organs and the six fu-organs because every living thing arises from earth. When earth qi is thick (abundant), things begin to grow, and when earth qi is thin (insufficient), things are doomed to death.

然土气之所以能厚者，全赖火气之来生也；胃之能化水谷者，亦赖火气之能化也。今胃中有火，宜乎生土，何以火盛而反致害乎？不知无火难以生土，而火多又能烁水。虽土中有火土不死，然亦必有水方不燥；使胃火太旺，必致烁干肾水，土中无水，则自润不足，又何以分润胞胎；土烁之极，火势炎蒸，犯心越神，儿胎受逼，安得不下坠乎。经所谓二阳之病发心脾者，正此义也。治法必须泄火滋水，使水气得旺，则火气自平，火平则汗狂燥渴自除矣。方用息焚安胎汤。

That earth qi can grow thick depends on the engendering of fire qi. That the stomach can transform water and grain depends on the transformation of fire qi. If there is fire in the stomach, a favorable condition for generating earth, how can fire in the stomach be exuberant and be harmful instead? It is challenging to generate Earth without fire, but fire, if excessive, will dry up water. Earth lives on as long as there is fire in it, but it is free from dryness only when there is also water in earth. Suppose stomach fire is over effulgent. It will inevitably dry up kidney water. If there is no water in earth, how can it spare any water to moisten the uterus when it has not enough to moisten even itself? When earth is burning intensely, the blaze flames and steams. It invades the heart and leads to mental aberration. The fetus is oppressed. How can it be prevented from sagging? This is just what is meant by the statement in the classic that, "Disease of the second yang (yangming) expands to the heart and spleen."

Treatment: Drain fire and enrich water. Once water qi is made effulgent, fire qi automatically becomes calm. Consequently, sweating, mania, agitation, and thirst are eliminated naturally. The formula to use is *Xī Fén Ān Taī Tān* (息焚安胎汤，Flames Quenching and Fetus Calming Decoction).

生地（一两，酒炒）　　　青篙（五钱）
白术（五钱，土炒）　　　茯苓（三钱）
人参（三钱）　　　　　　知母（二钱）
花粉（二钱）

shēng dì (rehmannia root), 1 liang (dry-fried with millet wine)

qīng hāo (Artemisia Apiacea), 5 qian

bái zhú (white atractylodes rhizome), 5 *qian* (dry-fried with earth)

fú líng (poria), 3 *qian*

rén shēn (ginseng), 3 *qian*

zhī mǔ (common anemarrhena rhizome), 2 *qian*

huā fěn (snakegourd root), 2 *qian*

水煎服。一剂而狂少平，二剂而狂大定，三剂而火尽解，胎亦安矣。此方药料颇重，恐人虑不胜，而不敢全用，又不得不再为嘱之。怀胎而火胜若此，非大剂何以能蠲，火不息则狂不止，而胎能安耶？况药料虽多，均是滋水之味，益而无损，勿过虑也。

Decoct the formula in water. When one *ji* is taken, mania is alleviated a little. When the second *ji* is taken, mania is mostly settled. After the third *ji* is taken, fire is resolved entirely, and the fetus is calm. This formula is a substantial dosage. In anticipation of some interns not daring to use it for fear patients cannot stand it, it is necessary to give some more assurance. When fire is overwhelming to such an extent in pregnancy, what can extinguish it except such a large dose? Unless the fire is put out, mania cannot be relieved. So how can the fetus be calm?

Furthermore, significant though the dosages are in quantity, the ingredients are but medicines to enrich water. They can do anything but harm. So there is no need to worry.

妊娠多怒堕胎

妇人有怀妊之后，未至成形，或已成形，其胎必堕。人皆曰气血衰微，不能固胎也，谁知是性急怒多，肝火大动而不静乎。夫肝本藏血，肝怒则不藏，不藏则血难固。盖肝虽属木，而木中实寄龙雷之火，所谓相火是也。相火宜静不宜动，静则安，动则炽。

Some women invariably miscarry when the fetus has or has not yet taken shape. Interns believe this is due to the declination of qi and blood failing to secure the fetus. Actually, this is because characteristic impetuosity and irascibility cause great stirring and restlessness of liver fire. The liver is responsible for storing blood. When one is angry, it fails to store, and then the blood becomes challenging to secure. Although the liver belongs to wood, there is dragon-thunderous fire hidden in wood, or in other words, ministerial fire. Ministerial fire prefers tranquility, not a disturbance. Given tranquility, it is calm. If stirred or agitated, it burns ragingly.

况木中之火，又易动而难静。人生无日无动之时，即无日非动火之时。大怒则火益动矣，火动而不可止遏，则火势飞扬，不能生气养胎，而反食气伤精矣。精伤则胎无所养，势必不坠而不已。经所谓少火生气，壮火食气，正此义也。治法宜平其肝中之火，利其腰脐之气，使气生夫血而血清其火，则庶几矣。方用利气泄火汤。

What is more, fire hidden in wood is easy to stir but challenging to be tranquil. In one's life, there is not a single day without disturbance. That means there is not a single day when fire is not stirred. Fire is all the more stirred in violent anger, and, when stirring, Fire becomes uncontrollable, and furious flames soar. Far from being able to engender qi or nourish the fetus, it consumes qi and damages essence. Once essence is damaged, the fetus has nothing to nourish it, which cannot but end in abortion. This is just what is meant by the classic statement that, "Mild fire promotes qi production. Vigorous fire consumes qi."

Treatment: calm the liver fire, soothe the qi of the lumbus, and navel. Once qi is made to engender blood and able to clear fire, recovery will be realized soon. The formula to use is *Lì Qì Xiè Huǒ Tāng* (利气泄火汤，Qi Soothing and Fire Purging Decoction).

人参（三钱） 　　　　白术（一两，土炒）

甘草（一钱） 　　　　熟地（五钱，九蒸）

当归（三钱，酒洗） 　　白芍（五钱，酒炒）

芡实（三钱，炒） 　　　黄芩（二钱，酒炒）

rén shēn (ginseng), 3 *qian*

bái zhú (white atractylodes rhizome), 1 *liang* (dry-fried with earth)

gān cǎo (licorice root), 1 *qian*

shú dì (prepared rehmannia root), 5 *qian* (fully steamed)

dāng guī (Chinese angelica), 3 *qian* (washed with millet wine)

bái sháo (white peony root), 5 *qian* (dry-fried with millet wine)

qiàn shí (euryale seed), 3 *qian* (dry-fried)

huáng qín (scutellaria root), 2 *qian* (dry-fried with millet wine)

水煎服。六十剂而胎不坠矣。此方名虽利气，而实补气也。然补气而不加以泄火之品，则气旺而火不能平，必反害其气也。故加黄芩于补气之中以泄火，又有熟地、归、芍以滋肝而壮水之主，则血不燥而气得和，怒气息而火自平，不必利气而气无不利，即无往而不利矣。

Decoct the formula in water. After sixty *ji* is taken, abortion is prevented. Although this formula is entitled "qi soothing" Decoction, it supplements qi. However, if fire-purging ingredients were not added to these qi-supplementing medicines, qi might become effulgent, and fire would remain restless. This would harm qi.

For this reason, *huáng qín* (黄芩，scutellaria root) is added to qi-supplementing medicines in order to purge fire. Besides, *shú dì* (熟地，prepared rehmannia root), *dāng guī* (当归，Chinese angelica), and *bái sháo* (白芍，white peony root) are used to nourish the liver and invigorate the water source (to inhibit exuberant yang). Thus, blood is free from dryness and qi is brought into harmony, angry qi is appeased, and fire calms down. Qi is relieved of inhibition without fail and without needing to use qi-activating medicine. There is no doubt about the effect.

Volume Six

Miscarriage

小产

Chapter Forty-eight
Miscarriage Due to Sexual Intercourse

行房小产

妊妇因行房癫狂,遂致小产,血崩不止。人以为火动之极也,谁知是气脱之故乎。大凡妇人之怀妊也,赖肾水以荫胎。水源不足,则火易沸腾。加以久战不已,则火必大动,再至兴酣颠狂,精必大泄。精大泄则肾水益涸,而龙雷相火益炽。水火两病,胎不能固而堕矣。胎堕而火犹未息,故血随火而崩下,有不可止遏之势。人谓火动之极,亦未为大误也。但血崩本于气虚,火盛本于水亏,肾水既亏,则气之生源涸矣;气源既涸,而气有不脱者乎? 此火动是标,而气脱是本也。经云:治病必求其本。本固而标自立矣。若只以止血为主,而不急固其气,则气散不能速回,而血何由止。不大补其精,则水涸不能速长,而火且益炽,不揣其本,而齐其末,山未见有能济者也。方用固气填精汤。

Miscarriage with persistent bleeding caused by sexual intercourse in pregnant women is supposedly due to excessive fire stirring. In fact, it is due to the collapse of qi. Being pregnant depends upon the nourishment the fetus receives from kidney water. When water does not have enough sources, fire will flame up. Added with long-time intercourse, fire will flare up, and essence will be drained. When the essence is exhausted, kidney water will be depleted.

Moreover, the dragon-thunderous ministerial fire will be more blazing. Both water and fire are not in a formal condition; the fetus cannot be secured, which then causes miscarriage. Fire does not cool down with the miscarriage, and blood comes down with fire unrestrained. People say it is the excessive stirring of fire, which is not a big mistake. However, bleeding is caused by qi deficiency, and exuberant fire is caused by water depletion. Now that the kidney water is depleted, the source of qi generation becomes exhausted. With the source exhausted, how can qi be expected not to collapse? Therefore, stirring fire is just *biao*, (the tip aspect, or branch), while qi collapsing is *ben*, (the root aspect). The classic states: "to treat the disease, it must be pursued to its *ben*." Once *ben* is secured, *biao* will be naturally normal. If stopping bleeding is considered the central task without securing qi on time, qi will disperse and not return soon. Then how can bleeding be stopped? If essence is not significantly supplemented, water, which has become exhausted, cannot proliferate. Then fire rages even more intensely. We have never seen anyone who can get a curative effect by treating the tips instead of focusing on the root. The formula to use is *Gù Qì Tián Jīng Tāng* (固气填精汤, Qi Securing and Essence Replenishing Decoction).

人参（一两）　　　　　　黄芪（一两，生用）

白术（五钱，土炒）　　　大熟地（一两，九蒸）

当归（五钱，酒洗）　　　三七（三钱，研末）

荆芥穗（二钱，炒黑）

rén shēn (ginseng), 1 *liang*

huáng qí (astragalus root), 1 *liang*（raw）

bái zhú (white atractylodes rhizome), 5 *qian* (dry-fried with earth)

shú dì (prepared rehmannia root), 1 *liang* (big ones, fully steamed)

dāng guī (Chinese angelica), 5 *qian* (washed with millet wine)

sān qī (pseudoginseng root), 3 *qian* (ground)

jīng jiè suì (fineleaf schizonepeta spike), 2 *qian* (charred)

水煎服。一剂而血止，二剂而身安，四剂则全愈。此方之妙，妙在不去清火，而惟补气补精，其奏功独神者，以诸药温润能除大热也。盖热是虚，故补气自能摄血，补精自能止血，意在本也。

Decoct the formula in water. When one *ji* is taken, bleeding is stopped. When the second *ji* is taken, the body is out of danger. After four *ji* is taken, complete recovery is effected. The subtlety of this formula lies in its supplementing qi and essence without clearing fire. What accounts for its miraculous effect is that various ingredients, which are warm and moistening, can eliminate intense heat. Because this heat is deficient heat, supplementing qi can gain the effect of controlling blood, and supplementing essence may stop bleeding. The formula aims at treating the root.

Chapter Forty-nine
Miscarriage Due to Wrenching and Contusion

跌闪小产

妊妇有跌扑闪挫，遂致小产，血流紫块，昏晕欲绝者。人皆曰瘀血作祟也，谁知是血室损伤乎。夫血室与胞胎相连，如唇齿之相依。胞胎有伤，则血室亦损，唇亡齿寒，理有必然也。然胞胎伤损而流血者，其伤浅；血室伤损而流血者，其伤深。伤之浅者，疼在腹；伤之深者，晕在心。同一跌扑损伤，而未小产与已小产，治各不同。未小产而胎不安者，宜顾其胎，而不可轻去其血；已小产而血大崩，宜散其瘀，而不可重伤其气。盖胎已堕，血既脱，而血室空虚，惟气存耳。倘或再伤其气，安保无气脱之忧乎。经云：血为营，气为卫。使卫有不固，则营无依而安矣。故必补气以生血，新血生而瘀血自散矣。方用理气散瘀汤。

Some pregnant women experience falls, contusion, or wrenching and subsequently suffer from miscarriage accompanied by bleeding with dark blood clots, dizziness, and faintness. Interns all declare this is due to blood stasis. In fact, it is the detriment of the blood chamber in the uterus which should be blamed. The blood chamber is connected with the fetus as the lips are to the teeth. When the fetus is hurt, the uterus must have been hurt too. Teeth are exposed to cold when lips are lost. However, for bleeding caused by damage to the uterus, the damage is superficial. The damage to the blood chamber causes bleeding, and the damage is deep-seated. Superficial damage gives pain in the abdomen, whereas deep-seated damage causes faintness (due to deficiency) of the heart. Similar injuries may cause miscarriage or not. The treatment should not be the same. If there is no miscarriage, but the fetus is restless, it is proper to attend to the fetus, and it is not advisable to activate the blood to resolve stasis blindly. If there is a miscarriage accompanied by severe bleeding, it is advisable to remove the blood stasis, but it is not permissible to inflict new injury to qi.

After the fetus has aborted and the blood has collapsed, the blood chamber is vacuous and empty and what is left is nothing but qi. If this qi were to be damaged, how can we avoid qi collapse? The classic states: "blood is the nutrient aspect, and qi is the defensive aspect." If the defensive aspect (qi) is insecure, the nutrient aspect cannot remain calm for having nothing to support it. Therefore, it is necessary to supplement qi to engender blood. When the new blood is engendered, static blood will be dispersed naturally. The formula to use is *Lǐ Qì Sàn Yū Tāng* (理气散瘀汤, Qi Regulating and Stasis Dissipating Decoction).

人参（一两）　　　　　　黄芪（一两，生用）

当归（五钱，酒洗）　　　茯苓（三钱）

红花（一钱）　　　　　　丹皮（三钱）

姜碳（五钱）

rén shēn (ginseng), 1 *liang*

huáng qí (astragalus root), 1 *liang* (raw)

dāng guī (Chinese angelica), 5 *qian* (washed with millet wine)

fú líng (poria), 3 *qian*

hóng huā (safflower), 1 *qian*

dān pí (tree peony bark), 3 *qian*

Jiāng tàn (prepared dried ginger), 5 *qian*

水煎服。一剂而流血止，二剂而昏晕除，三剂而全安矣。此方用人参、黄芪以补气，气旺则血可摄也；用当归、丹皮以生血，血生则瘀难留也；用红花、黑姜以活血，血活则晕可除也；用茯苓以利水，水利则血易归经也。

Decoct the formula in water. After one *ji* is taken, bleeding is stopped. After the second *ji* is taken, dizziness and faintness will disappear. When the third *ji* is taken, the body is completely recovered. This formula uses *rén shēn* (人参, ginseng) and Huangqi to supplement qi. When qi is exuberant, blood can be controlled. It uses *dāng guī* (当归, Chinese angelica) and *dān pí* (丹皮, cortex moutan) to engender blood so that the blood stasis will be removed. *Hóng huā* (红花, safflower) and *Jiāng tàn* (姜碳, prepared dried ginger) are used to promote blood circulation so that the dizziness and faintness will disappear. *Fú líng* (茯苓, poria) is used for draining water so that blood will return to its channels.

大便干结小产

妊妇有口渴烦躁，舌上生疮，两唇肿裂，大便干结，数日不得通，以致腹疼小产者。人皆曰大肠之火热也，谁知是血热烁胎乎。夫血所以养胎也，温和则胎受其益，太热则胎受其损。如其热久烁之，则儿在胞胎之中，若有探汤之苦，难以存活，则必外越下奔，以避炎气之逼迫，欲其胎之不堕也得乎。然则血荫乎胎，则血必虚耗。血者阴也，虚则阳亢，亢则害矣。且血乃阴水所化，血日荫胎，取给刻不容缓。而火炽阴水不能速生以化血，所以阴虚火动。阴中无非火气，血中亦无非火气矣，两火相合，焚逼胎儿，此胎之所以下坠也。

Some pregnant women suffer from thirst, vexation, sore and swollen tongue, cracked lips, dry stool, constipation lasting for several days, and subsequent abdominal pain and even miscarriage. Interns all declare this is due to fire heat of the large Intestine. Actually, it is due to hot blood burning the fetus. As a fetus-nourishing substance, blood benefits the fetus when it is warm but injures it when it is boiling. If blood remains hot for an extended period and burns, the fetus in the uterus will suffer such torment as if in boiling water, so much so that it becomes difficult for the fetus to survive. It has no other choice but to move out and run down to escape the flaming oppression. Then, how can abortion be avoided? Because it nourishes the fetus, blood is bound to be consumed and turns deficient during pregnancy. Blood belongs to yin. When blood becomes deficient, yang will become hyperactive. The hyperactivity of yang harms.

Furthermore, blood is transformed from yin water. As blood has to nourish the fetus every day, it demands a supply of blood urgently. Whereas, if fire is burning ragingly, yin water cannot be engendered quickly enough to transform blood. As a result, kidney yin becomes deficient, and fire is stirred. Because yin now is full of nothing but fire, and blood is full of nothing but fire, these two fires join each other to burn and press the fetus so that the fetus drops.

治法宜清胞中之火，补肾中之精，则可已矣。或疑儿已下坠，何故再顾其胞？血不荫胎，何必大补其水？殊不知火动之极，以致胎坠，则胞中纯是一团火气，此火乃虚火也。实火可泄，而虚火宜于补中清之，则虚火易散，而真水可生。倘一味清凉以降火，全不顾胞胎之虚实，势必至寒气逼人，胃中生气萧索矣。胃乃二阳，资养五脏者也。胃阳不生，何以化精微以生阴水乎。有不变为劳瘵者几希矣。方用加减四物汤。

Treatment: Clear fire from the uterus and supplement essence in the kidneys. Then everything will be alright.

It may be questioned why the uterus should be the primary concern since the fetus has aborted and why water should be significantly supplemented since it is the blood that fails to nourish the fetus. It should be understood that when fire stirs to such an extreme extent that it results in abortion, the uterus is filled with masses of fire qi. However, this fire is deficient fire. Excess fire allows for purging, but deficient fire requires clearing by way of supplementation. In this way, deficient fire is easy to dissipate, and kidney water will be engendered. Suppose cool and clearing ingredients are used exclusively to reduce fire without considering whether the uterus is deficient or replete. In that case, cold qi will undoubtedly be made to oppress menacingly. Thus, the vital qi is left in dire meagerness in the stomach. The stomach, the foot yangming, nourishes and provides supplementation for the five *zang*-organs. If the stomach yang stops being engendered, what else can transform the refined essence to engender yin water? Few cases can avoid changing into consumptive diseases if treated erroneously. The formula to use is *Jiā Jiǎn Sì Wù Tāng* (加减四物汤, Four Substances Variant Decoction).

熟地（五钱，九蒸）	白芍（三钱，生用）
当归（一两，酒洗）	川芎（一钱）
山栀子（一钱，炒）	山萸（二钱，蒸，去核）
山药（三钱，炒）	丹皮（三钱，炒）

shú dì (prepared rehmannia root), 5 *qian* (fully steamed)

bái sháo (white peony root), 3 *qian* (raw)

dāng guī (Chinese angelica), 1 *liang* (washed with millet wine)

chuān xiōng (Sichuan lovage root), 1 *qian*

shān zhī zǐ (gardenia), 1 *qian* (dry-fried)

shān yú (fructus corni), 2 *qian* (steamed, stoned)

shān yào (common yam rhizome), 3 *qian* (dry-fried)

dān pí (tree peony bark), 3 *qian* (dry-fried)

水煎服。四五剂而愈矣。丹皮性极凉血，产后用之，最防阴凝之害，慎之。

Decoct the formula in water. After four or five *ji* is taken, recovery is achieved. *Dān pí* (丹皮, tree peony bark) is by nature extremely capable of cooling blood and may result in the danger of congealing yin when employed in postpartum cases. Take care!

Chapter Fifty-one

Miscarriage with Aversion to Cold and Abdominal Pain

畏寒腹疼小产

妊妇有畏寒腹疼，因而堕胎者，人只知下部太寒也，谁知是气虚不能摄胎乎！夫人生于火，亦养于火，非气不充，气旺则火旺，气衰则火衰。人之所以坐胎者，受父母先天之真火也。先天之真火，即先天之真气以成之。故胎成于气，亦摄于气，气旺则胎牢，气衰则胎堕，胎日加长，而气日加衰，安得不堕哉！况又遇寒气外侵，则内之火气更微，火气微则长养无资，此胎之不能不堕也。使当其腹疼之时，即用人参、干姜之类补气祛寒，则可以疼止而胎安。无如人拘于妊娠之药禁而不敢用，因致堕胎，而仅存几微之气，不急救气，尚有何法？方用黄芪补气汤。

Some pregnant women experience miscarriage resulting from aversion to cold and abdominal pain. Interns know this is due to excessive cold in the lower *jiao*. Who would suspect that it is due to qi deficiency failing to contain the fetus? Human beings are given birth to and nurtured by fire, but fire cannot be replenished without qi. When qi is effulgent, fire is effulgent. When qi is debilitated, fire is debilitated. Because of receiving genuine fire (kidney fire) from its parents prenatally, the human fetus is conceived. The genuine innate fire (kidney fire)'s forming, and growth depends on innate genuine qi. Therefore, the fetus develops from and is contained by qi. When qi is effulgent, the fetus is secure. When qi is debilitated, the fetus falls. As the fetus grows day by day, so qi day by day becomes debilitated. How can the fetus be calm and not fall? What is more, if cold qi happens to invade from outside, internal fire qi becomes even more feeble. Enfeebled fire qi has no means to nurture the fetus for a long time. Therefore, the fetus cannot help but fall. If medicines such as *rén shēn* (人参, ginseng), *gān jiāng* (干姜, dried ginger rhizome) had been administered in time to supplement qi and the cold had been dispelled when the abdominal pain first began, the pain could have been relieved, and the fetus calmed.

However, interns blindly adhering to the medical prohibitions of pregnancy dare not employ these medicines. Now that there is only an iota of qi left, there are no other means but to rescue qi without delay. The formula to use is *Huáng Qí Bǔ Qì Tāng* (黄芪补气汤, Milkvetch Root Qi Supplementing Decoction)

黄芪（二两，生用）　　　　　　肉桂（五分，去粗皮，研末）

当归（一两，酒洗）

huáng qí (astragalus root), 2 *liang* (raw)

ròu guì (cinnamon bark), 5 *fen*

dāng guī (Chinese angelica), 1 *liang*

水煎服。五剂愈矣。倘认定是寒，大用辛热，全不补气与血，恐过于燥热，反致亡阳而变危矣。

Decoct the formula in water. When five *ji* has been taken, a recovery is effected. If the case is differentiated as a cold syndrome, and hot and pungent medicines are used in large amounts without medicines to supplement qi and blood, such a formula being too dry and hot would probably cause yang to collapse and turn the case critical.

Chapter Fifty-two
Miscarriage Due to Rage

大怒小产

妊妇有大怒之后，忽然腹疼吐血，因而堕胎，及堕胎之后，腹疼仍未止者。人以为肝之怒火未退也，谁知是血不归经而然乎。夫肝所以藏血者也。大怒则血不能藏，宜失血而不当堕胎，何为失血而胎亦随堕乎？不知肝性最急，血门不闭，其血直捣于胞胎，胞胎之系，通于心肾之间，肝血来冲，必断绝心肾之路；胎因心肾之路断，胞胎失水火之养，所以堕也。

Following intense anger, some pregnant women suddenly contract abdominal pain and vomit blood. Subsequently, they miscarry, after which the abdominal pain persists. Interns suppose this is due to the unappeased angry fire of the liver. Actually, it is caused by blood failing to return to the vessels. The liver stores blood. During intense anger, blood cannot be stored. As a result, blood should be lost, but abortion should not occur. Then, why does abortion follow the loss of blood? Because the liver is the most impetuous of all the organs by nature, blood will rush directly into the fetus if the blood gate is open. The collateral channel that connects the fetus passes between the heart and the kidneys. When liver blood comes surging, the passageway connecting the heart and the kidneys is unavoidably cut. As a result of this passageway being broken, the fetus can no longer be nurtured by water and fire. Therefore, the fetus falls.

胎既堕矣，而腹疼如故者，盖因心肾未接，欲续无计，彼此痛伤肝气，欲归于心而心不受，欲归于肾而肾不纳，故血犹未静而疼无已也。治法宜引肝之血，仍入于肝，而腹疼自已矣。然徒引肝之血而不平肝之气，则气逆而不易转，即血逆而不易归也。方用引气归血汤。

Once the fetus has fallen, why does abdominal pain continue as before? The reason lies in the disharmony between the heart and kidneys. They are inclined but have no means to resume their connection. This painfully hurts the liver qi, which is rejected when it comes to the heart and is denied reception when it comes to the kidneys. Therefore, blood is not yet tranquilized, and pain persists.

Treatment: Conduct liver blood back to the liver again. Then abdominal pain will disappear by itself. However, simply conducting liver blood without calming liver qi cannot easily succeed in regulating qi counter-flow or leading counter-flow of the blood back to the liver. The formula to use is *Yǐn Qì Guī Xuè Tāng* (引气归血汤, Qi Conducting and Blood Returning Decoction).

白芍（五钱，酒炒）	当归（五钱，酒洗）
白术（三钱，土炒）	甘草（一钱）
黑芥穗（三钱）	丹皮（三钱）
姜炭（五分）	香附（五分，酒炒）
麦冬（三钱，去心）	郁金（一钱，醋炒）

bái sháo (white peony root), 5 *qian* (dry-fried with millet wine)

dāng guī (Chinese angelica), 5 *qian* (washed with millet wine)

bái zhú, Bighead Atractylodes Rhizome, 3 *qian* (dry-fried with earth)

gān cǎo (licorice root), 1 *qian*

hēi jiè suì (charred schizonepeta), 3 *qian*

dān pí (cortex moutan), 3 *qian*

jiāng tàn (prepared dried ginger) , 5 *fen*

xiāng fù (cyperus), 5 *fen* (dry-fried with millet wine)

mài dōng (dwarf lilyturf tuber), *3 qian* (pith discarded)

yù jīn, (turmeric root tuber), 1 *qian*

水煎服。此方名为引气，其实仍是引血也，引血亦所以引气，气归于肝之中，血亦归于肝之内，气血两归，而腹疼自止矣。

Decoct in water and take orally. Though titled "qi-conducting", this formula is capable of conducting blood. To conduct blood, however, is also to conduct qi. When qi returns to the liver, blood returns to the liver too. When both qi and blood return, abdominal pain ceases by itself.

Volume Seven

Normal Delivery

正产

Chapter Fifty-three

Normal Delivery but the Placenta Does not Descend

正产胞衣不下

产妇有儿已下地，而胞衣留滞于腹中，二三日不下，心烦意躁，时欲昏晕。人以为胞衣之蒂未断也，谁知是血少干枯，粘连于腹中乎。世人见胞衣不下，未免心怀疑惧，恐其冲之于心，而有死亡之兆，然而胞衣究何能上冲于心也。但胞衣不下，瘀血未免难行，恐有血晕之虞耳。治法仍宜大补其气血，使生血以送胞衣，则胎衣自然润滑，润滑则易下，生气以助生血，则血生自然迅速，尤易催堕也。方用送胞汤。

After a fetus is born, the placenta in some women may remain stagnant within the abdomen and will not descend even after two or three days. They also feel vexation, agitation, and faint. Interns suppose this is due to the pedicle of the placenta failing to come off. In fact, it is dry, withered blood making the placenta adhere to the inside of the abdomen. Seeing that the placenta does not descend, people are usually full of worry and apprehension, fearing that the placenta might surge up to the heart, causing signs of death. However, is it possible for the placenta to surge up into the heart? When the placenta does not descend, static blood most probably moves with difficulty. Thus, blood dizziness may be induced.

Treatment: Greatly supplement qi and blood. When blood is generated to convey the placenta, the placenta will naturally be moistened and become slippery, which makes descending easy. When qi is generated to assist the generation of blood, blood will be generated soon, making it far easier to hasten the placenta's descending. The formula to use is *Sòng Bāo Tāng* (送胞汤, Placenta Delivering Decoction).

当归（二两，酒洗）　　　　　　川芎（五钱）
益母草（一两）　　　　　　　　乳香（一两，不去油）

没药（一两）　　　　　　　　　芥穗（三钱，炒黑）

麝香（五厘，研，另冲）

dāng guī (Chinese angelica), 2 *liang*

chuān xiōng (Sichuan lovage root), 5 *qian*

yì mǔ cǎo (motherwort), 1 *liang* (oil kept)

rǔ xiāng (frankincense), 1 *liang*

mò yào (myrrh), 1 *liang*

jiè suì (fineleaf schizonepeta spike), 3 *qian* (charred)

shè xiāng (musk), 5 *li*, (ground, dissolved in water and take separately)

水煎服，立下。此方以芎、归补其气血，以荆芥引血归经，用益母、乳香等药逐瘀而下胞衣，新血既生，则旧血难存；气旺上升，而瘀浊自降，尚有留滞之苦哉。夫胞衣是包儿之一物，非依于子，即依于母，子生而不随子俱下，以子之不可依也，故留滞于腹，若有回顾其母之心。母胞虽已生子，而其蒂间之气原未遽绝，所以留连欲脱而未脱，往往有存腹六七日不下，而竟不腐烂者，正以其尚有生气也。可见胞衣留腹，不能杀人，补之而自降耳。或谓胞衣既有生气，补气补血，则胞衣亦宜坚牢，何以补之而反降也？不知子未下，补则益于子；子已下，补则益于母。益子而胞衣之气连，益母而胞衣之气脱。此胞胎之气关，通则两合，闭则两开矣。故大补气血而胞衣反降也。

Decoct the formula in water and take it orally. The placenta will go down immediately. This formula uses *chuān xiōng* (川芎, Sichuan lovage root) and *dāng guī* (当归, Chinese angelica) to supplement qi and blood, *jīng jiè suì* (荆芥穗, fineleaf schizonepeta spike) to guide the blood to return to its vessels, *yì mǔ cǎo* (益母草, motherwort) and *rǔ xiāng* (乳香, frankincense), and other herbs to remove the stasis and move the placenta down. When new blood has been generated, old blood is impossible to remain. When qi is effulgent and begins to rise, stasis with turbidity begins to descend automatically. How can there be an affliction of retention and stagnation then? The placenta is what wraps the fetus. It is attached to either the fetus or the mother. It fails to follow the fetus going out because the fetus is unreliable. Therefore, it lingers behind in the abdomen as if it had filial compassion towards its mother. Although the fetus has left the uterus, the placenta's pedicle has not yet broken off its relationship with the mother's qi. Therefore, the placenta, though on the verge of coming off, is reluctant to do so.

In some cases, the placenta may be retained for six or seven days, but it does not putrefy. The reason is simple that it still maintains life qi. It is evident that a placenta retained in the abdomen cannot kill a person and that it will drop by itself when supplementation is applied. Since the placenta still possesses life qi, it should get firmer and stronger when qi and blood are supplemented. Why should the placenta drop (instead of rising)? Supplementation benefits the fetus before it is delivered but the mother after it is born. When it benefits the fetus, placenta qi becomes adhesive. When it benefits the mother, placenta qi deserts. There is a gate of qi within the uterus. When it is open, the mother and fetus are united. When it is shut, they depart from each other. Therefore, when qi and blood are significantly supplemented, the placenta will descend instead of becoming more firmly attached.

有妇人子下地五六日，而胞衣留于腹中，百计治之，竟不能下，而又绝无昏晕烦躁之状，人以为瘀血之粘连也，谁知是气虚不能推送乎。夫瘀血在腹，断无不作祟之理，有则必然发晕。今安然无恙，是血已净矣。血净宜清气升而浊气降。今胞衣不下，是清气下降而难升，遂至浊气上浮而难降。然浊气上升，又必有烦躁之病，今亦安然者，是清浊之气两不能升也。然则补其气不无浊气之上升乎？不知清升而浊降者，一定之理，未有清升而浊亦升者也。苟能于补气之中，仍分其清浊之气，则升清正所以降浊也。方用补中益气汤。

Some women still have the placenta retained in their abdomen five or six days after the fetus is delivered. Although various means are tried, it refuses to drop, but there are no fainting, vexation, or agitation signs. Interns suppose this is due to the adhesion of static blood. Actually, it is qi deficiency, and it fails to push and convey. If there were static blood in the abdomen, it is destined to cause trouble and cause fainting. However, in this case, there are not these kinds of problems. Proving that there is no static blood. When blood is clean, clear qi is supposed to ascend, while turbid qi descends. Because the placenta is retained, clear qi descends and has difficulty ascending. Then, turbid qi floats upward and is difficult to descend. With turbid qi ascending, however, there ought to occur vexation and agitation. However, in this case, there is no vexation and agitation. It is because neither clear nor turbid qi can ascend. However, if qi is supplemented, will not turbid qi be made to ascend? It is an invariable law that the clear ascends while the turbid descends. There is never such an occasion when the clear ascends, and the turbid also ascends. If clear and turbid qi is separated by supplementing qi, then the clear qi will be uplifted, resulting in the turbid qi moving downward. The formula to use is *Bǔ Zhōng Yì Qì Tāng* (补中益气汤, Center-Supplementing and Qi-Boosting Decoction).

人参（三钱）　　　　　生黄芪（一两）

柴胡（三分）　　　　　炙草（一分）

当归（五钱）　　　　　白术（五分，土炒）

升麻（三分）　　　　　陈皮（二分）

莱菔子（五分，炒，研）

rén shēn (ginseng), 3 *qian*

huáng qí (astragalus root), 1 *liang* (raw)

chái hú (bupleurum), 3 *fen*

zhì gān cǎo (prepared licorice root), 1 *fen*

dāng guī (Chinese angelica), 5 *qian*

bái zhú (white atractylodes rhizome), 5 *fen* (dryed-fried with earth)

shēng má (black cohosh rhizome), 3 *fen*

chén pí (aged tangerine peel), 2 *fen*

lái fú zǐ (radish seed), 5 *fen* (dryed-fried, ground)

水煎服。一剂而胞衣自下矣。夫补中益气汤乃提气之药也，并非推送之剂，何以能降胞衣如此之速也？然而浊气之不降者，由于清气之不升也。提其气则清升而浊降，浊气降则腹中所存之物，即无不随浊气而尽降，正不必再用推送之法也。况又加莱菔子数分，能理浊气，不至两相扞格，所以奏功之奇也。

Decoct the formula in water and take it orally. After one *ji* is taken and the placenta drops by itself. *Bǔ Zhōng Yì Qì Tāng* (补中益气汤, Center-Supplementing and Qi-Boosting Decoction) is a formula to raise qi rather than to push and convey it. Then why is it able to downbear the placenta so quickly? It is because when the clear qi does not ascend, the turbid qi can not descend. When qi is raised, the clear ascends, the turbid then can descend. With the descent of turbid qi, what is retained in the abdomen will also descend without fail. There is no need to apply the pushing-conveying method. What is more, *lái fú zǐ* (莱菔子, radish seed) can regulate turbid qi so that the two kinds of qi will not interfere with each other. Because of this, the effect is terrific.

Chapter Fifty-four
Normal Delivery But with qi Deficiency, Blood Fainting

正产气虚血晕

妇人甫产儿后，忽然眼目昏花，呕恶欲吐，中心无主，或神魂外越，恍若天上行云。人以为恶血冲心之患也，谁知是气虚欲脱而然乎。盖新产之妇，血必尽倾，血室空虚，止存几微之气；倘其人阳气素虚，不能生血，心中之血，前已荫胎，胎堕而心中之血亦随胎而俱堕，心无血养，所赖者几微之气以固之耳。今气又虚而欲脱，而君心无护，所剩残血欲奔回救主，而血非正血，不能归经，内庭变乱而成血晕之症矣。治法必须大补气血，断不可单治血晕也；或疑血晕是热血上冲，而更补其血，不愈助其上冲之势乎？不知新血不生，旧血不散，补血以生新血，正活血以逐旧血也。然血有形之物，难以速生，气乃无形之物，易于迅发，补气以生血，尤易于补血以生血耳。方用补气解晕汤。

Following delivery, some women suddenly have vertigo and blurred vision, retching, nausea, desire to vomit, and absence of governance in the heart or wandering spirit as if walking on the clouds in the sky. People suppose this is due to the trouble of lochia blood surging into the heart. Who would suspect that this is due to qi deficiency on the verge of collapse? During delivery, blood pours out. The blood chamber is empty, and only a tiny amount of qi is left. If the woman has innate yang qi deficiency, she is consistently unable to engender blood. The blood in the heart has been consumed in nourishing the fetus. With the delivery of the fetus, blood in the heart has run out with the fetus. Now that the heart is left with no blood to nourish, it has only the tiny amount of qi to rely on to secure it. What is worse, qi is also deficient and on the verge of collapse. There is nothing to protect the monarch organ (heart). The remnant blood is unable to return to the vessels and develops into blood fainting.

Treatment: Supplement qi and blood drastically. It is improper to treat blood fainting only. It may be questioned that if blood fainting is caused by hot blood upsurging, blood will be helped to surge up with more significant momentum when blood is supplemented. Old blood will not disperse unless new blood is engendered. Supplementing blood to engender new blood is as good as promoting blood circulation to dispel old blood. While blood, a kind of tangible substance, is difficult to engender quickly, qi, an intangible substance, is easy to engender quickly. Therefore, it is easier to supplement qi in order to engender blood than to supplement blood alone. The formula to use is *Bǔ Qì Jiě Yūn Tāng* (补气解晕汤，Qi Supplementing and Fainting Relieving Decoction).

人参（一两）　　　　　生黄芪（一两）

当归（一两）　　　　　黑芥穗（三钱）

姜炭（一钱）

rén shēn (ginseng), 1 *liang*

huáng qí (astragalus root), 1 *liang* (raw)

dāng guī (Chinese angelica), 1 *liang*

hēi jiè suì (charred fineleaf schizonepeta spike), 3 *qian*

jiāng tàn (prepared dried ginger), 1 *qian*

水煎服。一剂而晕止，二剂而心定，三剂而血生，四剂而血旺，再不晕矣。此乃解晕之圣药，用参、芪以补气，使气壮而生血也；用当归以补血，使血旺而养气也。气血两旺，而心自定矣。用荆芥炭引血归经，用姜炭以行瘀引阳，瘀血去而正血归，不必解晕而晕自解矣。一方之中，药止五味，而其奏功之奇而大如此，其神矣乎。原方极妙，不可加减。

Decoct the formula in water and take it orally. When one *ji* is taken, fainting is relieved. When the second *ji* is taken, the heart is stabilized. When the third *ji* is taken, blood is engendered. After the fourth *ji* is taken, blood is effulgent, and fainting will not recur. This is a divine formula for relieving fainting. *Rén shēn* (人参, ginseng) and *huáng qí* (黄芪, astragalus root) are used to supplement qi. When qi is effulgent, it may engender blood. *Dāng guī* (当归, Chinese angelica) is used to supplement blood. When blood is effulgent, it may nourish qi. When qi and blood are both flourishing, the heart will be in peace. *Jīng jiè tàn* (荆芥炭, charred fineleaf schizonepeta spike) is used to lead blood back to the vessels.

Jiāng tàn (姜炭, prepared dried ginger) is used to remove blood stasis and guide yang qi. When phlegm-blood is removed, healthy blood will come back to the vessels. Thus, the fainting is resolved automatically. How miraculous it is that a formula composed of but five ingredients are so wonderfully effective! There is no need to modify it.

Chapter Fifty-five
Normal Delivery But Blood Fainting & Inability to Speak

正产血晕不语

产妇有子方下地，即昏晕不语，此气血两脱也，本在不救，然救之得法，亦有能生者。山得岐天师秘诀，何敢隐而不宣乎？当斯之时，急用银针刺其眉心，得血出则语矣。然后以人参一两，煎汤灌之，无不生者。即用黄芪二两，当归一两，名当归补血汤，煎汤一碗灌之亦得生。万不可于二方之中，轻加附子。盖附子无经不达，反引气血之药，走而不守，不能专注于胞胎，不若人参、归、芪直救其气血之绝，聚而不散也。

As soon as the fetus has been delivered, some women have dizziness and fainting with an inability to speak. This is due to the collapse of both blood and qi. This is usually classified among hopeless cases, but if the rescue method is appropriate, survival is not an impossibility. At the critical juncture, one should acupuncture the midpoint between the eyebrows with a silver needle promptly. When blood is let out, the ability to speak will be recovered. After that, decoct *Rén shēn* (人参, ginseng) 1 *liang* and feed the decoction to the patient. The resurrection will be brought without fail.

Life can also be brought back by feeding a bowl of a decoction named *Dāng Guī Bǔ Xuè Tāng* (当归补血汤, Chinese Angelica Blood-Supplementing Decoction), comcessposed of 2 *liang* of *huáng qí* (黄芪, astragalus root) and 1 *liang* of *dāng guī* (当归, Chinese angelica).

On no account, *fù zǐ* (附子, prepared aconite root) should be added to these two decoctions. *Rén shēn* (人参, ginseng), *dāng guī* (当归, Chinese angelica), and *huáng qí* (黄芪, astragalus root) come straight to the rescue of expiring qi and blood and accumulate them and without dissipating them. While *fù zǐ* (附子, prepared aconite root) can reach every meridian and spurs medicines supplementing qi and blood to wander rather than maintain their due position, which results in that each of the herbs cannot dedicate to the uterus.

盖产妇昏晕，全是血室空虚，无以养心，以致昏晕。舌为心之苗，心既无主，而舌又安能出声耶？夫眉心之穴，上通于脑，下通于舌，而其系则连于心，刺其眉心，则脑与舌俱通，而心之清气上升，则瘀血自然下降矣，然后以参、芪、当归之能补气生血者，煎汤灌之，则气与血接续，又何至于死亡乎。

Generally speaking, dizziness and fainting in delivery are caused by the uterus's deficiency and weakness with nothing to nourish the heart. The tongue is the sprout of the heart. Once the heart has no governance, how can the tongue utter voice? The midpoint between the eyebrows has access to the brain above and the tongue below. At the same time, its collaterals connect with the heart. When this point is needled, both the brain and tongue are unobstructed, and the clear qi of the heart ascends. Thus static blood naturally descends. After that, decoct and take medicines capable of supplementing qi and engendering blood, such as *rén shēn* (人参, ginseng), *huáng qí* (黄芪, astragalus root) and *dāng guī* (当归, Chinese angelica), and qi and blood will be replenished. How can death possibly come?

虽单用参、芪、当归，亦有能生者，然终不若先刺眉心之为更妙。世人但知灸眉心之法，不知刺更胜于灸，盖灸法缓而刺法急，缓则难于救绝，急则易于回生。所谓急则治其标，缓则治其本者，此也。

Simple administration of *rén shēn* (人参, ginseng), *huáng qí* (黄芪, astragalus root) and *dāng guī* (当归, Chinese angelica) may be able to avert death in some cases. However, it is less effective than if preceded by needling the midpoint between the eyebrows. Interns are acquainted with the moxibustion method of the midpoint between the eyebrows, but they do not know that needling excels this process. Moxibustion is a slow method, while acupuncture is a quick method. It is difficult for such a slow method to rescue exhaustion syndrome, but it is easy for a quick method to bring back life. This is so-called "To treat the tip aspect first in an emergency, to treat the root aspect when it is not urgent."

Chapter Fifty-six
Normal Delivery But Lochiostasis Surging the Heart Causing Fainting and Mania

正产败血攻心晕狂

妇人有产后二三日，发热，恶露不行，败血攻心，狂言呼叫，甚欲奔走，拿提不定，人以为邪热在胃之过，谁知是血虚心不得养而然乎。夫产后之血，尽随胞胎而外越，则血室空虚，脏腑皆无血养，只有心中之血，尚存几微，以护心君。

Two or three days after delivery, some women suffer from fever, retention of lochia, lochiostasis surging the heart, manic ravings and shoutings, and, in severe cases, a desire to run about but have hesitation in movement. People suppose this is due to trouble caused by pathogenic heat in the stomach. Who would suspect that this is due to blood deficiency failing to nurture the heart? Blood has all gone with the fetus during the delivery, the blood chamber (uterus) becomes deficient. None of the *zang* (viscera) and *fu* (bowel) organs have any blood for nourishment, and only in the heart is there a tiny amount of blood left to protect the heart sovereign.

而脏腑失其所养，皆欲取给于心；心包为心君之宰相，拦绝各脏腑之气，不许入心，始得心神安静，是护心者全藉心包之力也。使心包亦虚，不能障心，而各脏腑之气遂直入于心，以分取乎心血，心包情急，既不能内顾其君，又不能外御乎众，于是大声疾呼，号鸣勤王，而其迹象反近于狂悖，有无可如何之势，故病状似热而实非热也。治法须大补心中之血，使各脏腑分取以自养，不得再扰乎心君，则心君泰然，而心包亦安矣。方用安心汤。

Because the *zang* and *fu* organs have nothing for nourishment, they are all inclined to turn to the heart for supplies. As premier of the heart sovereign, the *xinbao* (pericardium) intercepts qi of the *zang* and *fu* organs. It does not allow them to enter the heart so that calmness and tranquility of the heart spirit are ensured. Thus, the heart is protected entirely by the strength of the pericardium. If the pericardium is also deficient and unable to serve as shelter for the heart,

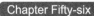
therefore the qi of the *zang* and *fu* organs will directly enter the heart to share blood in the heart. The pericardium is now in an urgent situation; it cannot look after its sovereign internally or defend against the pressing masses externally. It then raises its cries, giving signs bordering on mania and eccentricity and displaying helpless desperation. Therefore, this disease shows heat, but, practically speaking, it is not a heat syndrome. The treatment method must powerfully supplement the blood in the heart for the *zang* and *fu* organs to share in its nourishment and prevent them from harassing the heart anymore. Thus, the heart will become composed, and the pericardium will be quiet. The formula to use is *Ān Xīn Tāng* (安心汤, Heart Calming Decoction).

当归（二两）　　　　　　　川芎（一两）
生地（五钱，炒）　　　　　丹皮（五钱，炒）
生蒲黄（二钱）　　　　　　干荷叶（一片，引）

dāng guī (Chinese angelica), 2 *liang*

chuān xiōng (Sichuan lovage root), 1 *liang*

shēng dì (rehmannia root), 5 *qian* (dry-fried)

dān pí (tree peony bark), 5 *qian* (dry-fried)

pú huáng (cattail pollen), 2 *qian* (raw)

gān hé yè (lotus leaf), 1 piece (dried, as guiding herb)

水煎服。一剂而狂定，恶露亦下矣。此方用芎、归以养血，何以又用生地、丹皮之凉血，似非产后所宜。不知恶露所以奔心，原因虚热相犯，于补中凉之，而凉不为害，况益之以荷叶，七窍相通，引邪外出，不惟内不害心，且佐蒲黄以分解乎恶露也。但只可暂用以定狂，不可多用以取咎也。谨之！慎之！

Decoct the formula in water and take it orally. When one *ji* is taken, mania is settled, and lochia is discharged as well. This formula uses *chuān xiōng* (川芎, Sichuan lovage root) and *dāng guī* (当归, Chinese angelica) to nurture blood. However, why are *shēng dì* (生地, rehmannia root) and *dān pí* (丹皮, tree peony bark) added to cool blood? This seems inappropriate in a postpartum case. It is the attack of deficiency-heat that causes the lochia to rush upon the heart. Cooling in combination with supplementation does not harm.

What is more, with the help of *hé yè* (荷叶, lotus leaf), the formula frees all the seven orifices and leads pathogenic factors out. It can prevent pathogenic factors from harming the heart internally. Also, *pú huáng* (蒲黄, cattail pollen) is used to assist in decomposing the lochia. Although this formula can be used to settle mania temporarily, it should not be used too often lest it incurs trouble. Be cautious and discreet.

【服药后狂定，宜服加味生化汤。

当归（一两一钱，酒洗）　　　　　川芎（三钱）

桃仁（钱半，研）　　　　　　　　荆芥穗（一钱，炒炭）

丹皮（钱半）

服四剂妙。】

[After taking this decoction, mania is settled; it is proper to take *Jiā Wèi Shēng Huà Tāng* (加味生化汤, Supplemented Engendering and Transforming Decoction).

dāng guī (Chinese angelica), 1 *liang* and 1 *qian* (washed with millet wine)

chuān xiōng, Sichuan lovage root, 3 *qian*

táo rén (peach kernel), 1 *qian* and 5 *fen* (ground)

jīng jiè suì (fineleaf schizonepeta spike), 1 *qian* (charred)

dān pí (tree peony bark), 1 *qian* and 5 *fen*

It is advised to take 4 *ji*.]

Chapter Fifty-seven
Normal Delivery But Intestinal Prolapse

正产肠下

产妇肠下，亦危症也。人以为儿门不关之故，谁知是气虚下陷而不能收乎。夫气虚下陷，自宜用升提之药，以提其气。然新产之妇，恐有瘀血在腹，一旦提气，并瘀血升腾于上，则冲心之患，又恐变出非常，是气又不可竟提也。气既不可竟提，而气又下陷，将用何法以治之哉？盖气之下陷者，因气之虚也，但补其气，则气旺而肠自升举矣。惟是补气之药少，则气力薄而难以上升，必须以多为贵，则阳旺力强，断不能降而不升矣。方用补气升肠饮。

Prolapse of the intestines in the birthing woman is a critical condition. People suppose it to be due to the non-closure of the baby gate. Who would suspect collapse due to qi deficiency and failing to withdraw the intestine? In case of collapse due to qi deficiency, it is naturally proper to use herbs for ascending and lifting to lift qi. However, because for a woman who has just given birth, most likely, there is static blood in the abdomen, if qi is raised, static blood might be brought up with it to soar into the upper part of the body. This would cause the trouble of surging up into the heart, which is likely to cause extraordinary transmuted syndromes.

Therefore, qi-raising cannot be carried out in a big way. Then, what method can be adopted to treat it when qi has collapsed? Generally speaking, qi collapse is caused by qi deficiency. If it is supplemented, qi will become effulgent, and the intestine will rise by itself. However, taking only a small amount of qi supplementing medicinals will not make qi strong enough. In this case, a great quantity is necessary to make the yang qi effulgent and great in strength. The intestine will ascend naturally. The formula to use is *Bǔ Qì Shēng Cháng Yǐn* (补气升肠饮, Qi Supplementing and Intestine Lifting Decoction).

人参（一两，去芦）   生黄芪（一两）

当归（一两，酒洗）   白术（五钱，土炒）

川芎（三钱）　　　　　　　　升麻（一分，酒洗）

rén shēn (ginseng), 1 *liang* (with the little rhizomes on the top removed)

huáng qí (astragalus root), 1 *liang* (raw)

dāng guī (Chinese angelica) (raw), 1 *liang* (washed with millet wine)

bái zhú (white atractylodes rhizome), 5 *qian*

chuān xiōng (Sichuan lovage root), 3 *qian* (washed with millet wine)

shēng má (black cohosh rhizome), 1 *fen*

水煎服。一剂而肠升矣。此方纯于补气，全不去升肠，即如用升麻一分，亦不过引气而升耳。盖升麻之为用，少则气升，多则血升也，不可不知。又方用蓖麻仁四十九粒，捣涂顶心以提之，肠升即刻洗去，时久则恐吐血，此亦升肠之一法也。

Decoct the formula in water and take it orally. When one *ji* is taken, the intestine is lifted. This formula solely supplements qi without lifting medicinals. Even the employment of 1 *fen shēng má* (升麻, black cohosh rhizome) is merely to conduct and upbear qi. In terms of *shēng má* (升麻, black cohosh rhizome), a small amount lifts qi, while a large amount raises blood. This cannot be ignored.

Another formula uses 49 seeds of *bì má rén* (蓖麻仁, castor seed), pounded and applied on the patient's vertex as an up-raiser. As soon as the intestine is lifted, it must be washed off since long retention may cause vomiting of blood. This is an alternative method to up-lifting the intestines.

Volume Eight

After Delivery (Postpartum Disorders)

产后

产后少腹痛

妇人产后少腹疼痛，甚则结成一块，按之愈疼。人以为儿枕之疼也，谁知是瘀血作祟乎。夫儿枕者，前人谓儿头枕之物也。儿枕之不疼，岂儿生不枕而反疼，是非儿枕可知矣。既非儿枕，何故作疼？乃是瘀血未散，结作成团而作疼耳。

After delivery, some women have lower abdominal pain. If severe, it can lead to a mass formation, and pressure makes the pain worse. Interns suppose this is due to "fetus' pillow pain." Actually, this trouble is caused by blood stasis. The "fetus' pillow" was defined by our predecessors as the place where the fetus pillows its head. However, if there was no pain when the fetus was pillowing its head during gestation, how can one believe that pain arises owing to freedom from such pillowing after the delivery of the fetus? It is evident that the so-called "fetus' pillow" does not cause this pain. Then, what is the reason? It is caused by static blood, which, not yet dispersed, binds into lumps.

凡此等症，多是壮健之妇，血有余而非血不足也，似乎可用破血之药。然血活则瘀自除，血结则瘀作祟，若不补血而反败血，虽瘀血可消，毕竟耗损难免，不若于补血之中，以行逐瘀之法，则气血不耗，而瘀亦尽消矣。方用散结定疼汤。

This syndrome is usually seen in strong women whose blood is super-abundant rather than insufficient. Therefore, it seems proper to use blood-breaking medicinals. When blood is in good circulation, stasis is naturally eliminated. Whereas when blood binds, stasis causes trouble. However, if blood is vanquished instead of supplemented, though static blood is dispersed, consumption and depletion cannot be avoided. A better way is to integrate the method of dispelling stasis into that of supplementing blood. Thus, stasis is dispersed completely, while qi and blood have no consumption. The formula to use is *Sàn Jié Dìng Téng Tāng* (散结定疼汤, Mass Dissipating and Pain Relieving Decoction).

当归（一两，酒洗）　　　　川芎（五钱，酒洗）

丹皮（二钱，炒）　　　　　益母草（三钱）

黑芥穗（二钱）　　　　　　乳香（一钱，去油）

山楂（十粒，炒黑）　　　　桃仁（七粒，炒，研）

dāng guī (Chinese angelica), 1 *liang* (washed with millet wine)

chuān xiōng (Sichuan lovage root), 5 *qian* (washed with millet wine)

dān pí (tree peony bark), 2 *qian*

yì mǔ cǎo (motherwort) , 3 *qian*

hēi jiè suì (charred fineleaf schizonepeta spike), 2 *qian*

rǔ xiāng (frankincense), 1 *qian* (oil removed)

shān zhā (Chinese hawthorn fruit), 10 pieces (charred)

táo rén (*peach kernel*), 7 pieces (dry-fried, ground)

水煎。一剂而疼止而愈，不必再剂也。此方逐瘀于补血之中，消块于生血之内，妙在不专攻疼病而疼病止。彼世人一见儿枕之疼，动用元胡、苏木、蒲黄、灵脂之类以化块，又何足论哉。

Decoct the formula in water. When one *ji* is taken, the pain is relieved, and the patient is recovered. There is no need to take the second *ji*. This formula integrates stasis-dispelling with blood-supplementing and can disperse clots while engendering blood. Its subtlety lies in stopping pain without specifically attacking it. People nowadays tend to use such medicinals like *yuán hú* (元胡, corydalis tuber), *sū mù* (苏木, sappan wood), *pú huáng*(蒲黄, cattail pollen), *líng zhī* (灵脂, reishi mushroom) to transform clots whenever they meet "fetus' pillow pain." It is not worth comment.

妇人产后少腹疼痛，按之即止，人亦以为儿枕之疼也，谁知是血虚而然乎。夫产后亡血过多，血室空虚，原能腹疼，十妇九然。但疼有虚实之分，不可不辨。如燥糠触体光景，是虚疼而非实疼也。大凡虚疼宜补，而产后之虚疼，尤宜补焉。惟是血虚之疼，必须用补血之药。而补血之味，多是润滑之品，恐与大肠不无相碍。然产后血虚，肠多干燥，润滑正相宜也，何碍之有？方用肠宁汤。

Postpartum lower abdominal pain in women, relieved by pressure, is also supposed to be pain due to "fetus's pillow pain." Actually, it is caused by blood deficiency. After delivery, too much blood is lost, and the blood chamber is empty and deficient. It is natural for abdominal pain to occur, and nine out of ten women suffer from it. This pain, however, is divided into two types: deficiency and excess syndrome. Syndrome differentiation must be made. If the pain is like that of dry husks touching the body, it is a deficient pain rather than excessive pain. Generally speaking, supplementation is a better way to treat deficient pain, especially in postpartum deficient pain. blood deficient pain should be treated with blood-supplementing medicinals. However, blood supplements usually moisten and lubricate, and they may well interfere with the large intestine. While, in terms of postpartum blood deficiency, the large intestines are usually dry. Therefore, moistening and lubricating is just what is desired. What kind of interference can there be? The formula to use is *Cháng Níng Tāng* (肠宁汤, Intestine-quieting Decoction).

当归（一两，酒洗）　　　　熟地（一两，九蒸）

人参（三钱）　　　　　　　麦冬（三钱，去心）

阿胶（三钱，蛤粉炒）　　　山药（三钱，炒）

续断（二钱）　　　　　　　甘草（一钱）

肉桂（二分，去粗，研）

dāng guī (Chinese angelica), 1 *liang* (washed with millet wine)

shú dì huáng (prepared rehmannia root), 1 *liang* (fully steamed)

rén shēn (ginseng), 3 *qian*

mài dōng (dwarf lilyturf tuber), 3 *qian* (pith discarded)

ē jiāo (donkey-hide gelatin), 3 *qian* (dry-fried with clam shell powder)

shān yào (common yam rhizome), 3 *qian* (dry-fried)

xù duàn (himalayan teasel root), 2 *qian*

gān cǎo (licorice root), 1 *qian*

ròu guì, (cinnamon bark), 2 *fen* (ground)

水煎服。一剂而疼轻，二剂而疼止，多服更宜。此方补气补血之药也，然补气而无太郁之忧，补血而无太滞之患。气血既生，不必止疼而疼自止矣。

Decoct the formula in water and take it orally. When one *ji* is taken, pain is mitigated; when the second *ji* is taken, the pain is relieved. Continuing to take more *ji* is more profitable. This formula is made up of medicinals to supplement qi and blood, but it supplements qi without taking the risk of over-depressing qi; it supplements blood without the trouble of over-stagnating blood. When qi and blood are generated, pain is stopped without specifically stopping it.

产后气喘

妇人产后气喘，最是大危之症，苟不急治，立刻死亡。人只知是气血之虚也，谁知是气血两脱乎。夫既气血两脱，人将立死，何又能作喘？然此血将脱，而气犹未脱也。血将脱而气欲挽之，而反上喘。如人救溺，援之而力不胜，又不肯自安于不救，乃召号同志以求助，故呼声而喘作。其症虽危，而可救处正在能作喘也。

Postpartum dyspnea in women is severe. If not be treated in time, it causes immediate death. Interns only know it is because of qi and blood deficiency; actually, it is caused by the collapse of both blood and qi. Since both qi and blood collapse and the patient is about to die, why does the patient suffer from dyspnea? In fact, it is the blood that is on the verge of collapse, while qi has not yet collapsed. As the blood is about to desert, but qi is trying to hold it back, qi contrarily goes up to cause dyspnea. This is like trying to pick up a drowning person. One's strength is unequal to the task, but one cannot resign oneself to failure. Therefore, one turns to call upon others for aid, shouting. This is dyspnea. Critical as the case may be, it is curable because the woman can still have dyspnea.

盖肺主气，喘则肺气似盛而实衰，当是之时，血将脱而万难骤生，望肺气之相救甚急，若赤子之望慈母然。而肺因血失，止存几微之气，自顾尚且不暇，又何能提挈乎血，气不与血俱脱者几希矣，是救血必须补气也。方用救脱活母汤。

The lungs govern qi. When there is dyspnea, lung qi seems exuberant but is extremely weak. At this moment, blood, which is on the verge of deserting and is impossible to engender quickly, is looking very anxiously for the lung qi's coming to its rescue. While there is only a tiny amount of qi left in the lungs because of blood loss, the lungs cannot look after themselves. How can they help to lift blood? It is a rare case where qi does not desert the blood. Therefore, in order to rescue blood, it is necessary to supplement qi. The formula to use is *Jiù Tuō Huó Mǔ Tāng* (救脱活母汤, Collapse Rescuing and Mother Saving Decoction).

人参（二两）　　　　　当归（一两，酒洗）

熟地（一两，九蒸）　　枸杞子（五钱）

山萸（五钱，蒸，去核）　麦冬（一两，去心）

阿胶（二钱，蛤粉炒）　　肉桂（一钱，去粗，研）

黑芥穗（二钱）

rén shēn (ginseng), 2 *liang*

dāng guī (Chinese angelica), 1 *liang* (washed with millet wine)

shú dì (prepared rehmannia root), 1 *liang* (fully steamed)

gǒu qǐ (Chinese wolfberry fruit), 5 *qian*

shān yú (fructus corni), 5 *qian* (steamed, cored)

mài dōng (dwarf lilyturf tuber), 1 *liang* (pith discarded)

ē jiāo (donkey-hide gelatin), 2 *qian* (dry-fried with clam shell powder)

ròu guì (cinnamon bark), 1 *qian* (ground)

hēi jiè suì (charred fineleaf schizonepeta spike), 2 *qian*

水煎服。一剂而喘轻，二剂而喘减，三剂而喘定，四剂而全愈矣。此方用人参以接续元阳，然徒补其气而不补其血，则阳燥而狂，虽回生于一时，亦旋得旋失之道。即补血而不补其肝肾之精，则本原不固，阳气又安得而续乎。所以又用熟地、山萸、枸杞之类，以大补其肝肾之精，而后大益其肺气，则肺气健旺，升提有力矣。

Decoct the formula in water and take it orally. When one *ji* is taken, dyspnea eases. When the second *ji* is taken, it is relieved. When the third *ji* is taken, it is settled. When the fourth *ji* is taken, a complete recovery can be achieved. In this formula, *rén shēn* (人参, ginseng) is used to recruit primordial yang. However, to supplement qi without supplementing blood will make the yang dry and restless. It may succeed in bringing life back for the time being, but this will result in the loss following immediately upon the gains. Supplementing blood without thinking about supplementing the liver and kidneys' essence will result in original qi's insecurity. In that case, how can yang qi be secured and increased? Therefore, *Shú dì* (熟地, prepared rehmannia root), *shān yú* (山萸, fructus corni), *gǒu qǐ zǐ* (枸杞子, Chinese wolfberry fruit), and the like are used to supplement the essence of the liver and kidneys significantly and then boost the lung qi significantly. Thus, the lung qi becomes sturdy and effulgent and robust enough to rise.

特虑新产之后，用补阴之药，腻滞不行，又加肉桂以补命门之火，使火气有根，助人参以生气，且能运化地黄之类，以化精生血。若过于助阳，万一血随阳动，瘀而上行，亦非保全之策，更加荆芥以引血归经，则肺气安而喘速定，治儿其神乎。

Due to specific concern that the use of yin-supplementing medicinals for postpartum women may cause greasiness and stagnation, *ròu guì* (肉桂, cinnamon bark) is added for supplementing *mìng mén* (命门, gate of vitality) fire. This makes the fire qi have a root and assists *rén shēn* (人参, ginseng) in engendering qi. Furthermore, it can transport and transform medicinals like *dì huáng* (地黄, rehmannia root) in order to transform essence and engender blood. If yang is unduly assisted, blood may follow yang and become stirred up, and stasis may ascend with it. It is not a safe strategy. So, *hēi jiè suì* (黑芥穗, charred fineleaf schizonepeta spike) is added to guide blood back to the vessels. Thus, lung qi is calmed, and dyspnea is soon settled. This treatment is nearly divine.

Chapter Sixty
Postpartum Aversion to Cold and Body Shivering

产后恶寒身颤

妇人产后恶寒恶心，身体颤，发热作渴，人以为产后伤寒也，谁知是气血两虚，正不敌邪而然乎。大凡人之气不虚，则邪断难入。产妇失血既多，则气必大虚，气虚则皮毛无卫，邪原易入，正不必户外之风来袭体也，即一举一动，风即可乘虚而入之。

Some women suffer from an aversion to cold, shivering of the body, fever, and thirst after delivery. People suppose these are the results of postpartum cold damage. Who would suspect these are due to the dual deficiency of qi and blood and *zheng qi* (healthy qi) defeated by pathogenic factors? Generally, as long as the *zheng qi* (healthy qi) in the body is not deficient, pathogenic factors cannot invade. While when blood is lost in significant amounts, the woman after delivery will be severely deficient in *zheng qi* (healthy qi). If qi is deficient, the skin and hair are defenseless and pathogenic factors naturally find their way quite easily to invade. This does not need the external wind to attack the body. Given any moment, external wind may take advantage of deficiency to invade.

然产后之妇，风易入而亦易出。凡有外邪之感，俱不必祛风，况产妇之恶寒者，寒由内生也；发热者，热由内弱也；身颤者，颤由气虚也。治其内寒，而外寒自散；治其内弱，而外热自解；壮其元阳，而身颤自除。方用十全大补汤。

As for women after delivery, it is easy for the wind to invade and just as easy for it to leave the body. To treat such kind of invasion of external pathogenic factors, there is no need to expel wind. What is more, in birthing women, if there is an aversion to cold, the cold is generated from the interior. If there is a fever, the heat is due to internal weakness. Body shivering is due to qi deficiency. When internal cold is treated, external heat is resolved. When internal weakness is treated, the external cold will disperse naturally. When primordial yang is strengthened, shivering of the body is eliminated of itself. The formula to use is *Shí Quán Dà Bǔ Tāng* (十全大补汤, Perfect Major Supplementation Decoction).

人参（三钱）	白术（三钱，土炒）
茯苓（三钱，去皮）	甘草（一钱，炙）
川芎（一钱，酒洗）	当归（三钱，酒洗）
熟地（五钱，九蒸	白芍（二钱，酒炒）
黄芪（一两，生用）	肉桂（一两，去粗，研）

rén shēn (ginseng), 3 *qian*

bái zhú (white atractylodes rhizome), 3 *qian* (dry-fried with earth)

fú líng (poria), 3 *qian* (peeled)

gān cǎo (licorice root), 1 *qian* (dry-fried)

chuān xiōng (Sichuan lovage root), 1 *qian* (washed with millet wine)

dāng guī (Chinese angelica), 3 *qian* (washed with millet wine)

shú dì (prepared rehmannia root), 5 *qian* (fully steamed)

bái sháo (white peony root), 2 *qian* (dry-fried with millet wine)

huáng qí (astragalus root), 1 *liang* (raw)

ròu guì (cinnamon bark), 1 *liang* (ground)

水煎服。一剂而诸病悉愈。此方但补气与血之虚，而不去散风与邪之实，正以正足而邪自除也，况原无邪气乎。所以奏功之捷也。

（宜连服数剂，不可只服一剂。）

Decoct the formula in water and take it orally. When one *ji* is taken, all disorders will be resolved. This formula supplements deficiency of qi and blood without expelling wind and pathogenic factors. This is because when *zheng qi* (healthy qi) is strong, pathogenic factors are eliminated of themselves. Therefore, this formula offers a quick recovery.

(Several *ji* should be administrated in succession. Do not administer only one *ji*.)

产后恶心呕吐

妇人产后恶心欲呕，时而作吐。人皆曰胃气之寒也，谁知是肾气之寒乎。夫胃为肾之关，胃之气寒，则胃气不能行于肾之中；肾之气寒，则肾气亦不能行于胃之内。是肾与胃不可分而两之也。惟是产后失血过多，必致肾水干涸，肾水涸应肾火上炎，当不至胃有寒冷之虞，何故肾寒而胃亦寒乎？

Some women suffer from nausea, retching and vomiting sometimes. People all declare this is due to cold of the stomach. However, who would suspect cold of the kidney? As the stomach supplies nourishment for the kidneys and is the anchor of the kidneys, cold of the stomach leads to the failing of stomach qi to reach the kidneys. When the kidney is cold, the qi (kidney) cannot flow inside the stomach. The stomach and kidneys are inseparable. In terms of the postpartum condition, excessive blood loss is bound to lead to dried-up kidney water. Dried up kidney water will result in the flaming upward of kidney fire. It should not result in cold of the stomach. How then can the kidney cold lead to the stomach cold?

盖新产之余，水乃遽然涸去，虚火尚不能生，火既不生，而寒之象自现。治法宜补其肾中之火。然火无水济，则火在水上，未必不成火动阴虚之症。必须于水中补火，肾中温胃，而后肾无太热之患，胃有既济之欢也。方用温肾止呕汤。

Shortly after delivery, although water has just dried up abruptly, deficient fire is not yet engendered. So, cold symptoms naturally occur. The proper treatment should be to supplement the fire in the kidneys. However, when fire in the kidneys has no water to assist, the fire would be greater than water, and most likely, the syndrome of yin deficiency stirring fire may occur. Therefore, it is necessary to incorporate fire reinforcing into water supplementing and to integrate stomach-warming into kidney-warming. In such a way, the kidneys will be spared the trouble of excessive heat, and the stomach has the coordination (between water and fire). The formula to use is *Wēn Shèn Zhǐ Ou Tāng* (温肾止呕汤, Kidney Warming and Vomit Stopping Decoction).

熟地（五钱，九蒸）　　　　巴戟（一两，盐水浸）

人参（三钱）　　　　　　　白术（一两，土炒）

山萸（五钱，蒸，去核）　　炮姜（一钱）

茯苓（二钱，去皮）　　　　橘红（五分，姜汁洗）

白蔻（一粒，研）

shú dì huáng (prepared rehmannia root), 5 *qian* (fully steamed)

bā jǐ (morinda root), 1 *liang* (soaked in salt water)

rén shēn (ginseng), 3 *qian*

bái zhú (white atractylodes rhizome), 1 *liang* (dry-fried with earth)

shān yú (fructus corni), 5 *qian* (steamed, stoned)

páo jiāng (prepared dried ginger), 1 *qian*

fú líng (poria), 2 *qian* (peeled)

jú hóng (red tangerine peel), 5 *fen* (washed with ginger juice)

bái kòu (round cardamon), 1 piece (ground)

水煎服。一剂而呕吐止，二剂而不再发，四剂而全愈矣。此方补肾之药多于治胃之品，然而治肾仍是治胃也。所以肾气升腾而胃寒自解，不必用大热之剂，温胃而祛寒也。

Decoct the formula in water and take it orally. When one *ji* is taken, retching and vomiting are stopped. When the second *ji* is taken, they will not recur. After the fourth *ji* is taken, complete recovery is effected. In this formula, herbs for supplementing the kidneys are in greater amount than stomach-treating ingredients. Treating the kidneys is for treating the stomach. Therefore, when kidney qi ascends, the stomach cold is resolved naturally. There is no need to employ hot medicinals to warm the stomach to dispel cold.

【服此方必待恶露尽后。若初产一二日之内，恶心欲呕，乃恶露上冲，宜服加味生化汤：

全当归（一两，酒洗）　　　川芎（二钱）

炮姜（一钱）　　　　　　　东楂炭（二钱）

桃仁（一钱，研）

用无灰黄酒一盅，水三盅同煎。】

[This formula should not be administered till the lochia has run out entirely. If the retching and vomiting occur one or two days after the delivery, they should be due to up-surging of the lochia. It is proper to administer *Jiā Wèi Shēng Huà Tāng* (加味生化汤, Supplemented Engendering and Transforming Decoction):

dāng guī (Chinese angelica), 1 *liang* (washed with millet wine)

chuān xiōng (Sichuan lovage root), 2 *qian*

páo jiāng (prepared dried ginger), 1 *qian*

shān zhā tàn (Charred Chinese hawthorn fruit), 2 *qian*

táo rén (peach kernel), 1 *qian* (ground)

Decoct the above medicinals with a cup of rice or millet wine mixed with 3 cups of water.]

产后血崩

少妇产后半月，血崩昏晕，目见鬼神。人皆曰恶血冲心也，谁知是不慎房帏之过乎。夫产后业逾半月，虽不比初产之二三日，而气血初生，尚未全复，即血路已净，而胞胎之损伤未痊，断不可轻于一试，以重伤其门户。

Half a month after delivery, some young women suffer from postpartum profuse uterine bleeding with dizziness and fainting. All people believe it is due to lochia blood surging into the heart. Who would suspect it is caused by indiscreet sexual intercourse? Although the situation over half a month after delivery is different from two or three days after parturition, qi and blood, which are just beginning to be engendered, are not yet wholly recovered. Even though the blood passages (neck of uterus and vagina) are clean, the uterus has not yet completely recovered from damage or injury. Therefore, it is inadvisable to try sexual intercourse, which may cause new damage to the neck of the uterus.

无奈少娇之妇，气血初复，不知慎养，欲心大动，贪合图欢，以致血崩昏晕，目见鬼神，是心肾两伤，不特胞胎门户已也。明明是既犯色戒，又加酣战，以致大泄其精，精泄而神亦随之而欲脱。此等之症，乃自作之孽，多不可活。然于不可活之中，而思一急救之法。舍大补其气与血，别无良法也。方用救败求生汤。

However, when qi and blood are at the beginning of recovery, instead of taking good care of their health and controlling sexual desire, young and tender ladies seek the pleasure of intercourse. This finally leads to bleeding with dizziness and fainting. It not only damages the uterine neck but also hurts the heart and kidneys. Lust and energy-consuming intercourse drain the essence considerably. When essence is drained, and spirit has deserted, there is no other reasonable choice but to supplement qi and blood significantly. This is an emergency treatment. The formula to use is

Jiù Bài Qiú shēng Tāng (救败求生汤，Collapse Rescuing and Life Rekindling Decoction)

人参（二两）	当归（二两，酒洗）
白术（二两，土炒）	九蒸熟地（一两）
山萸（五钱，蒸）	山药（五钱，蒸）
枣仁（五钱，生用）	附子（一分或一钱，自制）

rén shēn (ginseng), 2 *liang*

dāng guī (Chinese angelica), 2 *liang*

bái zhú (white atractylodes rhizome), 2 *liang*

shú dì (prepared rehmannia root), 1 *liang*

shān yú (fructus corni), 5 *qian* (steamed)

shān yào (common yam rhizome), 5 *qian*

zǎo rén (spiney date seed), 5 *qian* (raw)

fù zǐ (prepared aconite root), 1 *fen* or 1 *qian*

水煎服。一剂而神定，二剂而晕止，三剂而血亦止矣。倘一服见效，连服三四剂，减去一半，再服十剂，可庆更生。此方补气以回元阳于无何有之乡，阳回而气回，自可摄血以归神，生精而续命矣。

Decoct the formula with water and drink. When one *ji* is taken, the spirit is stabilized. When the second *ji* is taken, fainting stops. When a third *ji* is taken, bleeding is stopped. If the first *ji* takes effect, administer three or four more *ji* in succession. And then, reduce the dosage by half and administer ten more *ji*. Finally, resurrection can be celebrated. This formula supplements qi to recover the original yang from withering away. Once yang is recovered, qi is recovered and is naturally able to contain the blood. qi can guide the spirit back and engender essence to resume life.

【亦有中气素虚，产后顷刻血崩不止，气亦随之而脱。此至危之证，十常不救者八九，惟用独参汤尚可救活一二。辽人参（去芦）五钱，打碎，急煎，迟则气脱不及待矣。煎成，徐徐灌之，待气回再煎一服灌之。其余治法参看血崩门。但产后不可用杭芍炭以及诸凉药。然此证皆系临产一二日前入房所致，戒之。】

[There are also cases where the central qi has become deficient all along. Profuse bleeding occurs immediately after delivery with qi collapse. This is a highly critical case. Failure to save life happens in eight or nine out of ten cases. The one or two saved cases are done entirely by *Dú Shēn Tāng*(独参汤，Pure Ginseng Decoction). 5 *qian* of Liaoning *rén shēn* (人参，ginseng) (with the little rhizomes on the top removed) stemmed, smashed, and decocted rapidly. If there is any delay, qi will collapse. After the decoction has been prepared, give it to the patient slowly. When qi is back, decoct and administer another *ji*. For other treatment methods, refer to the chapters entitled *xuebeng* (Profuse Uterine Bleeding). However, in postpartum cases, *háng sháo tàn* (杭芍炭，charred Hangzhou white peony root) and various cooling medicinals should not be used. Such cases are all caused by sexual intercourse one or two days before delivery. Refrain from this!]

Chapter Sixty-three

Postpartum Incessant Dribbling of Blood Due to the Uterus Damaged by Hand

产后手伤胞胎淋漓不止

妇人有生产之时，被稳婆手入产门，损伤胞胎，因而淋漓不止，欲少忍须臾而不能。人谓胞破不能再补也，孰知不然。夫破伤皮肤，尚可完补，岂破在腹内者，独不可治疗？或谓破在外可用药外治，以生皮肤；破在内，虽有灵膏，无可救补。

In the course of giving birth, some women's uterus is damaged by the midwife who has put her hand into the neck of the uterus. As a result, blood dribbles incessantly and cannot be stopped for a moment. People think that a broken uterus is not mendable, but in fact, it is. Since injured skin can be mended, why should injuries inside the abdomen alone not be treatable? Some may argue that the exterior injuries may be cured by external treatment with medicinals to engender the skin. While, for the internal wounds, there is no way to apply any salvaging or mending even though there exists a cure-all medicinal paste.

然破之在内者，外治虽无可施力，安必内治不可奏功乎？试思疮伤之毒，大有缺陷，尚可服药以生肌肉，此不过收生不谨，小有所损，并无恶毒，何难补其缺陷也？方用完胞饮。

For the internal wounds, it is true that external treatments are not possible, but does internal treatment necessarily fail to achieve effect in such cases? Think of the exterior trauma; even if there are big wounds with abscess or infection, they can be helped to grow flesh through administering medication. What kind of difficulty is there in healing the injury, which is but a slight detriment without any toxic infection and is caused merely by carelessness during parturition? The formula to use is *Wán Bāo Yǐn* (完胞饮，Uterus Renewing Decoction).

人参（一两）   白术（一两，土炒）

茯苓（三钱，去皮）	生黄芪（五钱）
当归（一两，酒炒）	川芎（五钱）
白芨末（一钱）	红花（一钱）
益母草（三钱）	桃仁（十粒，泡，炒，研）

rén shēn (ginseng), 1 *liang*

bái zhú (white atractylodes rhizome), 1 *liang*

fú líng (poria), 3 *qian*

huáng qí (astragalus root), 5 *qian* (raw)

dāng guī (Chinese angelica), 1 *liang* (dry-fried with millet wine)

chuān xiōng (Sichuan lovage root), 5 *qian*

bāi jǐ (hyacinthbletilla), 1 *qian* (ground)

hóng huā (safflower), 1 *qian*

yì mǔ cǎo, (motherwort), 3 *qian*

táo rén (peach kernel), 10 pieces (soaked, dry-fried, ground)

用猪羊胞一个，先煎汤，后煎药，饥服十剂全愈。夫胞损宜用补胞之药，何以反用补气血之药也？盖生产本不可手探试，而稳婆竟以手探，胞胎以致伤损，则难产必矣。难产者，因气血之虚也。产后大伤气血，是虚而又虚矣。因虚而损，复因损而更虚，若不补其气与血，而胞胎之破，何以奏功乎。今之大补其气血者，不啻饥而与之食，渴而与之饮也，则精神大长，气血再造，而胞胎何难补完乎？所以旬日之内便成功也。

Boil a pig or sheep uterus and then decoct the medicines in the soup. Take the decoction when the stomach is empty. After ten *ji* is taken, a complete cure is effected. In case of a damaged uterus, it is appropriate to use uterus-supplementing medicinals. So why are qi and blood supplementing medicinals used here instead? In the course of delivery, it is not permissible to probe with hands. However, the midwife has done it and has damaged the uterus. This must have been because of a difficult delivery. A problematic delivery is due to qi and blood deficiency. A problematic delivery consumes and damages qi and blood, which adds to the deficiency. The deficiency was the cause of damage, and this damage, in turn, has worsened this deficiency. Besides greatly supplementing qi and blood, what else is effective for a broken uterus? Greatly supplementing qi and blood is just like offering food to the hungry or drink to the thirsty. Thus the essence spirit will be greatly enhanced; qi and blood will be produced again. Therefore, what kind of difficulty is there in renewing the uterus? Hence, success is achieved in no more than ten days.

Chapter Sixty-four
Postpartum Swelling and Edema of the Four Limbs

产后四肢浮肿

产后四肢浮肿，寒热往来，气喘咳嗽，胸隔不利，口吐酸水，两胁疼痛。人皆曰败血流于经络，渗于四肢，以致气逆也，谁知是肝肾两虚，阴不得出之阳乎。夫产后之妇，气血大亏，自然肾水不足，肾火沸腾。然水不足则不能养肝，而肝木大燥，木中乏津，木燥火发，肾火有党，子母两焚，火焰直冲，而上克肺金，金受火刑，力难制肝，而咳嗽喘满之病生焉。肝火既旺而下克脾土，土受木刑，力难制水，而四肢浮肿之病出焉。

Some women suffer from postpartum swelling and edema of four limbs, alternating chills, fever, asthmatic breath, coughing, blocking of the chest and diaphragm, acid regurgitation, and bilateral hypochondria pain. People all declare those are due to puerperal lochiostasis running into meridians and collaterals and penetrating the limbs. This then results in qi counterflow. Who would suspect a dual deficiency of the liver and kidneys and failure of yin going out of yang?

During postpartum, women's qi and blood are seriously depleted. Naturally, kidney water is insufficient, and kidney fire is flaming and steaming heat. When water is insufficient, it is unable to nurture the liver. Then liver wood becomes excessively dry and lacking in fluid. Dry wood causes fire. In this case, kidney fire finds an assisting partner. Both the mother and fetus organs are burning. Flames surge straight up and restrain lung metal. The (lung) metal is impaired by the (wood) fire and unable to restrain the liver. Thus, the problems like coughing, asthmatic breath, and blocking of the chest and diaphragm arise. If the liver fire becomes effulgent and goes down to restrain spleen earth, (spleen) earth is impaired by (liver) wood and has no strength left to inhibit water. Consequently, edema of the limbs appears.

然而肝木之火旺，乃假象而非真旺也。假旺之气，若盛而实不足，故时而热时而寒，往来无定，乃随气之盛衰以为寒热，而寒非真寒，热亦非真热，是以气逆于胸隔之间而不舒耳。两胁者，肝之部位也。酸者，肝之气味也。吐酸胁疼痛，皆肝虚而肾不能荣之象也。治法宜补血以养肝，补精以生血。精血足而气自顺，而寒热咳嗽浮肿之病悉退矣。方用转气汤。

However, this effulgent fire of liver wood is only a false impression. It is not effulgent. Falsely effulgent qi seems exuberant, but it is in fact, insufficient. Therefore, sometimes, there occurs fever and sometimes cold. These come and go unpredictably depending on the waxing and waning of qi. This cold is not actually cold. This heat is not actual heat. They are the manifestations of unsoothed qi counter-flowing between the chest and the diaphragm. The lateral costal region is where the liver is located, and sour is the flavor of the liver. Acid regurgitation and bilateral hypochondria pain are manifestations of liver deficiency and the kidneys' lack of ability to nourish and supplement. The appropriate treatment is to supplement blood to nurture the liver and supplement the essence to engender blood. When essence and blood are abundant, qi becomes normal by itself. All problems like chills and fever, coughing, and edema will disappear. The formula to use is *Zhuǎn Qì Tāng* (转气汤, Qi Changing Decoction).

人参（三钱）　　　　　茯苓（三钱，去皮）
白术（三钱，土炒）　　当归（五钱，酒洗）
白芍（五钱，酒炒）　　熟地（一两，九蒸）
山萸（三钱，蒸）　　　山药（五钱，炒）
芡实（三钱，炒）　　　柴胡（五分）
故纸（一钱，盐水炒）

rén shēn (ginseng), 3 *qian*

fú líng (poria), 3 *qian* (peeled)

bái zhú (white atractylodes rhizome), 3 *qian* (dry-fried with earth)

dāng guī (Chinese angelica), 5 *qian* (washed with millet wine)

bái sháo (white peony root), 5 *qian* (dry-fried with millet wine)

shú dì (prepared rehmannia root), 1 *liang* (fully steamed)

shān yú (fructus corni), 3 *qian* (steamed)

shān yào (common yam rhizome), 5 *qian* (dry-fried)

qiàn shí (euryale seed), 3 *qian* (dry-fried)

chái hú (bupleurum), 5 *fen*

gù zhĭ (oroxylum seed), 1 *qian* (dry-fried with salt water)

水煎服。三剂效，十剂痊。此方皆是补血补精之品，何以名为转气耶？不知气逆由于气虚，乃是肝肾之气虚也。补肝肾之精血，即所以补肝肾之气也。盖虚则逆，旺则顺，是补即转也。气转而各症尽愈，阴出之阳，则阴阳无扞格之虞矣。

（方妙不可加减。白芍宜炒炭用。）

Decoct the formula in water and take it orally. Many sound effects can be seen after 3 *ji* is taken. Complete recovery can be achieved after taking 10 *ji*. This formula is composed of ingredients for supplementing blood and essence. Then why is it named *zhuan qi* (qi rectifying)? It should be understood that the counterflow of qi is the result of qi deficiency, or rather, deficiency of liver and kidney qi. Supplementing the essence and blood of the liver and kidneys is as good as supplementing the qi of the liver and kidneys. Deficiency leads to counterflow, while effulgence leads to normalization and good order. So supplementing is rectifying. Once qi is rectified, all the disorders will be rectified, and when yin may go out of yang, the trouble of interference between yin and yang will disappear.

[This formula is so perfect that it allows no modification. *Bái sháo* (白芍, white peony root) should be slightly charred.]

Chapter Sixty-five

Discharge of Fleshy Fiber After Delivery

产后肉线出

　　妇人有产后水道中出肉线一条，长二三尺，动之则疼痛欲绝。人以为胞胎之下坠也，谁知是带脉之虚脱乎。夫带脉束于任督之间，任脉前而督脉后，二脉有力，则带脉坚牢；二脉无力，则带脉崩坠。产后亡血过多，无血以养任督，而带脉崩坠，力难升举，故随溺而随下也。带脉下垂，每每作痛于腰脐之间，况下坠者而出于产门之外，其失于关键也，更甚，安得不疼痛欲绝乎？

　　方用两收汤。

Some women have a fleshy fiber or thread 2~3 chi (or feet) long-running out from the water passage (vagina). This fiber or thread gives a deadly pain when touched. People suppose this is the prolapsed *bao tai* (uterus). Who would suspect collapse due to *dai mai* (belt vessel) deficiency? As *dai mai* (belt vessel) bundles *ren mai* (conception vessel) and *du mai* (governor vessel). Renmai is in the front, and dumai is in the back. When *ren mai* and *du mai* are strong, *dai mai* is solid and firm. When they are weak, *dai mai* collapses and sags. Because of the excessive postpartum loss of blood, there is no blood to nourish *ren mai* and *du mai*. As *dai mai* collapses and sags, left with no strength to raise itself up, it follows the urine out. Sagging of *dai mai* usually gives pain in the lumber and umbilical regions. What is worse, *dai mai* has collapsed beyond the birth gate, too far away from its proper position. How can it not cause deadly pain? The formula to use is *Liǎng Shōu Tāng* (两收汤, Dual Withdrawing Decoction).

人参（一两）	白术（二两，土炒）
川芎（三钱，酒洗）	九蒸熟地（二两）
山药（一两，炒）	山萸（四钱，蒸）
芡实（五钱，炒）	扁豆（五钱，炒）
巴戟（三钱，盐水浸）	杜仲（五钱，炒黑）

白果（十枚，捣碎）

rén shēn (ginseng), 1 *liang*

bái zhú (white atractylodes rhizome), 2 *liang* (dry-fried with earth)

chuān xiōng (Sichuan lovage root), 3 *qian* (washed with millet wine)

shú dì (prepared rehmannia root), 2 *liang* (fully steamed)

shān yào (common yam rhizome), 1 *liang* (dry-fried)

shān yú (fructus corni), 4 *qian* (steamed)

qiàn shí (euryale seed), 5 *qian* (dry-fried)

biǎn dòu (hyacinth bean), 5 *qian* (dry-fried)

bā jǐ (morinda root), 3 *qian* (soaked in salt water)

dù zhòng (eucommia bark), 5 *qian* (charred)

bái guǒ (ginkgo nut), 10 pieces (smashed)

水煎服。一剂而收半，二剂而全收矣。此方补任督而仍补腰脐者，盖以任督连于腰脐也。补任督而不补腰脐，则任督无助，而带脉何以升举？惟两补之，则任督得腰脐之助，带脉亦得任督之力而收矣。

Decoct the formula in water and drink. When one *ji* is taken, about half of the discharge will be withdrawn. After Two *ji* is taken, it will be withdrawn entirely. This formula is designed to supplement *ren mai*, *du mai*, lumbus, and umbilicus because these two meridians are linked with the lumbus and umbilicus. If *ren mai* and *du mai* are supplemented to exclude the lumbus and umbilicus, these two meridians would have no backing. Then, how could *dai mai* be up-lifted? Only if dual supplementation is applied can *ren mai* and *du mai* get support from the lumbus and umbilicus. So, *dai mai* can withdraw by the strength of these two meridians.

（此方凡肾虚腰痛、遗尿皆可治，甚勿轻忽。）

(This formula can treat lumbago and enuresis due to kidney deficiency. It should not be underestimated.)

Chapter Sixty-six

Postartum Agalactosis Due to qi and Blood Deficiency

产后气血两虚乳汁不下

妇人产后绝无点滴之乳，人以为乳管之闭也，谁知是气与血之两涸乎。夫乳乃气血所化而成也，无血固不能生乳汁，无气亦不能生乳汁。然二者之中，血之化乳，又不若气之所化为尤速。新产之妇，血已大亏，血本自顾不暇，又何能以化乳？乳全赖气之力，以行血而化之也。今产后数日，而乳不下点滴之汁，其血少气衰可知。气旺则乳汁旺，气衰则乳汁衰，气涸则乳汁亦涸，必然之势也。世人不知大补气血之妙，而一味通乳，岂知无气则乳无以化，无血则乳无以生。不几向饥人而乞食，贫人而索金乎？治法宜补气以生血，而乳汁自下，不必利窍以通乳也。方名通乳丹。

After delivery, some women do not have a drop of breast milk. People suppose this is due to blocked milk ducts. Who would suspect it is due to the drying up of both qi and blood? Milk is transformed from qi and blood. Milk cannot be produced without blood, neither can it be produced without qi.

In comparison, the blood's transforming into milk is less quick than the transformation of qi. For women who have just given birth, blood is too depleted to transform into milk. It entirely depends on the strength of qi to promote blood circulation and help to transform milk. Several days after delivery, the breasts have secreted not a drop of milk, revealing a deficiency of blood and debility of qi. When qi is effulgent, milk is effulgent. When qi is debilitated, milk is depleted. When qi is dried up, milk is dried up. This is an inescapable tendency. However, people who do not know the importance of greatly supplementing qi and blood tend to promote lactation blindly.

Nevertheless, without qi, milk cannot be transformed; without blood, milk cannot be generated. It is just like begging for food from a hungry man or asking for money from a poor man. The proper treatment is to supplement qi and generate blood, and breast milk will be secreted soon. There is no need to promote lactation. The formula to use is *Tōng Rǔ Dān* (通乳丹，Lactation Promoting Pills)

人参（一两）　　　　　　生黄芪（一两）

当归（二两，酒洗）　　　麦冬（五钱，去心）

木通（三分）　　　　　　桔梗（三分）

七孔猪蹄（二个，去爪壳）

rén shēn (ginseng), 1 *liang*

huáng qí (astragalus root) Radices Paeoniae Alba, 1 *liang* (raw)

dāng guī (Chinese angelica), 2 *liang* (washed with millet wine)

mài dōng (dwarf lilyturf tuber), 5 *qian* (pith removed)

mù tōng (akebia stem), 3 *fen*

jié gěng (platycodon root), 3 *fen*

zhū tí (pork trotter), 2,(claw case removed)

水煎服。二剂而乳如泉涌矣。此方专补气血以生乳汁，正以乳生于气血也。产后气血涸而无乳，非乳管之闭而无乳者可比。不去通乳而名通乳丹，亦因服之乳通而名之。今不通乳而乳生，即名生乳丹亦可。

Decoct the formula in water and take it orally. When two *ji* are taken, the patient will have milk gushing like a spring. This formula exclusively supplements qi and blood to produce breast milk. This is because there are no other producers of milk other than qi and blood. There is no comparison between the absence of breast milk due to postpartum drying up of qi and blood, and that due to blocked milk ducts. Though not composed of medicinals to unblock the milk duct, this formula is called Lactation Promoting Pills. Because it does not unblock the milk duct but produces milk, it is all right to call it *Shēng Rǔ Dān* (生乳丹，Milk Producing Pills).

产后郁结乳汁不通

少壮之妇，于生产之后，或闻丈夫之嫌，或听翁姑之诮，遂致两乳胀满疼痛，乳汁不通。人以为阳明之火热也，谁知是肝气之郁结乎。夫阳明属胃，乃多气多血之府也。乳汁之化，原属阳明。然阳明属土，壮妇产后，虽云亡血，而阳明之气实未尽衰，必得肝木之气以相通，始能化成乳汁，未可全责之阳明也。盖乳汁之化，全在气而不在血。

After delivery, some young women experience breast distention, fullness, and pain with galactostasis. People suppose this is due to fire heat of the *yang ming* meridian. Who would suspect depression caused by liver qi stagnation? The *yang ming* pertains to the stomach, a house abundant in both qi and blood. Transformation of breast milk is the responsibility of the *yangming*, which pertains to earth. In a constitutionally strong woman, even though the blood has collapsed after delivery, the qi of the *yang ming* is, practically speaking, not utterly debilitated. However, it cannot transform milk unless its flow is freed by the liver qi (wood). Therefore, *yangming* is but partly at fault. The transformation of milk does not depend on the blood but entirely upon qi.

今产后数日，宜其有乳，而两乳胀满作痛，是欲化乳而不可得，非气郁而何？明明是羞愤成郁，土木相结，又安能化乳而成汁也。治法宜大舒其肝木之气，而阳明之气血自通，而乳亦通矣，不必专去通乳也。方名通肝生乳汤。

Several days after delivery, breast milk should have been secreted. Distention, fullness, and pain in the breasts show a tendency but failure to transform milk. What else could cause this if not stagnated qi? It is apparent that there exists depression exacerbated by shame and indignation and that earth and wood are bound by each other. How can milk be transformed to produce a flow? The appropriate treatment is to soothe the liver (wood) qi greatly. Thus, qi and blood of the *yang ming* are naturally freed, and milk will flow unimpeded. There is no need to unblock it. The formula to use is *Tōng Gān Shēng Rǔ Tāng* (通肝生乳汤 Liver Freeing and Milk Producing Decoction).

白芍（五钱，醋炒）　　　当归（五钱，酒洗）

白术（五钱，土炒）　　　熟地（三分）

甘草（三分）　　　　　　麦冬（五钱，去心）

通草（一钱）　　　　　　柴胡（一钱）

远志（一钱）

bái sháo (white peony root), 5 *qian* (dry-fried with vinegar)

dāng guī (Chinese angelica), 5 *qian* (washed with millet wine)

bái zhú (white atractylodes rhizome), 5 *qian* (dry-fried with earth)

shú dì (prepared rehmannia root), 3 *fen*

gān cǎo (licorice root), 3 *fen*

mài dōng (dwarf lilyturf tuber), 5 *qian* (plumule removed)

tōng cǎo (rice paper plant pith), 3 *fen*

chái hú (bupleurum), 1 *qian*

yuǎn zhì (thin-leaf milkwort root), 1 *qian*

水煎服。一剂即通，不必再服也。

（麦冬用小米炒，不惟不寒胃，且得米味一直引入胃中；而化乳愈速。）

Decoct the formula in water and take it orally. After one *ji* is taken, the breast milk flows. There is no need for a second ji. [*Mài dōng*(麦冬, dwarf lilyturf tuber), when stir-fried with millets, far from cooling the stomach, will directly lead the medicinals into the stomach by the flavor of the grain. Thus, the transformation of milk will be quick.]

Volume Nine

Postpartum Disorders I

产后篇　上卷

Chapter Sixty-eight

An Overview of Postpartum Disorders

产后总论

凡病起于血气之衰，脾胃之虚，而产后尤甚。是以丹溪先生论产后，必大补气血为先，虽有他症，以末治之，斯言尽治产之大旨。若能扩充立方，则治产可无过矣。

Diseases originating from the declination of qi and blood or deficiency of the spleen and stomach tend to aggravate the patient after delivery. For that reason, in dealing with postpartum disorders, Master Zhu Danxi advocated giving priority to significantly supplementing qi and blood. Other problems are subordinate. This statement embraces all the principles of handling postpartum disorders. Applying it to the design of formulas, one will be free from errors in handling parturient-related cases.

夫产后忧惊劳倦，气血暴虚，诸症乘虚易入。如有气毋专耗散，有食毋专消导。热不可用芩连，寒不可用桂附。寒则血块停滞，热则新血崩流。

After delivery, worry, panic, tiredness, fatigue, and sudden deficiency of qi and blood provide a chance for various symptoms to take advantage of the deficiency and enter the body. If there is depression due to qi stagnation, do not apply consuming-dissipation methods.

If there is food accumulation, do not use medicines to help digestion and remove food accumulation.

In the case of heat, do not use herbs like *huáng qín* (黄芩, scutellaria root) and *huáng lián* (黄连, coptis rhizome).

In the case of cold, do not use medicines like *ròu guì* (肉桂, cinnamon bark) and *fù zǐ* (附子, prepareded aconite root).

Cold leads to blood clots, stoppage, and stagnation. Heat leads to new blood flooding.

至若中虚外感，见三阳表症之多，似可汗也，在产后而用麻黄，则重竭其阳；见三阴里症之多，似可下也，在产后而用承气，则重亡阴血。

As to external contraction with central deficiency, if the patient shows more evidence of an exterior syndrome of the three yang meridians, it seems that using diaphoresis is suitable. Using *má huáng* (麻黄, ephedra) after delivery will result in severe exhaustion of yang.

If the patient presents more evidence of an interior syndrome of the three-yin meridians, it seems that using purgation is suitable. However, using *Chéng Qì Tāng* (承气汤, Purgative Decoction) after delivery will result in the severe loss of yin (blood).

耳聋胁痛，乃肾虚恶露之停，休用柴胡。谵语出汗，乃元弱似邪之症，非同胃实。厥由阳气之衰，无分寒热，非大补不能回阳而起弱；痉因阴血之亏，不论刚柔，非滋荣不能舒筋而活络。乍寒乍热，发作无期，症似疟也，若以疟治，迁延难愈；言论无伦，神不守舍，病似邪也，若以邪治，危亡可待。

In the case of deafness and lateral costal pain caused by retention of lochia due to kidney deficiency, do not use *chái hú* (柴胡, bupleurum).

Delirium with perspiration, weakness of primordial qi, similar to the invasion of pathogenic factors, should not be treated as stomach excess.

In the case of syncope, which is due to the weakness of yang, be it cold or hot, to recover yang, and start convalescence from weakness, there is no other choice but to apply drastic tonification.

In the case of spasm, which is due to depletion of yin blood, be it hard or soft, to relax the tendon and activate the collateral, there is no other choice but to nourish and tonify.

Alternating chills and fever with attacks at irregular intervals are similar to the manifestations of malaria, but if treated as malaria, they will remain recurrent and refractory.

Incoherent speech and being restless as well as abstracted looks like an invasion of pathogenic factors. If it is treated as dispelling pathogenic factors, crisis and death are to be expected.

去血过多而大便燥结，肉苁蓉加于生化，非润肠承气之能通，去汗过多而小便短涩，六君子倍加参，芪，必生津助液之可利。加参生化汤频服，救产后之危；

长生活命丹屡用，苏绝谷之人。

Retention of dry feces due to excessive blood loss can be treated by adding *ròu cōng róng* (肉苁蓉, desert cistanche) to *Shēng Huà Tāng* (Engendering and Transforming Decoction). They are beyond the intestine-moistening and *Chéng Qì Tāng* (承气汤, Purgative Decoction).

In the case of short urine or dysuria due to excessive sweating, *Liù Jūn Zǐ Tāng* (六君子汤, Six Gentlemen Decoction) with a double amount of *rén shēn* (人参, ginseng) and *huáng qí* (黄芪, astragalus root) is capable of engendering fluid and assisting humor to effect disinhibition.

Jiā Shēn Shēng Huà Tāng (加参生化汤, Engendering and Transforming Decoction Added with Ginseng), taken at short intervals, can rescue postpartum crises.

Cháng Shēng Huó Mìng Dān (长生活命丹, Life-Saving Pills), taken frequently, can resurrect a patient who has stopped taking in food.

颓疝脱肛，多是气虚下陷，补中益气之方。口噤拳挛，乃因血燥类风，加参生化之剂。产户入风而痛甚，服宜羌活养荣汤。玉门伤凉而不闭，洗宜蛇莬萸硫散。怔忡惊悸，生化汤加以定志。

Severe indirect hernia and prolapse of the rectum, usually due to collapse caused by qi deficiency, are indications of *Bǔ Zhōng Yì Qì Tāng* (补中益气汤, Center-Supplementing and Qi-Boosting Decoction.)

Trismus and hypertonicity of the fists caused by dry blood and quasi-wind (stroke) are indications of *Jiā Shēn Shēng Huà Tāng* (加参生化汤, Engendering and Transforming Decoction Plus Ginseng).

For severe pain in the birth gate due to the inroads of wind, it is proper to administer *Qiāng Huó Yǎng Róng Tāng* (羌活养荣汤, Notoptetygium Root Nutrient-Nourishing Decoction).

Postpartum laceration of the perineum due to attacking of cold is best treated by washing with *Shé Tù Yú Liú Sǎn** (蛇莬萸硫散, Cnidium Fruit, Dodder Seed, Medicinal Evodia Fruit and Sulphur Powder).

To treat palpitation, *Shēng Huà Tāng* (生化汤, Engendering and Transforming Decoction) can stabilize the mind.

似邪恍惚，安神丸助以归脾。因气而闷满虚烦，生化汤加木香为佐；因食而嗳酸恶食，六君子加神曲、麦芽为良。苏木、莪术，大能破血；青皮、枳壳，最消满胀。

To treat absent-mindedness as if spellbound, *Ān Shén Wán* (安神丸, Spirit-Calming Pill) should be helped by *Guī Pí Tāng* (归脾汤, Spleen-Restoring Decoction).

In the case of oppression, fullness, deficiency, and vexation due to qi stagnation, *mù xiāng* (木香, common aucklandia root) can be added as an assistant to *Shēng Huà Tāng* (生化汤, Engendering and Transforming Decoction).

To treat oxyrygmia (acid reflux) and anorexia due to indigestion, it is better to add *shén qū* (神曲, medicated leaven) and *mài yá* (麦芽, germinated barley) to *Liù Jūn Zǐ Tāng* (六君子汤, Six Gentlemen Decoction).

Sū mù (苏木, sappan wood) and *é zhú* (莪术, curcumae rhizome) are particularly capable of breaking blood.

Qīng pí (青皮, green tangerine peel) and *zhǐ qiào* (枳壳, bitter orange) are most capable of resolving flatulency with fullness.

一应耗气破血之剂，汗吐宣下之法，止可施诸壮实，岂宜用于胎产。大抵新产后，先问恶露如何，块痛未除，不可遽加参术。腹中痛止，补中益气无疑。至若亡阳脱汗，气虚喘促，频服加参生化汤，是从权也。又如亡阴火热，血崩厥晕，速煎生化原方，是救急也。

All qi-consuming, blood-stasis-breaking medicinals and methods such as diaphoresis, emetic, diffusion, and purgation, are usually applied in excess syndromes but not in cases of pregnancy or postpartum.

In terms of a case shortly after delivery, it is necessary above all to inquire about the lochia as a rule.

If there is abdominal after-pain due to blood stasis not yet relieved, do not use *rén shēn* (人参, ginseng) and *bái zhú* (白术, white atractylodes rhizome) hastily. If the abdominal pain has relieved, tonifying the middle and benefiting qi is definitely the proper way.

For a case of depletion of yang due to profuse sweating at a critical stage and asthma due to qi deficiency, take *Jiā Shēn Shēng Huà Tāng*（加参生化汤, Engendering and Transforming Decoction Plus Ginseng）frequently. It serves as an expedient measure. However, where yin depletion with fire heat and metrorrhagia with syncope and dizziness are concerned, boil *Shēng Huà Tāng* (生化汤, Engendering and Transforming Decoction) without delay for emergency treatment.

王太仆云：治下补下，治以急缓。缓则道路达而力微，急则气味厚而为重。

故治产当遵丹溪而固本，服法宜效太仆以频加。

Grand Servant Wang (Wang Bing) said, "to treat the lower, supplement the lower with swift treatment. The slow method clears roads but is small in strength, while the swift method is thick in flavor and massive in strength". Therefore, it is proper to follow Zhu Danxi to reinforce the body base to treat postpartum disorders. As to the administration method, it is proper to follow Grand Servant Wang (Wang Bing) on administering in short intervals.

凡付生死之重寄，须着意于极危；欲求俯仰之无亏，用存心于爱物。此虽未尽产症之详，然所闻一症，皆援近乡治验为据，亦未必无小补云。

Being entrusted with a matter of life and death, one should always focus on and anticipate the most critical condition. If one wants to feel no qualms as a doctor, one should never lose his or her sympathy and kindness for the patient. Although this work does not cover all postpartum disorders, it will hopefully be valuable since each case study is supported by the evidence of clinical experience gathered from the nearby residents.

*

Shé Tù Yú Liú Sǎn: *liú huáng* (硫磺, sulphur) 4 *liang*, *wú zhū yú* (吴茱萸, medicinal evodia fruit) 1.5 *liang*, *tù sī zǐ* (菟丝子, dodder seed) 1.6 *liang*, *shé chuáng zǐ* (蛇床子, cnidium fruit) 1 *liang*. Grind the medicinals into powder, decoct it in water, use the decoction wash the birth gate.

Chapter Sixty-nine

Indications and Contraindications of Antenatal & Postpartum Disorders I

产前后方证宜忌 一

正产
Normal Delivery

正产者，有腹或痛或止，腰胁酸痛；或势急而胞未破，名弄胎。服八珍汤加香附自安。有胞破数日而痛尚缓，亦服上药俟之。

In a normal delivery, intermittent abdominal pain with lumbar and lateral costal aching pain or urgency with the placenta still intact is called playing fetus (excessive fetus movement in late pregnancy). Take *Bā Zhēn Tāng* (Eight Precious Ingredients Decoction) with *xiāng fù* (香附, cyperus), and it will surely calm the fetus. In case of mild pain lingering several days after breaking the placenta, administer the above medicinals and wait.

伤产
Premature Delivery

伤产者，胎未足月，有所伤动，或腹痛脐痛，或服催生药太早，或产母努力太过，逼儿错路，不能正产。故临月必举动从容，不可多睡，饱食饮酒，但觉腹中动转，即正身仰卧，待儿转顺。与其临时费力，不如先时慎重。

In premature delivery, injury or stirring of the fetus before full term, abdominal and umbilicus pain, too early administration of birth-hastening medicinals (oxytocin), or overexertion of the mother may force the fetus to deviate from its position to render natural delivery impossible. Therefore, in the month when childbirth is due, the mother should behave in a leisurely way and refrain from oversleeping, overeating, and drinking wine. When feeling the fetus turning in the womb, the mother should lie on her back to wait for the fetus to turn in position. It is better to be cautious in advance than to have trouble in the end.

调产
Balancing or Adjusting Delivery

调产者，产母临月，择稳婆，办器用，备参药。产时不可多人喧闹，二人扶身，或凭物站。心烦，用滚水调白蜜一匙，独活汤更妙；或饥，服糜粥少许，勿令饥渴。有生息未顺者，只说有双胎，或胎衣不下，勿令产母惊恐。

In terms of adjusting delivery, when childbirth is due, choose the midwife, ready the necessary instruments and utensils, and have medicinals like *rén shēn* (人参, ginseng) in-store. During delivery, the presence of many people making noise is not allowed. The birthing woman can be supported by two persons or stand against something. In case of heart vexation, take a spoonful of honey dissolved in boiling water, but it is better to administer *Dú Huó Tāng* (独活汤, Double Teeth Pubescent Angelica Root Decoction)*. When hungry, take some porridge. Do not let the mother go hungry or thirsty. In case of difficult delivery, say it is due to twins or non-descension of the placenta. The birthing mother should be kept free from panic.

*

Duhuo Tang (Doubleteeth Pubescent Angelica Decoction), in the original book, the composition of this formula is not mentioned. In other books, the formula has different ingredients. However, the main ingredients are *dú huó*,(独活, double teeth pubescent angelica root), *qiāng huó* (羌活, notoptetygium root), *fáng fēng*(防风, saposhnikovia root), *rén shēn* (人参, ginseng), *chuān xiōng*（川芎, Sichuan lovage root）, and the rest of the ingredients.

Chapter Seventy

Indications and Contraindications of
Antenatal & Postpartum Disorders Ⅱ

产前后方证宜忌 二

催生
Hastening Parturition

催生者，因坐草太早，困倦难产，用八珍汤，稍佐以香附、乳香，以助血气。胞衣早破，浆血已干，亦用八珍汤。

In terms of hastening parturition, in the case of an extended delivery time or fatigue and sleepiness due to complex delivery, administer Bazhen Tang (Eight Precious Ingredients Decoction) with a small amount of *xiāng fù* (香附, cyperus) and *rǔ xiāng* (乳香, frankincense) to assist blood and qi. *Bā Zhēn Tāng*（八珍汤，Eight-Gem Decoction）can also be used in the case of an early broken placenta with blood already dried out.

冻产
Frozen Delivery

冻产者，天寒血气凝滞，不能速生，故衣裳宜厚，产室宜暖，背心、下体尤要。

Frozen delivery means the delivery cannot be smooth because of the cold weather, which causes the stagnation of blood and qi. Therefore, the birthing woman should be warmly clothed and placed in a warm chamber. The chest and upper back, as well as the lower body, should be kept particularly warm.

热产
Hot Delivery

热产者，暑月宜温凉得宜。若产室人众，热气蒸逼，致头痛、面赤、昏晕等症，宜饮清水少许以解之。然风雨阴凉，亦当避之。

In hot months, the delivery room temperature should be adjusted to the appropriate comfort of the patient. If the room is crowded, hot, steaming air may cause headache, red facial complexion, fainting, in addition to other symptoms. It is appropriate to drink a little cool water to relieve. It is, however, necessary to keep off wind, rain, and shady coolness.

难产
Difficult Delivery

难产者，交骨不开，不能生产也，服加味芎归汤，良久即下。

小川芎（一两）	当归（一两）
败龟板（一个，酒炙）	妇人发灰一握（须用生过男妇者，为末）

水一盏，煎七分服。

For a difficult delivery due to failure of the interlocking bones to open, administer *Jiā Wèi Xiōng Guī Tāng* (加味芎归汤，Supplemented Sichuan Lovage Root and Chinese Angelica Decoction). After a while, the fetus will come down.

xiǎo chuān xiōng (Sichuan lovage root), 1 *liang* (small ones)

dāng guī (Chinese angelica), 1 *liang*

guī bǎn (tortoise plastron), 1 piece (liquid-fried with millet wine)

fù rén fà huī (charred hair of women), a handful

Boil in a big cup of water down to 7/10 of a cup and take.

Chapter Seventy-one

Indications and Contraindications of Antenatal & Postpartum Disorders Ⅲ

产前后方证宜忌 三

下胞
Descending the Placenta

胞衣不下，用滚酒送下失笑散一剂，或益母丸，或生化汤送鹿角灰一钱，或以产母发入口作吐，胞衣即出。有气虚不能送出者，腹必胀痛，单用生化汤。

| 全当归（一两） | 川芎（三钱） |
| 白术（一钱） | 香附（一钱） |

加人参三钱更妙，用水煎服。

As for the fetal placenta that does not descend, use one *ji* of *Shī Xiào Sǎn* (失笑散, Sudden Smile Powder), and take it with warm millet wine. Alternatively, use one *ji* of *Yì Mǔ Wán* (Motherwort Pill) or one *ji* of *Shēng Huà Tāng* (生化汤, Engendering and Transforming Decoction) with 1 *qian* of *lù jiǎo huī* (鹿角灰, degelatinated deer antler ash) mixed in. Alternatively, provoke vomiting by putting the mother's hair in her mouth, and the placenta will be discharged. The inability to bring the placenta forth due to qi deficiency must be accompanied by abdominal distention and pain. Use only *Shēng Huà Tāng* (生化汤, Engendering and Transforming Decoction):

dāng guī (Chinese angelica), 1 *liang* (whole)

chuān xiōng (Sichuan lovage root), 3 *qian*

bái zhú (white atractylodes rhizome), 1 *qian*

xiāng fù (cyperus), 1 *qian*

It will be better if 3 *qian* of *rén shēn* (人参, ginseng) is added. Decoct the formula in water and take.

一方，用蓖麻子二两，雄黄二钱，研膏，涂足下涌泉穴，衣下，急速洗去。

Another method is to grind *bì má zǐ* (蓖麻子, castor seed), 2 *liang*, and *xióng huáng* (雄黄, realgar) 2 *qian* into a paste and apply it to *yǒng quán xué* (涌泉穴, KI 1) on the soles of the feet. As soon as the placenta drops, wash the paste off.

平胃散：

南苍术（米泔水浸炒）	厚朴（姜炒）
陈皮（二钱）	炙草（二钱）

共为粗末，或水煎，或酒煎，煎成时加朴硝二钱，再煎一二沸，温服。

失笑散：五灵脂、蒲黄，俱研为细末，每服三钱，热酒下。

Píng Wèi Sǎn (平胃散, Stomach-Calming Powder):

cāng zhú (atractylodes rhizome), 2 *qian*

hòu pò, magnolia bark, 2 *qian* (dry-fried with ginger)

chén pí (aged tangerine peel), 2 *qian*

zhì cǎo (prepared licorice root), 2 *qian*

Powder coarsely 2 *qian* of each of the above and decoct in either water or millet wine. After the mixture is boiled down to the desired degree, put in 2 *qian* of *pò xiāo* (朴硝, mirabilite) and continue boil for 1 minute. To be taken warm.

Shī Xiào Sǎn (失笑散, Sudden Smile Powder):

wǔ líng zhī (五灵脂, flying squirrel faeces) and *pú huáng* (蒲黄, cattail pollen), both are ground fine. Take 3 *qian* once, down with warm millet wine.

治产秘验良方
Secret, Proven, Effective Formula for Birthing

治横生逆产，至数日不下，一服即下。有未足月，忽然胎动，一服即安。或临月先服一服，保护无虞。更能治胎死腹中，及小产伤胎无乳者，一服即如原体。

This formula treats transverse birth or inverted delivery when labor has lasted for several days, but the fetus is not yet born. One *ji* will bring down the fetus. In case of sudden stirring of the fetus before maturation, one *ji* will calm it down. Administering one *ji* towards delivery ensures safety. This formula is particularly effective in treating fetal death within the abdomen and miscarriage damage of the fetus, and absence of breast milk (agalactosis). Take one *ji*, and it will effect a perfect recovery.

全当归（一钱五分）	川芎（一钱五分）

川贝母（一钱，去心）　　　　荆芥穗、黄芪（各八分）

厚朴（姜炒）　　　　　　　　蕲艾（七分）

红花（七分）　　　　　　　　菟丝子（一钱二分）

甘草（五分）　　　　　　　　羌活（六分，面炒）

枳壳（六分，面炒）　　　　　白芍（一钱二分，冬月不用）

dāng guī (Chinese angelica), 1 *qian* and 5 *fen* (whole)

chuān xiōng (Sichuan lovage root), 1 *qian* and 5 *fen*

chuān bèi mǔ (Sichuan fritillaria bulb) , 1 *qian* (hearts removed)

jīng jiè suì (fineleaf schizonepeta spike), 8 *fen*

huáng qí (astragalus root), 8 *fen*

hòu pò (magnolia bark), 7 *fen* (dry-fried with ginger)

qí ài (mugwort leaf), 7 *fen* (produced in Qizhou)

hóng huā (safflower), 7 *fen*

tù sī zǐ (dodder seed), 1 *qian* and *2 fen*

gān cǎo (licorice root), 5 *fen*

qiāng huó (notoptetygium root), 6 *fen* (dry-fried with wheat flour)

zhǐ qiào (bitter orange), 6 *fen* (dry-fried with wheat flour)

bái sháo (white peony root), 1 *qian* and 2 *fen* (excluded in winter)

上十三味，只用十二味，不可加减。安胎去红花，催生去蕲艾。用井水盅半，姜三片为引，热服。渣用水一盅，煎半盅，热服。如不好，再用水一盅，煎半盅，服之即效，不用二剂。

Of these 13 ingredients, 12 are used in practice, and the formula does not allow for any modification. To calm the fetus, subtract *hóng huā* (红花, safflower). To hasten birth, subtract *qí ài* (蕲艾, mugwort leaf). Boil in one and a half cups of clean water and take warm with three slices of Ginger as conductor. Then, the dregs are to be boiled in a cup of water down to 1/2, and the decoction is to be taken warm. If no effect is brought, boil the dregs in 1 cup of water down to half again. After this is taken, the effect will indeed be achieved. There is no need to administer a second *ji*.

催生兔脑丸
Cui sheng Tu Nao Wan
(Birth Hastening Rabbit Brain Pills)

治横生、逆产神效。

腊月兔脑髓（一个）　　　　　母丁香（一个）

乳香（一钱，另研）　　　　　麝香（一分）

兔脑为丸，芡实大，阴干密封，用时以温酒送下一丸。

This formula offers a miraculous effect for transverse birth and inverted delivery.

tù nǎo (rabbit brain), 1 *head* (killed in the 12th month, lunar calender)

mǔ dīng xiāng (mother clove), 1 piece

rǔ xiāng (frankincense), 1 *qian* (ground)

shè xiāng* (musk), 1 *fen*

Make into pills the size of *qiàn shí* (芡实, euryale seed), dry in the shade, and seal tightly. When necessary, take one pill with warm millet wine.

*

shè xiāng (麝香, musk) is illegal to buy or sell in China now.

夺命丹
Duo Ming Dan
(Life Clutching Elixir)

临产未产时，目反口噤，面黑唇青，口中吐沫，命在须臾。若脸面微红，子死母活，急用。

蛇蜕（烧灰不存性）　　　　　蚕故子（烧灰不存性）

发灰（一钱）　　　　　　　　乳香（五分）

共为细末，酒下。

At the point of delivery, if the patient exhibits up-turned eyes, clenched jaw, a black facial complexion, green-blue lips, and foaming at the mouth corner, life is at stake. If the facial complexion is tinged with faint red, the fetus will die, and the mother will survive.

Immediately administer:

shé tuì (snake slough), (burnt without preserving its nature)

Cán gù zǐ (silkworm slough), (burnt without preserving its nature)

fà huī (charred hair), 1 *qian*

rǔ xiāng (frankincense), 5 *fen*

Powder fine and chase down with millet wine.

加味芎归汤
Jiawei Xionggui Tang (Supplemented Sichuan Lovage Rhizome and Chinese Angelica Decoction)

加味芎归汤：

治子宫不收，产门不闭

人参（二钱）	黄芪（一钱）
当归（二钱）	升麻（八分）
川芎（一钱）	炙草（四分）

五味子（十五粒）

再不收，加半夏八分，白芍八分酒妙（炒）。

Treats non-contraction and postpartum non-closure of the uterus.

rén shēn (ginseng), 2 *qian*

huáng qí (astragalus root), 1 *qian*

dāng guī (Chinese angelica), 2 *qian*

shēng má (black cohosh rhizome), 8 *fen*

chuān xiōng (Sichuan lovage root), 1 *qian*

zhì cǎo (prepared licorice root), 4 *fen*

wǔ wèi zǐ (Chinese magnolivine fruit), 15 pieces

If the uterus still refuses to contract, add *bàn xià* (半夏, pinellia rhizome) 8 *fen* and *bái sháo* (白芍, white peony root) 8 *fen* (dry-fried with Chinese millet wine).

Chapter Seventy-two

Indications and Contraindications of Antenatal & Postpartum Disorders Ⅳ

产前后方证宜忌 四

新产治法
Treatment for the Newly Birthed

生化汤先连进二服。若胎前素弱妇人,见危症热症堕胎,不可拘帖数,服至病退乃止。若产时劳甚,血崩形脱,即加人参三四钱在内,频服无虞。若气促亦加人参,加参于生化汤者,血块无滞,不可以参为补而弗用也。有治产不用当归者,见偏之甚。此方处置万全,必无一失。世以四物汤治产,地黄性寒滞血,芍药微酸无补,伐伤生气,误甚。

Firstly, administer 2 *ji* of *Shēng Huà Tāng* (生化汤, Engendering and Transforming Decoction) in succession. If the woman was weak before delivery or manifests a critical or hot condition or in case of miscarriage, administer this decoction till recovery. The number of *ji* may be unlimited.

In a case of labor leading to profuse bleeding or form desertion (body looks very thin and weak, loses weight quickly), add 3~4 *qian* of *rén shēn* (人参, ginseng). Administering this decoction at short intervals will ensure safety. In case of shortness of breath, also add *rén shēn* (人参, ginseng). Adding *rén shēn* (人参, ginseng) to *Shēng Huà Tāng* (生化汤, Engendering and Transforming Decoction) prevents blood clots from stagnation. It is wrong not to use *rén shēn* (人参, ginseng), thinking that it is a supplementing medicinal. Some doctors exclude *dāng guī* (当归, Chinese angelica) when treating postpartum cases. This view is highly one-sided. This formula is well designed, and there is no danger of anything going wrong.

People who treat postpartum cases with *Sì Wù Tāng* (四物汤, Four Substances Decoction) are quite wrong. This is because *dì huáng* (地黄, rehmannia root), being cold in nature, stagnates blood, while *Sháo yào* (芍药, peony root), slightly sour, offers no supplementation but attacks and damages qi.

产后用药十误
Ten Mistakes in Using Medicinals After Delivery

一因气不舒而误用耗气顺气等药，反增饱闷，陈皮用至五分，禁枳实、厚朴。

1. Even though qi is not soothed, it is a mistake to use qi-consuming or qi-normalizing medicinals, making stuffiness and oppression worse. *Chén pí* (陈皮, aged tangerine peel) is limited to 5 *fen*. *Zhǐ shí* (枳实, immature bitter orange) and *hòu pò* (厚朴, magnolia bark) are contraindicated.

二因伤气而误用消导，反损胃气，至绝谷，禁枳壳、大黄、蓬、棱、曲、朴。

2. Even though there is damage to qi, it is a mistake to use digestion promoting medicinals, which only damages stomach qi, even possibly to the extent of inability to take in any food. Consequently, *zhǐ qiào* (枳壳, bitter orange), *dà huáng* (大黄, rhubarb root and rhizome), *Péng é zhú* (蓬莪术, curcumae rhizome), *sān léng* (三棱, *common burr reed tuber*), *shén qū* (神曲, medicated leaven), *hòu pò* (厚朴, magnolia bark) are contraindicated.

三因身热而误用寒凉，必致损胃增热，禁芩、连、栀、柏、升、柴。

3. Even though there is a fever, it is a mistake to use cold and cooling medicinals, damaging the stomach and increasing heat. *Huáng qín* (黄芩, scutellaria root), *huáng lián* (黄连, coptis rhizome), *zhī zǐ* (栀子, gardenia), *huáng bǎi* (黄柏, amur cork-tree bark), *shēng má* (升麻, black cohosh rhizome), and *chái hú* (柴胡, bupleurum) are contraindicated.

四因日内未曾服生化汤，勿用参、芪、术，以致块痛不消。

4. If one has not administered *Shēng Huà Tāng* recently, *rén shēn* (人参, ginseng), *huáng qí* (黄芪, astragalus root), *bái zhú* (白术, white atractylodes rhizome) should not be taken because they will make pain due to blood clots challenging to relieve.

五毋用地黄以滞恶露。

5. Do not use *dì huáng* (地黄, rehmannia root) since it stagnates the lochia.

六毋用枳壳、牛膝、枳实以消块。

6. To dissipate blood clots, do not use *zhǐ qiào* (枳壳, bitter orange), *niú xī* (牛膝, two-toothed achyranthes root), or *zhǐ shí* (枳实, immature bitter orange).

七便秘毋用大黄、芒硝。

7. In case of constipation, do not use *dà huáng* (大黄, rhubarb root and rhizome), or *máng xiāo* (芒硝, sodium sulphate).

八毋用苏木、棱、蓬以行块, 芍药能伐气, 不可用。

8. To move blood clots, do not use *sū mù* (苏木, sappan wood), *sān léng* (三棱, *common burr reed tuber*), and *péng é zhú* (蓬莪术, curcumae rhizome). *Sháo yào* (芍药, peony root) should not be used since it is capable of attacking qi.

九毋用山楂汤以攻块定痛, 而反损新血。

9. Do not use *shān zhā Tāng* (山楂汤, Chinese Hawthorn Fruit Decoction) to attack blood clots or relieve pain. It will, on the contrary, damage new blood.

十毋轻服济坤丹以下胎下胞。

10. Administer *Jì Kūn Dān* (济坤丹, Woman Aiding Pill) cautiously.

产后危疾诸症, 当频服生化汤, 随症加减, 照依方论。

In treating various critical postpartum conditions, it is proper to administer *Shēng Huà Tāng* (生化汤, Engendering and Transforming Decoction) at short intervals with appropriate modification according to the symptoms.

Chapter Seventy-three
Indications and Contraindications of Antenatal & Postpartum Disorders V

产前后方证宜忌 五

产后寒热
Alternate Chills and Fever After Delivery

凡新产后，荣卫俱虚，易发寒热；身痛腹痛，决不可妄投发散之剂，当用生化汤为主，稍佐发散之药。产后脾虚，易于停食，以致身热，世人见有身热，便以为外感，遽然发汗，速亡甚矣，当于生化汤中加扶脾消食之药。大抵产后先宜补血，次补气。

Shortly after delivery, because of dual deficiency of nutrient qi and defense qi, women are liable to alternate chills and fever as well as body and abdominal pain. It is impermissible to use dispersing and distributing formulas without warrant. *Shēng Huà Tāng* (生化汤，Engendering and Transforming Decoction) should be used as a basis with a small amount of dispersing and distributing herbs as assistants. After delivery, as the spleen is deficient and liable to food retention, fever may result. Whenever they see fever, people nowadays tend to ascribe this to external contraction and rashly use diaphoresis. This accelerates collapse tremendously. It is proper to add spleen-supporting and food-dispersing medicinals to *Shēng Huà Tāng* (生化汤，Engendering and Transforming Decoction). Generally speaking, after delivery, it is necessary to supplement blood first and then qi.

若偏补气而专用参、芪，非善也。产后补虚，用参、芪、芎、归、白术、陈皮、炙草，热轻则用茯苓淡渗之药，其热自除，重则加干姜。或云大热而用姜何也？曰此热非有余之热，乃阴虚内生热耳。盖干姜能入肺分，利肺气，又能入肝分，引众药生血，然必与阴血药同用之。产后恶寒发热腹痛者，当主恶血。若腹不痛，非恶血也。

However, it is not wise to use *rén shēn* (人参, ginseng) and *huáng qí* (黄芪, astragalus root) to supplement qi solely. To supplement postpartum deficiency, use *rén shēn* (人参, ginseng), *huáng qí* (黄芪, astragalus root) *chuān xiōng* (Sichuan lovage root), *dāng guī* (当归, Chinese angelica), *bái zhú* (白术, white atractylodes rhizome), *chén pí* (陈皮, aged tangerine peel), and *zhì gān cǎo* (炙甘草, prepared licorice root). If there is slight heat, use herbs of a bland taste that eliminate dampness, such as *fú líng* (茯苓, poria), the heat will disappear. In case of severe heat, add *gān jiāng* (干姜, dried ginger rhizome).

It may be questioned what good it is to use *gān jiāng* (干姜, dried ginger rhizome) in the presence of great heat? The answer is that it is not an excess heat but heat generated by yin deficiency in the interior. *gān jiāng* (干姜, dried ginger rhizome) can enter the lung channel to disinhibit the lung qi and enter the liver channel to conduct various medicinals to engender blood. It must be used, however, in combination with yin and blood medicinals. Postpartum aversion to cold with fever, if accompanied by abdominal pain, should be ascribed to lochiostasis. If there is no abdominal pain, it should not be ascribed to lochiostasis.

产后寒热，口眼歪邪，此乃气血虚甚，以大补为主，左手脉不足，补血药多于补气药；右手脉不足，补气药多于补血药。切不可用小续命等发散之药。

Postpartum alternating chills and fever accompanied with facial palsy are due to severe deficiency of qi and blood. Thus, great supplementation should be mainly used. If the pulse on the left wrist is weak, blood-supplementing medicinals should be used more than qi-supplementing medicinals. However, if the pulse on the right wrist is weak, more medicinals should be used to supplement qi than to supplement blood. Do not, at any rate, use dispersing and distributing formulas such as *Xiǎo Xù Mìng Tāng* (小续命汤, Minor Life Reinforcing Decoction).

胎前患伤寒疫症疟疾堕胎等症
Cold Damage, Epidemic Diseases, or Malaria Before Birth

胎前或患伤寒、疫症、疟疾，热久必致堕胎，堕后愈增热，因热消阴血，而又继产失血故也。治者甚勿妄论伤寒、疟疫未除，误投栀子豉汤、柴、芩、连、柏等药。虽或往来潮热，大小便秘，五苓、承气等药，断不可用。只重产轻邪，大补气血，频服生化汤。如形脱气脱，加生脉散以防血晕。盖川芎味辛能散，干姜能除虚火，虽有便秘烦渴等症，只多服生化汤，自津液生而二便通矣。若热用寒剂，愈虚中气，误甚。

If there is Cold Damage, Epidemic Diseases, or Malaria before birth, the enduring fever will inevitably result in miscarriage. Fever will increase because it consumes Yin blood and abortion also brings about blood loss. The practitioner must guard against misusing *Zhī Zǐ Chǐ Tāng* (栀子豉汤, Gardenia and Prepared Soybean Decoction) or medicinals such as *chái hú* (柴胡, bupleurum), *huáng qín* (黄芩, scutellaria root), *huáng lián* (黄连, coptis rhizome), *huáng bǎi* (黄柏, amur cork-tree bark), to name a few. This is due to the miscalculation that cold damage or epidemic disease have not yet been eliminated. Even if there is intermittent tidal fever, constipation, and dysuria, *Wǔ Líng Sǎn* (五苓散, Five Substances Powder with Poria), *Chéng Qì Tāng* (承气汤, Purgative Decoction), or the like is prohibited. It is necessary to emphasize the treatment of postpartum conditions and the treatment of external pathogenic factors subordinate to them.

Thus the proper method is to supplement qi and blood significantly by administering *Shēng Huà Tāng* (生化汤, Engendering and Transforming Decoction) at short intervals. In case of the collapse of both form (body appearance due to weakness or weight loss) and qi, add *shēng mài Sǎn* (生脉散, Pulse-Engendering Powder) to prevent postpartum fainting due to hemorrhage. *chuān xiōng* (川芎, Sichuan lovage root) is pungent in flavor and capable of dissipating; *Gān jiāng* (干姜, dried ginger rhizome) can eliminate the deficient fire. Therefore, even in the case of constipation and polydipsia, administer more *Shēng Huà Tāng* (生化汤, Engendering and Transforming Decoction), and fluids will naturally be engendered and urination and defecation freed. If cold formulas are used for heat, central qi is made even more deficient. This is a severe fault.

· Chapter Seventy-four ·
Treatment Methods for Various Postpartum Symptoms Ⅰ

产后诸症治法 一

血块
Blood Clots

此症勿拘古方，妄用苏木、蓬、棱，以轻人命。其一应散血方、破血药俱禁用。虽山楂性缓，亦能害命，不可擅用。惟生化汤系血块圣药也。

To treat this syndrome, do not blindly adhere to the ancient formulas. Indiscreet use of *sū mù* (苏木, sappan wood), *sān léng* (三棱, *common burr reed tuber*), and *péng é zhú* (蓬莪术, curcumae rhizome) means trifling with lives. All the blood-dissipating formulas and blood-stasis-breaking medicinals are prohibited. Moderate as *shān zhā* (山楂, Chinese hawthorn fruit) is, it can take life and, therefore, should not be used unless warranted. The only divine formula to treat blood clots is *Shēng Huà Tāng* (生化汤, Engendering and Transforming Decoction).

生化汤原方：

当归（八钱）	川芎（三钱）
桃仁（十四粒，去皮尖，研）	黑姜（五分）
炙草（五分）	用黄酒，童便各半，煎服。

Shēng Huà Tāng (生化汤, Engendering and Transforming Decoction)

dāng guī (Chinese angelica), 8 *qian*

chuān xiōng (Sichuan lovage root), 3 *qian*

táo rén (peach kernel), 14 pieces, skinned, tip-nipped

hēi jiāng (prepared dried ginger), 5 *fen*

zhì cǎo (prepared licorice root), 5 *fen*

Decoct the formula in millet wine and take orally.

又益母丸、鹿角灰，就用生化汤送下一钱。外用烘热衣服，暖和块痛处，虽大暑亦要和暖块痛处。有气不运而晕迷厥，切不可妄说恶血抢心，只服生化汤为妙。俗有生地、牛膝行血；山棱、蓬术败血；山楂、沙糖消块；蕲艾、椒酒定痛，反致昏晕等症，切不可妄用。二、三、四日内，觉痛减可揉，乃虚痛也，宜加参生化汤。

Another therapy: Take *Yì Mǔ Wán* (益母丸, Motherwort Pill) and 1 *qian* of *lù jiǎo huī* (鹿角灰, degelatinated deer antler ash) with *Shēng Huà Tāng* (生化汤, Engendering and Transforming Decoction).

As an external treatment, heat cloths by fire to warm the place of the painful lump. This should be done even during the time of severe summer heat. Be sure not to ascribe coma and fainting due to non-movement of qi obtrusively. This causes postpartum lochiostasis, which attacks the heart. Only *Shēng Huà Tāng* (生化汤, Engendering and Transforming Decoction) is desirable under this condition.

There is a widespread belief that *shēng dì* (生地, rehmannia root), *niú xī* (牛膝, two-toothed achyranthes root) have the function of moving blood. Also, *sān léng* (三棱, *common burr reed tuber*), and *é zhú* (莪术, curcumae rhizome) can break blood clots. *shān zhā* (山楂, Chinese hawthorn fruit) and granulated sugar can resolve masses. *Qí ài* (蕲艾, mugwort leaf) and *jiāo jiǔ* (椒酒, pricklyash peel wine) can relieve pain. On the contrary, they cause such disorders as dizziness and fainting and should not be introduced unless warranted. If the pain feels better after two, three, or four days and can be relieved by massage, this is deficient pain. It is appropriate to administer *Jiā Shēn Shēng Huà Tāng* (加参生化汤, Engendering and Transforming Decoction Plus Ginseng).

如七日内，或因寒凉食物，结块痛甚者，加入肉桂八分于生化汤内。如血块未消，不可加参、芪，用之则痛不止。总之，慎勿用峻利药，勿多饮姜椒艾酒。频服生化汤，行气助血，外用热衣以暖腹。如用红花以行之，苏木、牛膝以攻之则误。

If the lumps (blood clots) give severe pain within seven days due to cold food, add eight *fen ròu guì* (肉桂, cinnamon bark) to *Shēng Huà Tāng* (生化汤, Engendering and Transforming Decoction). Do not add *rén shēn* (人参, ginseng) and *huáng qí* (黄芪, astragalus root) before these blood lumps are resolved. Otherwise, the pain will become enduring.

As an aside, be sure not to use harshly disinhibiting medicinals, do not take much vinum made from *gān jiāng* (干姜, dried ginger rhizome), *huā jiāo* (花椒,

pricklyash peel), and *Qí ài* (蕲艾, mugwort leaf). Just take *Shēng Huà Tāng* (生化汤, Engendering and Transforming Decoction) frequently to move qi and assist blood. Moreover, externally, use heated clothes to warm the abdomen. It is wrong to use *hóng huā* (红花, safflower) to promote circulation and use *sū mù* (苏木, sappan wood) as well as *niú xī* (牛膝, two-toothed achyranthes root) to attack it.

其胎气胀, 用乌药、香附以顺之, 枳壳、厚朴以舒之, 甚有青皮、枳实、苏子以下气定喘, 芩、连、栀子、黄柏以退热除烦。至于血结更甚, 反用承气汤下之而愈结; 汗多小便短涩, 反用五苓散通之而愈秘。非徒无益, 而又害之也。

肉桂一作三分。

In fetal qi distention, use *wū yào* (乌药, combined spicebush root) and *xiāng fù* (香附, cyperus) to soothe it. Using *zhǐ qiào* (枳壳, bitter orange) and *hòu pò* (厚朴, magnolia bark) relieves it.

In a severe case of asthma, use *qīng pí* (青皮, green tangerine peel), *zhǐ shí* (枳实, immature bitter orange), and *sū zǐ* (苏子, perilla fruit) to descend qi and relieve it.

To relieve fever and anxiousness use *huáng qín* (黄芩, scutellaria root), *huáng lián* (黄连, coptis rhizome), *zhī zǐ* (栀子, gardenia), and *huáng bǎi* (黄柏, amur cork-tree bark).

If there is more severe blood binding, inappropriately using *Chéng Qì Tāng* (承气汤, Purgative Decoction) to purge it will make the binding more serious.

If there is profuse sweating with short, inhibited urination, inappropriate use of *Wǔ Líng Sǎn* (五苓散, Five Substances Powder with Poria) to free the blockage will make this stoppage more serious. This formula is ineffectual and can even make the illness grow worse.

ròu guì (肉桂, cinnamon bark) is 3 *fen* in another edition.

凡儿生下, 或停血不下, 半月外尚痛, 或外加肿毒, 高寸许, 或身热, 减饮食, 倦甚, 必用生化汤加三棱、蓬术、肉桂等, 攻补兼治, 其块自消。如虚甚, 食少泄泻, 只服此帖定痛, 且健脾胃, 进食止泻, 然后服消块汤。

Generally speaking, after the fetus is delivered, and the mother has a case of blood retention, which is still giving pain half a month later, with swelling which rises to 1 *cun* or so in height, or has a fever with reduced appetite and severe fatigue, there is no other choice but to administer *Shēng Huà Tāng* (生化汤, Engendering and Transforming Decoction). However, it must be given with the addition of *sān léng* (三棱，common burr reed tuber), *péng zhú* (蓬术，curcumae rhizome), and *ròu guì* (肉桂，cinnamon bark), and other ingredients to attack and supplement simultaneously. Then the blood lump will disappear by itself.

In a case of severe deficiency with reduced appetite and diarrhea, take this decoction only to stop the pain. It is additionally capable of strengthening the spleen and stomach, promoting digestion, and stopping diarrhea. Afterward, administer *Xiāo Kuài Tāng* (消块汤，Lumps Resolving Decoction).

加味生化汤：治血块日久不消，半月后方可用之。

川芎（一钱）	当归（三钱）
黑姜（四分）	桃仁（十五粒）
三棱（六分，醋炒）	元胡（六分）
肉桂（六分）	炙草（四分）

Jiā Wèi Shēng Huà Tāng (加味生化汤，Supplemented Engendering and Transforming Decoction):

Used to treat blood lumps that do not resolve for long time. It may be used up to two weeks after delivery.

chuān xiōng (Sichuan lovage root), 1 *qian*

dāng guī (Chinese angelica), 3 *qian*

hēi jiāng (prepared dried ginger), 4 *fen*

táo rén (peach kernel), 15 pieces

sān léng (common burr reed tuber), 6 *fen* (dry-fried with vinegar)

yuán hú (corydalis tuber), 6 *fen*

ròu guì (cinnamon bark), 6 *fen*

zhì cǎo (prepared licorice root), 4 *fen*

Chapter Seventy-five

Treatment Methods for Various Postpartum Syndrome Ⅱ

产后诸症治法 二

血晕
Blood Fainting

分娩之后，眼见黑花，头眩昏晕，不省人事者，一因劳倦甚而气竭神昏，二因大脱血而气欲绝，三因痰火乘虚泛上而神不守。当急服生化汤二三帖，外用韭菜细切，纳有嘴瓶中，用滚醋二盅冲入瓶内，急冲产母鼻中，即醒。若偏信古方，认为恶血抢心，而轻用散血之剂；认为疫火，而用无补消降之方，误甚矣。

After delivery, some patients suffer from dizziness and blurred vision, fainting, and loss of consciousness. The following reasons cause this:

1. Qi exhaustion and unconsciousness due to over-fatigue.

2. Impending qi exhaustion due to excessive loss of blood.

3. Spirit failing to keep (to its abode) due to phlegm fire taking advantage of qi deficiency and invading the upper (*jiao*).

For these cases, 2 or 3 *ji* of *Shēng Huà Tāng* (生化汤, Engendering and Transforming Decoction) should be administered immediately. As an external treatment, finely shred *jiǔ cài* (韭菜, Chinese chives), put it in a bottle with a small opening, pour in 2 small cups of boiling vinegar, and let the steam flow into the nose of the birthing mother quickly. Then the patient will come round. If interns mistakenly diagnose it as the lochia attacking the heart and treat it with blood dissipating formulas, or consider it as pestilence fire and use formulas for dispersing and descending, it is a grave mistake.

如晕厥，牙关紧闭，速煎生化汤，挖开口，将鹅毛探喉，酒盏盛而灌之。如灌下腹中渐温暖，不可拘帖数。外用热手在单衣上，从心揉按至腹，常热火暖之一两时。服生化汤，四帖完即神清。始少缓药，方进粥，服至十剂而安。故犯此者，速灌药火暖，不可弃而不救。若在冬月，妇人身欠暖，亦有大害。临产时必预煎生化汤，预烧秤锤硬石子，候儿下地，连服二三帖。又产妇枕边行醋韭投醋瓶之法，绝无晕症。又儿生时，合家不可喜子而慢母，产母不可顾子忘倦，又不可产讫即卧，或忿怒逆气，皆致血晕。慎之，慎之！

Treatment: In a case of loss of consciousness with clenched teeth, boil some *Shēng Huà Tāng* (生化汤, Engendering and Transforming Decoction) immediately, pry the teeth, probe the throat with a goose quill, and then feed the decoction with a small cup of millet wine. If the abdomen gets warmer as the decoction is administered, continue the administration without regard to *ji*'s amount.

Externally, press and rub the patient through thin clothes from the heart down to the abdomen with a frequently warm hand heated by fire. In 2 to 4 hours, when 4 *ji* of *Shēng Huà Tāng* (生化汤, Engendering and Transforming Decoction) is taken, the patient will have a clear state of mind. Then, slow down the administration of the decoction and feed a little porridge. When 10 *ji* taken, the patient is safe.

Therefore, in case of such an attack, feed the decoction promptly and keep the patient warm. It is not permitted to give up and abandon rescue efforts. If the woman's body cannot be kept warm in the winter months, there will be a severe danger. Near the time of labor, it is necessary to have *Shēng Huà Tāng* (生化汤, Engendering and Transforming Decoction) prepared and stones heated (for warmth). After the fetus is delivered, take 2 or 3 *ji* in succession. Fainting can be prevented by the method of pouring vinegar into chives. What is more, when the fetus is delivered, the family should not be too delighted to neglect the mother. Nor should the mother so indulge in the infant as to forget her own fatigue. The mother should not lie down upon finishing delivery or get angry to provoke qi's counterflow. Any one of the above may lead to blood fainting. Be cautious!

加味生化汤：治产后三血晕症。

川芎（三钱）	当归（六钱）
黑姜（四分）	桃仁（十粒）
炙草（五分）	荆芥（四分，炒黑）

Jiā Wèi Shēng Huà Tāng (加味生化汤, Supplemented Engendering and Transforming Decoction) treats the three types of blood fainting.

chuān xiōng (Sichuan lovage root), 3 *qian*

dāng guī (Chinese angelica), 6 *qian*

hēi jiāng (prepared dried ginger), 4 *fen*

táo rén (peach kernel), 10 pieces

zhì cǎo (prepared licorice root), 5 *fen*

jīng jiè (schizonepeta), 4 *fen* (charred)

大枣，水煎服。劳倦甚而晕，及血崩气脱而晕，并宜速灌两服。如形色脱，或汗出而脱，皆急服一帖，即加人参三四钱，（一加肉桂四分），决不可疑参为补而缓服。痰火乘虚泛上而晕，方内加橘红四分；虚甚加人参二钱；肥人多痰，再加竹沥七分，姜汁少许。总不可用棱术破血等方。其血块痛甚，兼送益母丸，或鹿角灰、或元胡散，或独胜散、上消血块方，服一服即效，不必易方。从权救急。

Decoct the formula in water with *dà zǎo* (大枣, Chinese date) and take it orally. If there is fainting either due to severe fatigue or qi exhaustion caused by excessive blood loss, it is proper to administer 2 *ji* instantly.

In the case of either form and complexion desertion (very thin and easy to lose weight) or absence of sweat due to excessive perspiration, administer 1 *ji* immediately with 3~4 *qian* of *rén shēn* (人参, ginseng), [4 *fen ròu guì* (肉桂, cinnamon) in a variant edition]. Do not delay administering *rén shēn* (人参, ginseng) because of its supplementing function[1].

In the case of fainting due to phlegm fire taking advantage of qi deficiency, add four *fen jú hóng* (橘红, red tangerine peel) to the formula. In the case of a severe qi deficient syndrome, add 2 *qian* of *rén shēn* (人参, ginseng). For the overweight patient who is abundant in phlegm, add, in addition, 7 *fen zhú lì* (竹沥, bamboo sap) and a little ginger juice.

In no case should a blood-breaking formula composed of *sān léng* (三棱, *common burr reed tuber*), *é zhú* (莪术, curcumae rhizome), or the like be employed. Therefore, in the case of a painful lump (blood clot) pain, additionally administer *Yì Mǔ Wán* (益母丸, Motherwort Pill), *lù jiāo huī* (鹿角灰, degelatinated deer antler ash), *Yuán Hú Sǎn* (元胡散, Corydalis Tuber Powder)[2], *Dú Shèng Sǎn* (独胜散, Unique Conquering Powder)[3] or.

Take only one of the above blood lump-dispersing supplements to Shenghua Tang, and the effect will be achieved. There is no need to change to another supplement halfway. First-aid measures should be taken per the conditions.

加参生化汤：治产后形色脱晕，或汗多脱晕。

人参（三钱，有倍加至五钱者）　　川芎（二钱）

当归（五钱） 炙草（四分）

桃仁（十粒） 炮姜（四分）

大枣

水煎服。

Jiā Shēn Shēng Huà Tāng (加参生化汤, Engendering and Transforming Decoction Plus Ginseng): treats postpartum fainting with form and complexion desertion ot sweating desertion due to excessive perspiration.

rén shēn (ginseng), 3 *qian*, (may be increased to 5 *qian*)

chuān xiōng (Sichuan lovage root), 2 *qian*

dāng guī (Chinese angelica), 5 *qian*

zhì cǎo (prepared licorice root), 4 *fen*

táo rén (peach kernel), 10 pieces

páo jiāng (prepared dried ginger), 4 *fen*

dà zǎo (Chinese date)

Decoct the formula in water and take it orally.

脉脱形脱，将绝之症，必服此方，加参四五钱，频频灌之。产后血崩血晕，兼汗多，宜服此方。无汗不脱，只服本方，不必加参。左尺脉脱，亦加参。此方治产后危急诸症，可通用，一昼一夜，必须服三四剂。若照常症服，岂能接将绝之气血，扶危急之变症耶！产后一二日，血块痛虽未止，产妇气血虚脱，或晕或厥、或汗多、或形脱，口气渐凉，烦渴不止，或气喘急，无论块痛，从权用加参生化汤。病势稍退，又当减参，且服生化汤。

In the case of pulse collapse and form collapse, there is no other choice but to take this formula with *rén shēn* (人参, ginseng) 4~5 *qian* added.

Administer the decoction at short intervals. It is appropriate to take this formula for profuse postpartum bleeding and blood fainting with profuse sweating.

If there is no sweating and no collapse, administer only the primary formula with no need to add *rén shēn* (人参, ginseng). If the *chi* pulse on the left hand is collapsing, *rén shēn* (人参, ginseng) should be added too. This formula can be used to treat various postpartum critical and acute conditions. It is necessary to take three to four *ji* in one day and night. Taking the usual dose can not rescue qi and blood, which are on the border of exhaustion.

Jiā Shēn Shēng Huà Tāng (加参生化汤, Engendering and Transforming Decoction Plus Ginseng) could be used as first aid one or two days after delivery if the birthing mother with blood lump pain has not been relieved. Additionally, they may also have qi and blood collapse, dizziness, fainting, profuse sweating, form (body) collapse with breath getting cold, constant polydipsia, or rapid short breathing. When the condition abates a little, it is necessary to subtract *rén shēn* (人 参, ginseng) but continue to take Shenghua Tang.

加减法：血块痛甚加肉桂七分；渴加麦冬一钱，五味十粒；汗多加麻黄根一钱；如血块不痛，加炙黄芪一钱以止汗；伤饭食面食，加炒神曲一钱，麦芽五分炒；伤肉食，加山楂五个，砂仁四钱（炒）。

Methods of modifying:

In the case of severe lump pain, add seven *fen* of *ròu guì* (肉桂, cinnamon bark).

In the case of thirst, add 1 *qian* of *mài dōng* (麦冬, dwarf lilyturf tuber) and ten pieces of *wǔ wèi zǐ* (五味子, Chinese magnolivine fruit).

In cases of profuse sweating, add 1 *qian má huáng gēn* (麻黄根, ephedra root).

If there is no lump (blood clot) pain, add 1 *qian zhì huáng qí* (炙黄芪, honey-fried radix astragali) to stop sweating.

In cases of indigestion for food made from wheat flour, add 1 *qian* stir-fried *shén qū* (神曲, medicated leaven) and 5 *fen* dry-fried *mài yá* (麦芽, germinated barley).

In cases of indigestion from eating meat, add five pieces of *shān zhā* (山楂, Chinese hawthorn fruit) and 4 *qian* of *shā rén* (砂仁, villous amomum fruit).

*

[1] Usually, tonics like Ginseng are taken slowly day by day, while under this emergency, it should be administered as soon as possible.

[2] *Yuán Hú Sǎn* (corydalis tuber Powder) is composed of *yuán hú* (元胡, corydalis tuber), *dāng guī* (当归, Chinese angelica), *pú huáng* (蒲黄, cattail pollen), *chì sháo* (赤芍, red peony root), *ròu guì* (肉桂 cinnamon bark), each 1 *qian*; *Jiāng huáng* (姜黄, turmeric root tuber), *mù xiāng* (木香, common aucklandia root), *rǔ xiāng* (乳香, frankincense), *mò yào* (没药, myrrh), each 7 *fen*; *Zhì cǎo* (炙草, prepared licorice root), 5 *fen*; and *shēng jiāng* (生姜, Ginger), three slices.

[3] *Dú Shèng Sǎn* (独胜散, Unique Conquering Powder) is ground *wǔ líng zhī* (五灵脂, flying squirrel faeces), 2 *liang*.

Chapter Seventy-six

Treatment Methods for Various Postpartum Symptoms Ⅲ

产后诸症治法 三

厥症
Syncope

妇人产有用力过多，劳倦伤脾，故逆冷而厥，气上胸满，脉去形脱，非大补不可，岂钱数川芎、当归能回阳复神乎。必用加参生化汤倍参，进二剂，则气血旺而神自生矣，厥自止矣。若服药而反渴，另有生脉散、独参代茶饮，救脏之燥。如四肢逆冷，又泻痢类伤寒阴症，又难用四逆汤，必用倍参生化汤加附子一片，可以回阳止逆，又可以行参、归之力。立二方于下分先后。

In the course of delivery, some women overexert themselves. Overstraining impairs the spleen. As a result, syncope occurs with cold limbs. As qi ascends to fill up the chest, the pulse disappears, and form collapses (body looks very thin and weak, loses weight quickly). There is no other choice but to supplement the blood significantly. A few *qian* of *chuān xiōng* (川芎, Sichuan lovage root) and *dāng guī* (当归, Chinese angelica) will not be sufficient to restore yang and spirit. It is necessary to use *Jiā Shēn Shēng Huà Tāng* (加参生化汤, Engendering and Transforming Decoction Plus Ginseng), but with a double amount of ginseng.

When Two *ji* is taken, qi and blood become effulgent, and the spirit recovers. Syncope comes to an end. Suppose the patient feels thirsty after taking the formula. In that case, *Shēng Mài Sǎn* (生脉散, Pulse Engendering Powder) and *Dú Shēn Tāng* (独参汤, Pure Ginseng Decoction) can be taken as tea to rescue the organs from dryness.

If the patient exhibits cold limbs with diarrhea due to yin syndrome with cold damage, *Sì Nì Tāng* (四逆汤, Frigid Extremities Decoction) is unsuitable. It is necessary to use *Shēng Huà Tāng* (生化汤, Engendering and Transforming Decoction) with a double amount of ginseng. A slice of *fù zǐ* (附子, prepared aconite root) should be added to restore yang and rescue from (body) collapse. It can also assist the function of ginseng and *dāng guī* (当归, Chinese angelica). The two formulas are given below.

加参生化汤：治产后发厥，块痛未止，不可加芪、术。

川芎（二钱）　　　　　　当归（四钱）

炙草（五分）　　　　　　炮姜（四分）（一作黑姜）

桃仁（十粒，去皮尖，研）　人参（二钱）

枣，水煎。

进二服。

Jiā Shēn Shēng Huà Tāng (加参生化汤, Engendering and Transforming Decoction Plus Ginseng): treats postpartum syncope. Before lump pain is relieved, do not add *huáng qí* (黄芪, asastragalus root) and *bái zhú* (白术, white atractylodes rhizome).

chuān xiōng (Sichuan lovage root), 2 *qian*

dāng guī (Chinese angelica), 4 *qian*

zhì cǎo (prepared licorice root), 5 *fen*

páo jiāng (prepared dried ginger), 4 *fen*

táo rén (peach kernel), 10 pieces (skinned, tip-nipped, ground)

rén shēn (ginseng), 2 *qian*

dà zǎo (Chinese date)

Decoct the formula in water and take 2 *ji*.

滋荣益气复神汤：治产后发厥，块痛已除可服此方。

人参（三钱）　　　　　　黄芪（一两，蜜炙）

白术（一钱，土炒）　　　当归（三钱）

炙草（四分）　　　　　　陈皮（四分）

五味（十粒）　　　　　　川芎（一钱）

熟地（一钱）　　　　　　麦芽（一钱）

枣一枚

水煎服。

Zī Róng Yì Qì Fù Shén Tāng (滋荣益气复神汤, Constitution Enriching, Qi Reinforcing, and Spirit Restoring Decoction): treats postpartum syncope when lump pain is already relived.

rén shēn (ginseng), 3 *qian*

huáng qí (astragalus root), 1 *liang*, honey-fried

bái zhú (white atractylodes rhizome), 1 *qian*, dry-fried with earth

dāng guī (Chinese angelica),3 *qian*

zhì cǎo (prepared licorice root), 4 *fen*

chén pí (aged tangerine peel), 4 *fen*

wǔ wèi (Chinese magnolivine fruit), 10 pieces

chuān xiōng (Sichuan lovage root), 1 *qian*

shú dì (prepared rehmannia root), 1 *qian*

mài yá, (germinated barley), 1 *qian*

dà zǎo (Chinese date; jujube), 1 piece

Decoct the formula in water and take it orally.

手足冷，加附子五分；汗多，加麻黄根一钱，熟枣仁一钱；妄言妄见，加益智、柏子仁、龙眼肉；大便实，加肉苁蓉二钱。大抵产后晕厥二症相类，但晕在临盆，症急甚于厥，宜频服生化汤几帖，块化血旺，神清晕止，若多气促形脱等症，必加参、芪。厥在分娩之后，宜倍参生化汤，止厥以复神，并补气血也，非如上偏补气血而可愈也。要知晕有块痛，芪、术不可加；厥症若无块痛，芪、术、地黄，并用无疑也。

If the patient has cold hands and feet, add 5 *fen* of *fù zǐ* (附子，prepared aconite root) to the formula.

If there is profuse sweating, add 1 *qian* of *má huáng gēn* (麻黄根，ephedra root) and 1 *qian* of *shú zǎo rén* (熟枣仁，prepared spiney date seed).

If the patient has ravings with hallucinations, add *yì zhì* (益智，sharp leaf glangal fruit), *bǎi zǐ rén* (柏子仁，oriental arborvitael), *Lóng Yǎn Ròu* (龙眼肉，Longan) to the formula.

In case of constipation, add 2 *qian* of *ròu cōng róng* (肉苁蓉，desert cistanche) to the formula.

Generally speaking, postpartum blood fainting and syncope are similar. However, fainting may happen in the delivery process, and its signs are more acute than those of syncope. It is proper to administer *Shēng Huà Tāng* (生化汤，Engendering and Transforming Decoction) in quick succession. Blood clot lumps will be resolved, and blood will become effulgent. The spirit will become clear, and fainting will be stooped. If there are signs of rapid short breathing and form collapse, it is vital to add ginseng and *huáng qí* (黄芪，astragalus root) to the formula.

Syncope usually happens after delivery. *Shēng Huà Tāng* (生化汤，Engendering and Transforming Decoction) with a double amount of Ginseng is required to stop syncope and restore the spirit and supplement qi and blood. It cannot be relieved by merely supplementing qi and blood, as said above. If there is lump pain accompanied by fainting, *huáng qí* (黄芪，astragalus root) and *bái zhú* (白术，white atractylodes rhizome) should not be used. In case there is syncope without lump pain, using *huáng qí* (黄芪，astragalus root), *bái zhú* (白术，white atractylodes rhizome) and *shú dì* (熟地，prepared rehmannia root) in combination goes without question.

Chapter Seventy-seven
Treatment Methods for Various Postpartum Symptoms Ⅳ

产后诸症治法 四

血崩
Profuse Uterine Bleeding

产后血大来，审血色之红紫，视形色之虚实。如血紫有块，乃当去其败血也，止留作痛，不可论崩。如鲜红之血，乃是惊伤心不能生血，怒伤肝不能藏血，劳伤脾不能统血，俱不能归经耳。当以崩治，先服生化汤几帖，则行中自有补。若形脱汗多气促，宜服倍参生化汤几帖以益气，非棕灰之可止者。如产后半月外崩，又宜升举大补汤治之，此症虚极，服药平稳，未见速效，须二十帖后，诸症顿除。

In postpartum hematorrhea, doctors should distinguish if the blood is red or purple and determine if the patient's body and complexion are deficient or excess. If the blood is purple and contains clots, it is necessary to remove the lochiostasis. The stagnation and retention of lochiostasis are the cause of pain. This should not be regarded as *xue beng* (profuse uterine bleeding). If the blood is bright red, this indicates not engendering blood due to the heart's being damaged by fright. Not being able to store blood is due to the liver being damaged by anger. Not being able to govern blood is due to the spleen being damaged by overwork. These are all cases of blood failing to return to the vessels and should be treated as *xue beng* (profuse uterine bleeding).

First, a few *ji* of *Shēng Huà Tāng* (生化汤，Engendering and Transforming Decoction) should be administered. Supplementation will be achieved through moving the blood. Suppose there are symptoms like body collapse, profuse sweating, and hasty breathing. In that case, it is proper to administer several *ji* of *Shēng Huà Tāng* (生化汤，Engendering and Transforming Decoction) with a double amount of ginseng to boost qi.

It is not bleeding that can be stopped by *zōng huī*(棕灰, trachycarpus stiple fiber ash).

If *xue beng* (profuse uterine bleeding) occurs half a month after delivery, the appropriate formula is *Shēng Jǔ Dà Bǔ Tāng* (升举大补汤, Up-lifting and Great Supplementing Decoction). Because this is a severe deficient syndrome, rapid effects cannot be expected after taking this decoction. The various signs will be eliminated after 20 *ji* have been administered.

生血止崩汤：治产后血崩。

川芎（一钱）　　　当归（四钱）

黑姜（四分）　　　　　　炙草（五分）

桃仁（十粒）　　　　　　荆芥（五分，炒黑）

乌梅（五分，火段灰）　　蒲黄（五分，炒）

枣，水煎。

忌姜、椒、热物，生冷。

（凡止崩用荆芥，俱宜炒黑。）

Shēng Xuè Zhǐ Bēng Tāng (生血止崩汤, Blood Engendering and Bleeding Stopping Decoction): treat postpartum profuse uterine bleeding.

chuān xiōng (Sichuan lovage root), 1 *qian*

dāng guī (Chinese angelica), 4 *qian*

hēi jiāng (prepared dried ginger), 4 *fen*

zhì cǎo (prepared licorice root), 5 *fen*

táo rén (peach kernel), 10 pieces

Jīng jiè (schizonepeta), 5 *fen* (charred)

wū méi (smoked plum), 5 *fen* (calcined)

pú huáng (cattail pollen), 5 *fen* (dry-fried)

Decoct the formula in water with *dà zǎo* (大枣, Chinese date).

Ginger, pepper, hot, cold, and raw foods are contraindicated.

[When *Jīng jiè* (荆芥, schizonepeta) is used for treating *xue beng* (profuse uterine bleeding), it should always be charred.]

鲜红血大来，荆芥穗炒黑、白芷各五分。血竭形败，加参三四钱；汗多气促，亦加参三四钱；无汗，形不脱，气促，只服生化汤，多服则血自平。有言归、芎但能活血，甚误。

Variations by Symptoms:

In the case of enormous running of bright red blood, add charred *jīng jiè suì* (荆芥穗, fineleaf schizonepeta spike), *bái zhǐ* (白芷, angelica root), each 5 *fen* to the formula.

If there is blood exhaustion and deterioration of the body, add 4 *qian* of *rén shēn* (人参, ginseng) to the formula.

In case there is profuse sweating and distressed rapid breathing, add *rén shēn* (人参, ginseng) 3~4 *qian*.

In case there is no sweating, no body collapse but distressed rapid breathing, administer *Shēng Huà Tāng* (生化汤, Engendering and Transforming Decoction).

After taking a sufficient number of *ji*, the bleeding will stop. Some interns say that *dāng guī* (当归, Chinese angelica) and *chuān xiōng* (川芎, Sichuan lovage root) can only quicken the blood. It is totally wrong.

升举大补汤: 滋荣益气。如有块动, 只服前方, 芪、术勿用。

黄芪（四分）	白术（四分）
陈皮（四分）	人参（二钱）
炙草（四分）	升麻（四分）
当归（二钱）	熟地（二钱）
麦冬（一钱）	川芎（一钱）
白芷（四分）	黄连（三分, 炒）

荆芥穗（四分, 炒黑）

Shēng Jǔ Dà Bǔ Tāng (升举大补汤, Up-lifting and Great Supplementing Decoction): enriching construction and boosting qi. In case of lump moving, only administer the above formula, do not use *huáng qí* (黄芪, astragalus root) and *bái zhú* (白术, white atractylodes rhizome).

huáng qí (astragalus root), 4 *fen*

bái zhú (white atractylodes rhizome), 4 *fen*

chén pí (aged tangerine peel), 4 *fen*

rén shēn (ginseng), 2 *qian*

zhì cǎo (prepared licorice root), 4 *fen*

shēng má (black cohosh rhizome), 4 *fen*

dāng guī (Chinese angelica), 2 *qian*

shú dì (prepared rehmannia root), 2 *qian*

mài dōng, dwarf lilyturf tuber, 1 *qian*

chuān xiōng, (Sichuan lovage root), 1 *qian*

bái zhǐ (angelica root), 4 *fen*

huáng lián (coptis rhizome), 3 *fen* (dry-fried)

jīng jiè suì (schizonepeta), 4 *fen* (charred)

汗多，加麻黄根一钱，浮麦炒一小撮；大便不通，加肉苁蓉一钱，禁用大黄；气滞，磨木香三分；痰，加贝母六分，竹沥、姜汁少许；寒嗽，加杏仁十粒，桔梗五分，知母一钱；惊，加枣仁、柏子仁各一钱；伤饭，加神曲、麦芽各一钱；伤肉食，加山楂、砂仁各八分，俱加枣，水煎。身热不可加连、柏，伤食怒气，均不可专用耗散无补药。凡年老虚人患崩，宜升举大补汤。

Variations by symptoms:

If there is profuse sweating, add 1 *qian má huáng gēn* (麻黄根，ephedra root) and a pinch of *fú xiǎo mài* (浮小麦，blighted wheat, dry-fried) to the formula.

In case there is constipation, add 1 *qian ròu cōng róng* (肉苁蓉，desert cistanche) to the formula. *Dà huáng* (大黄，rhubarb root and rhizome) is prohibited.

If there is qi stagnation, add 3 *fen* ground *mù xiāng* (木香，common aucklandia root) to the formula.

If there is phlegm, add 6 *fen bèi mǔ* (贝母，fritillaria bulb), a little *zhú lì* (竹沥，Bamboo Sap), and Ginger juice.

In case there is cold coughing, add ten seeds of *xìng rén* (杏仁，apricot kernel), *jié gěng* (桔梗，platycodon root) 5 *fen*, and *zhī mǔ* (知母，common anemarrhena rhizome) 1 *qian*.

If the patient has been frightened, add *zǎo rén* (枣仁，spiney date seed) and *bǎi zǐ rén* (柏子仁，oriental arborvitael), each 1 *qian* to the formula.

For dyspepsia, add *shén qū* (神曲，medicated leaven), Maiya (Germinated Barley), each 1 *qian*. For the dyspepsia of meat food, add *shān zhā* (山楂，Chinese hawthorn fruit) and *shā rén* (砂仁，villous amomum fruit), each 8 *fen* to the formula.

All these are added with *zǎo* (枣，Chinese date). Decocted in water.

Even though there is body heat, *huáng lián* (黄连，coptis rhizome) and *huáng bǎi* (黄柏，amur cork-tree bark) should not be used.

Even though there is dyspepsia or the patient is angry, do not use consuming, dissipating medicines without supplementing medicines. As for an older woman suffering from *xue beng* (profuse uterine bleeding), *Shēng Jǔ Dà Bǔ Tāng* (升举大补汤，Up-lifting and Great Supplementing Decoction) is recommended.

Chapter Seventy-eight

Treatment Methods for Various Postpartum Symptoms Ⅴ

产后诸症治法 五

气短似喘
Shortness of Breath Similar to Dyspnea

因血脱劳甚，气无所恃，呼吸止息，违其常度。有认为痰火，反用散气化痰之方，误人性命，当以大补血为主。如有块，不可用参、芪、术；无块，方可用本方去桃仁，加熟地并附子一片；足冷，加熟附子一钱，及参、术、陈皮，接续补气养荣汤。

Because of blood collapse (severe blood deficiency) and severe fatigue, qi may lose its support and, the breath may deviate from its average pace. Interns suppose this is due to phlegm fire and mistakenly treat it with a qi-dissipating, phlegm-transforming formula. This will put the patients' life in danger. It is necessary to mainly and significantly supplement blood.

If there are lumps, do not use *rén shēn* (人参, ginseng), *huáng qí* (黄芪, astragalus root), and *bái zhú* (白术, white atractylodes rhizome). Only when there are no lumps, the following formula is applicable. In that case, *táo rén* (桃仁, *peach kernel*) is left out, and a slice of *shú dì* (熟地, prepared rehmannia root) and *fù zǐ* (附子, prepared aconite root) are added.

In case cold feet present, add 1 *qian fù zǐ* (prepared aconite root) in addition to *rén shēn* (人参, ginseng), *bái zhú* (白术, white atractylodes rhizome), and *chén pí* (陈皮, aged tangerine peel). Then continue with *Bǔ Qì Yǎng Róng Tāng* (补气养荣汤, Qi Supplementing and Nourishing Decoction).

加参生化汤：治分娩后即患短气者。有块不可加芪、术。

川芎（二钱）　　　　　　　　当归（四钱）

炙草（五分）　　　　　　　　黑姜（四分）

桃仁（十粒，去皮尖，研）　　　人参（二钱）

引加枣一枚，连进二三帖后，再用后方。

Jiā Shēn Shēng Huà Tāng (加参生化汤，Engendering and Transforming Decoction Plus Ginseng): Treats shortness of breath immediately following delivery. If there are lumps, do not use *huáng qí* (黄芪，astragalus root) and *bái zhú* (白术，white atractylodes rhizome).

chuān xiōng (Sichuan lovage root), 2 *qian*

dāng guī (Chinese angelica), 4 *qian*

zhì gān cǎo (prepared licorice root), 5 *fen*

hēi jiāng (prepared dried ginger), 4 *fen*

táo rén (peach kernel), 10 pieces, (peel and tip removed) *rén shēn* (ginseng), 2 *qian*

Add 1 piece of *dà zǎo* (枣，Chinese date) as guider. After 2~3 *ji* have been taken, take the following formula.

补气养荣汤：治产后气短促，血块不痛，宜服此方。

黄芪（一钱）　　　　　　　　白术（一钱）

当归（四钱）　　　　　　　　人参（三钱）

陈皮（四分）　　　　　　　　炙草（四分）

熟地（二钱）　　　　　　　　川芎（二钱）

黑姜（四分）

Bǔ Qì Yǎng Róng Tāng (补气养荣汤，Qi Supplementing and Nourishing Decoction): Treats postpartum shortness of breath. It is proper to administer this formula when there are blood lumps in bleeding but no pain:

huáng qí (astragalus root), 1 *qian*

bái zhú (white atractylodes rhizome), 1 *qian*

dāng guī (Chinese angelica), 4 *qian*

rén shēn (ginseng), 3 *qian*

chén pí (aged tangerine peel), 4 *qian*

zhì cǎo (prepared licorice root), 4 *fen*

shú dì (prepared rehmannia root), 2 qian

chuān xiōng (Sichuan lovage root), 2 *qian*

hēi jiāng (prepared dried ginger), 4 *fen*

如手足冷，加熟附子一钱；汗多，加麻黄根一钱，浮麦一小撮；渴，加麦冬一钱，五味子十粒；大便不通，加肉苁蓉一钱，麻仁一撮；伤面饭，加炒神曲一钱，炒麦芽一钱；伤肉食，加山楂、砂仁各五分。

按：麦芽有回乳之害，用者慎之！

黄芪、白术一作各二钱。凡止汗用浮麦宜炒。

Formula Variations:

In case of cold hands and feet, add 1 *qian* of *shú fù zǐ* (熟附子，prepared aconite root).

In case of profuse sweating, add one small handful of *fú mài* (浮麦，blighted wheat).

If the patient is thirsty, add a *qian* of *mài dōng* (麦冬，dwarf lilyturf tuber) and *wǔ wèi zǐ* (五味子，Chinese magnolivine fruit) 10 pieces.

In case of constipation, add 1 qian *ròu cōng róng* (肉苁蓉，desert cistanche) and a handful of *má rén* (麻仁，hemp seed).

In case of indigestion of cooked wheaten food, add dry-fried *shén qū* (神曲，medicated leaven) 1 *qian*, dry-fried *mài yá* (麦芽，germinated barley).

In case of indigestion of meat food, add *shān zhā* (山楂，Chinese hawthorn fruit) and *shā rén* (砂仁，villous amomum fruit) 5 fen, respectively.

dry-fried *mài yá* (麦芽，germinated barley) has the function of delectation. It should be used cautiously. The dosage of Huangqi and *bái zhú* (白术，white atractylodes rhizome) are given as 2 *qian* each in a variant edition. If there is sweating, it is proper to use dry-fried *fú mài* (浮麦，blighted wheat).

Chapter Seventy-nine

Treatment Methods for Various Postpartum Symptoms VI

产后诸症治法 六

妄言妄见
Wild Talk and Hallucinations

由气血虚，神魂无依也。治当论块痛有无缓急。若块痛未除，先服生化汤二三帖，痛止，继服加参生化汤，或补中益气汤，加安神定志丸调服之。若产日久，形气俱不足，即当大补气血，安神定志，服至药力充足，其病自愈。勿谓邪祟，若喷以法水惊之，每至不救。屡治此症，服药至十数帖方效。病虚似邪，欲除其邪，先补其虚，先调其气，次论诸病。此古人治产后虚症，及年老虚喘，弱人妄言。所当用心也。

For qi and blood deficiency, the spirit and ethereal soul have nothing on which to rely. To treat it, doctors should, firstly, differentiate whether the lump pain is acute or not. If the lump pain is not relieved, take *Shēng Huà Tāng* (生化汤, Engendering and Transforming Decoction) 2 to 3 *ji*. When the pain is gone, take *Jiā Shēn Shēng Huà Tāng* (加参生化汤, Engendering and Transforming Decoction Plus Ginseng) or *Bǔ Zhōng Yì Qì Tāng* (补中益气汤, Center-Supplementing and Qi-Boosting Decoction), combined with *Ān Shén Dìng Zhì Wán* (安神定志丸, Spirit Quieting and Mind Stabilizing Pill).

If the body and spirit are both deficient long after delivery, it is imperative to supplement qi and blood significantly, calm the spirit and stabilize the mind. When these medicinals have built up sufficient strength, the disease will automatically be eliminated. Do not believe that the patient is obsessed with an evil spirit. Spraying holy water can frighten the patient and makes the disease incurable. We have treated many cases where the effect can not be seen until more than a dozen *ji* is administered. This disease is due to deficiency, although it looks like obsession by evil spirits. To remove the evils, supplementing deficiency and regulating qi should be the first step. Then, other symptoms are treated. This is the ancient's approach in treating a postpartum deficiency, deficient panting of the aged, and crazy talk of a weak person. It deserves careful consideration.

安神生化汤：治产后块痛未止，妄言妄见症，未可用芪、术。水煎。

川芎（一钱）	柏子仁（一钱）
人参（一、二钱）	当归（二、三钱）
茯神（二钱）	桃仁（十二粒）
黑姜（四分）	炙草（四分）
益智（八分，炒）	陈皮（三分）
枣	

Ān Shén Shēng Huà Tāng (安神生化汤，Spirit Quieting, Engendering and Transformation Decoction): treats the conditions of postpartum lump pain not relieved yet, accompanied by crazy talk and Hallucinations. *huáng qí* (黄芪，astragalus root) and *bái zhú* (白术，white atractylodes rhizome) must not be used:

chuān xiōng (Sichuan lovage root), 1 *qian*

bǎi zǐ rén (oriental arborvitael), 1 *qian*

rén shēn (ginseng), 1~2 *qian*

dāng guī (Chinese angelica), 2~3 *qian*

fú shén (Indian bread with hostwood), 2 *qian*

táo rén (peach kernel), 12 pieces

hēi jiāng (prepared dried ginger), 4 *fen*

zhì cǎo (prepared licorice root), 4 *fen*

yì zhì (sharp leaf glangal fruit), 8 *fen* (dry-fried)

chén pí (aged tangerine peel), 3 *fen*

zǎo (Chinese date)

Decoct the formula in water.

滋荣益气复神汤：块痛已止，妄言妄见，服此方即愈。水煎服。

黄芪（一钱）	白术（一钱）
麦冬（一钱）	川芎（一钱）
柏子仁（一钱）	茯神（一钱）
益智（一钱）	陈皮（三分）
人参（二钱）	熟地（二钱）

炙草（四分）　　　　　　　五味子（十粒）

枣仁（十粒）　　　　　　　莲子（八枚）

元肉（八个）　　　　　　　枣

Zī Róng Yì Qì Fù Shén Tāng (滋荣益气复神汤，Construction Nourishing, qi Boosting, and Spirit Recovering Decoction): If lump pain has already been relieved, take this formula, crazy talk and hallucinations will be resolved immediately:

huáng qí (astragalus root), 1 *qian*

bái zhú (white atractylodes rhizome), 1 *qian*

mài dōng (dwarf lilyturf tuber), 1 *qian*

chuān xiōng (Sichuan lovage root), 1 *qian*

bǎi zǐ rén (oriental arborvitael), 1 *qian*

fú shén (Indian bread with hostwood), 1 *qian*

yì zhì (sharp leaf glangal fruit),1 *qian*

chén pí (aged tangerine peel), 3 *fen*

rén shēn (ginseng), 2 *qian*

shú dì (prepared rehmannia root), 2 *qian*

zhì cǎo (prepared licorice root), 4 *fen*

wǔ wèi zǐ (Chinese magnolivine fruit), 10 pieces

zǎo rén (spiney date seed), 10 pieces

lián zǐ (lotus seed), 8 pieces

yuán ròu (longan aril), 8 pieces

zǎo (Chinese date)

The formula is decocted in water and taken orally.

产后血崩、血脱、气喘、气脱，神脱、妄言，虽有血气阴阳之分，其精散神去一也。比晕后少缓，亦危症也。若非厚药频服，失之者多矣。误论气实痰火者，非也。新产有血块痛，并用加参生化汤，行中有补，斯免滞血血晕之失也。其块痛止，有宜用升举大补汤，少佐黄连，坠火以治血脱，安血归经也；有宜用倍参补中益气汤，少佐附子，助参以治气脱，摄气归渊也；有宜用滋荣益气复神汤，少佐痰剂，以清心火，安君主之官也。

Although there are differentiations of qi and blood, yin and yang, postpartum hematorrhea, blood collapse, shortness of breath, qi collapse, spirit collapse, and wild talk, all have in common a dispersed essence spirit. They are a little less acute than blood fainting but are no less critical. Unless potent formulas are administered in quick succession, many deaths will occur. It is misleading to allege that qi repletion and phlegm fire are responsible for these.

In case of blood lump pain shortly after delivery, administer *Jiā Shēn Shēng Huà Tāng* (加参生化汤，Engendering and Transforming Decoction Plus Ginseng) simultaneously. As supplementation is realized, blood stagnation and blood fainting are prevented. After lump pain is relieved, it is proper to use *Shēng Jǔ Dà Bǔ Tāng* (升举大补汤，Up-lifting and Great Supplementing Decoction) with a small amount of *huáng lián* (黄连，coptis rhizome) to downbear fire and treat blood collapse, as well as to calm blood so that it may return to the vessels.

Sometimes *Bǔ Zhōng Yì Qì Tāng* (补中益气汤，Center-Supplementing and Qi-Boosting Decoction) with double amount of ginseng is used with a small amount of *fù zǐ* (附子，prepared aconite root) to assist ginseng in treating qi collapse and containing qi to return to the place in where it should stay. Sometimes, *Zī Róng Yì Qì Fù Shén Tāng* (滋荣益气复神汤，Construction Nourishing, qi Boosting, and Spirit Recovering Decoction) is used, added with a small amount of phlegm eliminating medicinals as assistant to clear heart fire and to calm the office of the monarch (the heart).

Chapter Eighty

Treatment Methods for Various Postpartum Symptoms Ⅶ

产后诸症治法 七

伤食
Food Damage (Dyspepsia)

新产后禁膏粱，远厚味。如饮食不节，必伤脾胃。治当扶元，温补气血，健脾胃。审伤何物，加以消导诸药。生化汤加神曲、麦芽以消面食；加山楂、砂仁以消肉食。如寒冷之物，加吴萸、肉桂；如产母虚甚，加人参、白术。又有块，然后消补并治，无有不安者。屡见治者不重产后之弱，惟知速消伤物，反损真气，益增满闷。可不慎哉。

Shortly after delivery, one should abstain from greasy foods and intense flavors. Dietary irregularities inevitably damage the spleen and stomach. Therefore, treatment should support the original qi, warm and supplement qi and blood, and strengthen the spleen and stomach. Find out what substance is the cause of the damage, and add certain food-stagnation-removing medicinals.

To disperse cereal foods, add *shén qū* (神曲, medicated leaven) and *mài yá* (麦芽, germinated barley) in *Shēng Huà Tāng* (生化汤, Engendering and Transforming Decoction). Add *shān zhā* (山楂, Chinese hawthorn fruit) and *shā rén* (砂仁, villous amomum fruit) to disperse meat food.

In a case of indigestion due to eating cold foods, add *wú zhū yú* (吴茱萸, medicinal evodia fruit) and *ròu guì* (肉桂, cinnamon bark).

If the woman giving birth is severely weak, add ginseng and *bái zhú* (白术, white atractylodes rhizome).

If there are lumps, in addition, dispersion and supplementation can be used simultaneously afterward. The effect will show without fail. Unfortunately, it is common that interns give no importance to postpartum weakness and know no better than to rapidly disperse food stagnation, only to damage the original qi and make fullness and oppression all the more serious. How can caution not be taken?

加味生化汤：治血块未消，服此以消食。

川芎（二钱）　　　　　　当归（五钱）

黑姜（四分）　　　　　　炙草（五分）

桃仁（十粒）

问伤何物，加法如前，煎服。

Jiā Wèi Shēng Huà Tāng (加味生化汤, Supplemented Engendering and Transforming Decoction): this formula is taken to disperse food stagnation when blood clots are not eliminated yet.

chuān xiōng (Sichuan lovage root), 2 *qian*

dāng guī (Chinese angelica), 5 *qian*

hēi jiāng (prepared dried ginger), 4 *fen*

zhì cǎo (prepared licorice root), 5 *fen*

táo rén (peach kernel), 10 pieces

Make certain of what has caused the indigestion and add medicines as above. Decoct the formula in water and take orally.

健脾消食生化汤：治血块已除，服此消食。

川芎（一钱）　　　　　　人参（二钱）

当归（二钱）　　　　　　白术（一钱半）

炙草（五分）

审伤何物，加法如前。

如停寒物日久，脾胃虚弱，恐药不能运用，可用揉按，炒神曲熨之更妙。凡伤食误用消导药，反绝粥几日者，宜服此方。

Jiàn Pí Xiāo Shí Shēng Huà Tāng (健脾消食生化汤, Spleen Strengthening, Food Dispersing, Engendering and Transforming Decoction): take this formula to disperse food stagnation after blood clots are eliminated.

chuān xiōng (Sichuan lovage root), 1 *qian*

rén shēn (ginseng), 2 *qian*

dāng guī (Chinese angelica), 2 *qian*

bái zhú (white atractylodes rhizome), 1 and a half *qian*

zhì cǎo (prepared licorice root), 5 *fen*

Per what may have caused the damage, add medicines as above. If cold foods have been retained for a long time resulting in spleen and stomach deficiency, medicines may fail to work. It is necessary to use pressing and rubbing. It is better to warm with dry-fried *shén qū* (神曲，medicated leaven).

Suppose the patient cannot even take in porridge for several days due to misuse of food-stagnation-removing medicine to treat food damage. In that case, it is always proper to administer this formula.

长生活命丹：人参三钱，水一盅半，煎半盅。先用参汤一盏，以米饭锅焦研粉三匙，渐渐加参汤、焦锅粉，引开胃口。煎参汤用新罐或铜勺，恐闻药气要呕也。如服寒药伤者，加姜三大片煎汤。人参名活命草，锅焦名活命丹，此方曾救活数十人。

Cháng Shēng Huó Mìng Dān (长生活命丹，Life-Saving Pill):

Ginseng 3 *qian*, decocted in one and a half cups of water, with a half cup of decoction left. Cooked rice crust ground into powder, mixed with a bit of ginseng decoction.

The mixture is administered gradually to arouse the patient's appetite. Ginseng should be decocted in a new gallipot or big copper spoon (not a used pot for decocting herbal medicine) in case that the patient has nausea when she smells the medicine. If nausea is caused by taking cold medicine, add three pieces of ginger. Just as Ginseng is called a life-saving herb, cooked rice crust is called a life-saving pill. This formula has saved the lives of dozens of persons.

Chapter Eighty-one

Treatment Methods for Various Postpartum Symptoms Ⅷ

产后诸症治法 八

忿怒
Indignation

产后怒气逆，胸膈不利，血块又痛，宜用生化汤去桃仁。服时磨木香二分在内，则块化怒散，不相悖也。若轻产重气，偏用木香、乌药、枳壳、砂仁之类，则元气反损，益增满闷。又加怒后即食，胃弱停闷。当审何物，治法如前。慎勿用木香槟榔丸、流气引子之方，使虚弱愈甚也。

木香生化汤：治产后血块已除，因受气者。

川芎（二钱）	当归（六钱）
陈皮（三分）	黑姜（四分）

服时磨木香二分在内。此方减桃仁，用木香、陈皮。前有减干姜者，详之。

In the case of postpartum anger leading to qi counterflow and inhibited chest and diaphragm with lump pain, it is proper to administer *Shēng Huà Tāng* (Engendering and Transforming Decoction) with *táo rén* (桃仁, peach kernel) deleted. It should be taken with 2 *fen* of ground *mù xiāng* (木香, common aucklandia root) mixed in. The transformation of lumps and the dispersion of anger can be realized in a compatible way. Suppose the emphasis is given to qi and neglecting the postpartum condition. If medicinals such as *mù xiāng* (木香, common aucklandia root), *wū yào* (乌药, combined spicebush root), *zhǐ qiào* (枳壳, bitter orange), and *shā rén* (砂仁, villous amomum fruit) are used as essential ingredients. In that case, the original qi will be damaged, and fullness and oppression will become more serious. Suppose, additionally, a meal is eaten right after the indignation, which results in a weak stomach, food stagnation, and oppression. In that case, the doctor should make sure what food has caused the damage and treat it with the same method as above.

Mù Xiāng Bīng Láng Wán (Costus Root and Areca Pill) or *Liú Qì Yǐn Zǐ* (流气引子, Qi Flowing Drink)* should not be employed since these will make the deficiency and weakness more serious.

Mù Xiāng Shēng Huà Tāng (木香生化汤, Common Aucklandia Root Engendering and Transforming Decoction): treat postpartum suffering from indignation with blood lumps already eliminated.

　chuān xiōng (Sichuan lovage root), 2 *qian*

　dāng guī (Chinese angelica), 6 *qian*

　chén pí (aged tangerine peel), 3 *fen*

　hēi jiāng (prepared dried ginger), 4 *fen*

Before taking the formula, add 2 *fen* ground *mù xiāng* (木香, common aucklandia root). This formula is a variant of *Shēng Huà Tāng* (生化汤, Engendering and Transforming Decoction), with *táo rén* (桃仁, peach kernel) left out, with *mù xiāng* (木香, common aucklandia root) and *chén pí* (陈皮, aged tangerine peel) added. In the preceding section, there is also a variation with *hēi jiāng* (黑姜, prepared dried ginger) left out.

健脾化食散气汤：治受气伤食，无块痛者。

白术（二钱）　　　　　　当归（二钱）

川芎（一钱）　　　　　　黑姜（四分）

人参（二钱）　　　　　　陈皮（三钱）

审伤何物，加法如前。

Jiàn Pí Huà Shí Sàn Qì Tāng (健脾化食散气汤, Spleen Strengthening, Food Transforming, and Qi Dispersing Decoction): treats food damage (indigestion) due to indignation without lump pain.

　bái zhú (white atractylodes rhizome), 2 *qian*

　dāng guī (Chinese angelica), 2 *qian*

　chuān xiōng (Sichuan lovage root), 1 *qian*

　hēi jiāng (prepared dried ginger), 4 *fen*

　rén shēn (ginseng), 2 *qian*

　chén pí (aged tangerine peel), 3 *qian*

Per what food may have caused the indigestion, add and subtract as above.

大抵产后忿怒气逆及停食二症，善治者，重产而轻怒气消食，必以补气血为先。佐以调肝顺气，则怒郁散而元不损；佐以健脾消导，则停食行而思谷矣。若专理气消食，非徒无益，而又害之。

陈皮一作三分。又有炙草四分，存参。

Generally speaking, to treat the two postpartum conditions of qi counterflow caused by indignation and food stagnation, a good physician should always focus on the postpartum condition. The excellent physician should prioritize the supplementation of qi and blood, use liver regulating and qi soothing medicinals as assistants, and subordinate the dispersing of angry qi and transforming of food. Then, qi stagnation will be dissipated, and the original qi will suffer no damage. When spleen strengthening and food stagnation removing herbs are used as assistants, stagnant food is moved, and a desire for food comes back. If one merely focuses on qi regulating and food stagnation removing, harm rather than good is done.

In a variant edition, *chén pí* (陈皮, aged tangerine peel) is 3 *fen*, add *zhì cǎo* (炙草, prepared licorice root) 4 *fen*. Ginseng shoud be kept.

木香摈榔丸为行气导滞方、攻积泄热方，流气引子为理气和血，化湿畅中方剂。

*

Mù Xiāng Bīng Láng Wán (Costus Root and Areca Pill) is a formula for moving Qi, removing food stagnation, attacking accumulation, and discharging heat.

Liú Qì Yǐn Zǐ (流气引子, Qi Flowing Drink) is a formula for regulating Qi, harmonizing blood, transforming dampness, and freeing the middle energizer.

Chapter Eighty-two

Treatment Methods for Various Postpartum Symptoms Ⅸ

产后诸症治法 九

类疟
Quasi-Malaria

产后寒热往来,每日应期而发,其症似疟,而不可作疟治。夫气血虚而寒热更作,元气虚而外邪或侵,或严寒,或极热,或昼轻夜重,或日晡寒热,绝类疟症。治当滋荣益气,以退寒热。有汗宜急止,或加麻黄根之类。只头有汗而不及于足,乃孤阳绝阴之危症,当加地黄、当归之类。如阳明无恶寒,头痛无汗,且与生化汤,加羌活、防风、连须葱白数根以散之。其柴胡清肝饮等方,常山、草果等药,俱不可用。

滋荣养气扶正汤:治产后寒热有汗,午后应期发者。水煎。

人参（二钱）	炙黄芪（一钱）
白术（一钱）	川芎（一钱）
熟地（一钱）	麦冬（一钱）
麻黄根（一钱）	当归（三钱）
陈皮（四分）	炙草（五分）
枣	

After delivery, some women suffer from alternating fever and chills. It attacks daily at fixed intervals like malaria, but it should not be treated as malaria. It occurs because of qi and blood deficiency that fever and chills attack in an alternating way, and it is because of original qi deficiency that external evils invade. Thus, the patient shows severe cold, or extreme heat, feels better at day but worse at night, or has later afternoon tidal fever. This is all perfectly similar to malaria.

Treatment: Nourish construction and boost qi to reduce cold and fever. If sweating is present, it is imperative to stop it without delay. Medicines such as *má huáng gēn* (麻黄根，ephedra root) may sometimes be used.

When sweat only appears on the head and fails to reach the feet, it is an acute syndrome of solitary yang with expiring yin. Medicines such as *dì huáng* (地黄，rehmannia root), *dāng guī* (当归，Chinese angelica) should be used. If the *yangming* meridian has no sign of aversion to cold but with headache and absence of sweating, administer *Shēng Huà Tāng* (生化汤，Engendering and Transforming Decoction). Add to it *qiāng huó* (羌活，notoptetygium root), *fáng fēng* (防风，saposhnikovia root), *lián xū* (连须，scallion with fibrous root) for dissipating.

Formulas such as *Chái Hú Qīng Gān Yǐn* (柴胡清肝饮，Bupleurum Liver Clearing Decoction) and medicines like *cháng shān* (常山，dichroa root), *cǎo guǒ* (草果，tsaoko fruit) are all prohibited.

Zī Róng Yǎng Qì Fú Zhèng Tāng (滋荣养气扶正汤，Construction Nourishing, Qi Boosting, and Healthy-Qi Reinforcing Decoction) treats postpartum fever and chills with sweating that regularly attacks in the afternoon.

rén shēn (ginseng), 2 *qian*

huáng qí (astragalus root), 1 *qian* (honey-fried)

bái zhú (white atractylodes rhizome),1 *qian*

chuān xiōng (Sichuan lovage root), 1 *qian*

shú dì (prepared rehmannia root), 1 *qian*

mài dōng (dwarf lilyturf tuber), 1 *qian*

má huáng gēn (ephedra root), 1 *qian*

dāng guī (Chinese angelica), 3 *qian*

chén pí (aged tangerine peel), 4 *fen*

zhì gān cǎo (prepared licorice root), 5 *fen*

Decoct the formula with *zǎo* (枣，Chinese date) in water.

加减养胃汤：治产后寒热往来，头痛无汗类疟者。

炙草（四分）	白茯苓（一钱）
半夏（八分，制）	川芎（一钱）
陈皮（四分）	当归（三钱）
苍术（一钱）	藿香（四分）
人参（一钱）	

姜引煎服。

有痰加竹沥、姜汁、半夏、神曲，弱人兼服河车丸。凡久疟不愈，兼服参术膏以助药力。

参术膏：

白术一斤，米泔浸一宿，锉焙，人参一两。用水六碗，煎二碗，再煎二次，共汁六碗，合在一处，将药汁又熬成一碗，空心米汤化半酒盏。

Jiā Jiǎn Yǎng Wèi Tāng (加减养胃汤, Stomach Nourishing Variant Decoction) treats postpartum quasi-malaria with alternating fever and chills, headache, and absence of sweating.

zhì cǎo (prepared licorice root), 4 *fen*

bái fú líng (poria), 1 *qian*

bàn xià (pinellia rhizome), 8 *fen* (prepared)

chuān xiōng (Sichuan lovage root), 1 *qian*

chén pí (aged tangerine peel), 4 *fen*

dāng guī (Chinese angelica), 2 *qian*

cāng zhú (atractylodes rhizome), 1 *qian*

huò xiāng (agastache), 4 *fen*

rén shēn (ginseng), 1 *qian*

Decoct the formula with Ginger as guide.

Formula Variations:

If the patient has phlegm, add zhú lì (竹沥, bamboo sap), ginger Juice, *bàn xià* (半夏, pinellia rhizome), *shén qū* (medicated leaven).

If the patient is weak, take *Hé Chē Wan* (河车丸, Human Placenta Pill) simultaneously.

If the patient suffers from this problem for a long time, take *Shēn Zhú Gāo* (Ginseng and White Atractylodes Rhizome Extract) simultaneously to aid the strength of the Decoction.

Shēn Zhú Gāo (Ginseng and White Atractylodes Rhizome Extract):

bái zhú (white atractylodes rhizome), 1 *ji* (soaked in rice-washed water for one night, filed and dry-fried)

rén shēn (ginseng), 1 *liang*

Decoct the two medicines in 6 bowls of water down to two bowls of Decoction. Decoct the formula in this way another two times in order to get six bowlfuls of decoction. Put the six bowls of decoction together and boil it down to one bowlful. Dissolve half a cup of this extract in thin millet congee and take it on an empty stomach.

Chapter Eighty-three

Treatment Methods for Various Postpartum Symptoms X

产后诸症治法 十

类伤寒二阳症
Quasi-Cold Damage Symptoms of Two Yang (Meridians)

产后七日内，发热头痛恶寒，毋专论伤寒为太阳症；发热头痛胁痛，毋专论伤寒为少阳症。二症皆由气血两虚，阴阳不和而类外感。治者慎勿轻产后热门，而用麻黄汤以治类太阳症；又勿用柴胡汤以治类少阳症。且产母脱血之后，而重发其汗，虚虚之祸，可胜言哉。昔仲景云：亡血家不可发汗。丹溪云：产后切不可发表。二先生非谓产后真无伤寒之兼症也，非谓麻黄汤、柴胡汤之不可对症也，诚恐后辈学业偏门而轻产，执成方而发表耳。谁知产后真感风感寒，生化中芎、姜亦能散之乎。

Within seven days after delivery, when a woman suffers from headache and aversion to cold, this cannot be classified as a *taiyang* syndrome causing cold damage (exogenous febrile disease). Nor can fever, headache, and lateral costal pain be classified as a *shaoyang* syndrome of damage by cold. These two symptoms are both subsumed under external invasion, but actually, they are caused by both postpartum qi and blood deficiency and disharmony between yin and yang. Therefore, physicians should not overlook the postpartum heat syndrome and use *Má Huáng Tāng* (麻黄汤, Ephedra Decoction) to treat a quasi-*taiyang* syndrome or *(Xiǎo) Chái Hú Tāng* [（小）柴胡汤, Minor Bupleurum Decoction] to treat a quasi-*shaoyang* syndrome. What is more, if the woman giving birth who has suffered from blood desertion (severe blood deficiency) receives a sweating treatment, evacuating what is already deficient may bring unpredictable and disastrous consequences. *Zhang Zhongjing* said, "Patients with blood desertion cannot be treated by diaphoresis." *Zhu Danxi* said, "Exterior relieving should never be applied to postpartum cases for any reason." These two masters do not mean that there are no postpartum complications due to cold damage or that *Má Huáng Tāng* (麻黄汤, Ephedra Decoction) and *(Xiǎo) Chái Hú Tāng* [（小）柴胡汤, Minor Bupleurum Decoction] are not appropriate for their indicated symptoms. They worry about the beginners in later generations who may take a one-sided view and overlook the postpartum condition and instead stick to proven classical formulas and apply exterior relieving. In case of an actual invasion of wind or cold, *Shēng Huà Tāng* (生化汤, Engendering and Transforming Decoction) added with *chuān xiōng* (川芎, Sichuan lovage root) and *gān jiāng* (干姜, dried ginger rhizome) can dissipate them.

加味生化汤：治产后三日内发热头痛症。

川芎（一钱）	防风（一钱）
当归（三钱）	炙草（四分）
桃仁（十粒）	羌活（四分）

Jiā Wèi Shēng Huà Tāng (加味生化汤, Supplemented Engendering and Transforming Decoction): treats fever and headache within three days after delivery.

chuān xiōng (Sichuan lovage root), 1 *qian*

fáng fēng (saposhnikovia root), 1 *qian*

dāng guī (Chinese angelica), 3 *qian*

zhì cǎo (prepared licorice root), 4 *fen*

táo rén (peach kernel), 10 pieces

qiāng huó (notoptetygium root), 4 *fen*

查刊本去桃仁。然必须问有块痛与否，方可议去。服二帖后，头仍痛，身仍热，加白芷八分、细辛四分。如发热不退，头痛如故，加连须葱五个、人参三钱。产后败血不散，亦能作寒作热，何以辨之？曰：时有刺痛者，败血也；但寒热无他症者，阴阳不和也。刺痛用当归，乃和血之药。若乃积血而刺痛者，宜用红花、桃仁、归尾之类。

一本无桃仁，有黑姜四分。

In another version, there is no *táo rén* (桃仁, peach kernel). The deletion can only be discussed when we make sure whether the patient has lump pain. If headache and body heat continue after two *ji* are taken, add 8 *fen bái zhǐ* (白芷, angelica root) and 4 *fen xì xīn* (细辛, asarum).

If fever and headache remain the same as before, add five stalks of *xū cōng* (须葱, scallion with fibrous root) and 3 qian of Ginseng. Since postpartum lochia is not dispersed, it can also cause alternating fever and chills. How can this be differentiated? The answer is that intermittent, pricking pain indicates lochiostasis, while only alternating fever and chills without complications indicate disharmony between yin and yang. In case of pricking pain, use *dāng guī* (当归, Chinese angelica), which is a blood harmonizing medicinal. On the other hand, if the pricking pain is caused by accumulated blood stasis, it is proper to use *Hóng Huā* (Safflower), *táo rén* (桃仁, *peach kernel*), and *guī wěi* (归尾, Chinese angelica extremity).

In another edition, there is no *táo rén* (桃仁, *peach kernel*), but add *hēi jiāng* (黑姜, prepared dried ginger) 4 *fen*.

Chapter Eighty-four

Treatment Methods for Various Postpartum Symptoms XI

产后诸症治法 十一

类伤寒三阴症
Quasi-Cold Damage Symptoms of Three Yin Meridians

潮热有汗,大便不通,毋专论为阳明症;口燥咽干而渴,毋专论为少阴症;腹满液干,大便实,毋专论为太阴症;又汗出谵语便闭,毋专论为肠胃中燥粪宜下症。数症多由劳倦伤脾,运化稽迟,气血枯槁,肠腑燥涸,乃虚症类实,当补之症,治者勿执偏门轻产,而妄议三承气汤,以治类三阴之症也。

Tidal fever with sweating and constipation should not necessarily be differentiated as *yangming* syndrome. Dry mouth and throat with thirst should not necessarily be differentiated as *shaoyin* syndrome. Abdominal fullness with desiccated fluids and solid stools should not be differentiated as *taiyin* syndrome.

Sweating, incoherent speech, and constipation should not necessarily be differentiated as a syndrome of dry stool in the stomach and intestines, which would indicate that a purgative formula can be used. These symptoms are, in most cases, caused by damage of the spleen by taxation and fatigue, retarded transportation and exhausted qi and blood, and dried up intestines and bowels. These are deficient symptoms that are similar to excess symptoms and which require supplementation. Physicians should not adhere to a one-sided view and overlook the postpartum condition, nor rashly suggest the three *Chéng Qì Tāng*s (承气汤, Purgative Decoctions)[1] to treat these three quasi-yin syndromes.

间有少壮产后妄下,幸而无妨;虚弱产妇亦复妄下,多致不救。屡见妄下成膨,误导反结。又有血少,数日不通,而即下致泻不止者,危哉。

《妇人良方》云:产后大便秘,若计其日期,饭食数多,即用药通之,祸在反掌。必待腹满觉胀，欲去不能者，反结在直肠，宜用猪胆汁润之。若日期虽久，饮食如常，腹中如故，只用补剂而已。若服苦寒疏通，反伤中气，通而不止，或成痞满，误矣。

There are indeed a few cases of young, strong women who luckily are not harmed after being blindly treated with purgative formulas. After giving birth, most weak patients, after being treated with purgative formulas, develop incurable diseases. It is often seen that harsh purgatives lead to inflation (ectatic). Inappropriate abduction (guiding out accumulation) results in binding. Moreover, constipation lasts for several days due to a shortage of blood, having been abruptly turned to unstoppable diarrhea by purgatives. This is quite dangerous. It is stated in the *Fù Rén Liáng Fāng* (妇人良方, Fine Formulas for Women)[2]: "If postpartum constipation lasts for a few days with a lot of food intake, and is treated with purgative medicinals to relax the bowels, disastrous consequences will be inevitable. Not until the abdomen is felt full and distended, with a desire but cannot move the bowels, when accumulation has occurred in the rectum, it is proper to moisten the intestine with pig bile. If food is taken in as usual and there is no abnormal condition in the abdomen, though constipation has lasted long, nothing but supplementing medicines should be used. If bitter and cold medicines are used to dredge, central qi will be, on the contrary, damaged. Though it is dredged, constipation may not be relieved. Alternatively, stuffiness and fullness might develop." What a mistake!

养正通幽汤：治产后大便秘结类伤寒三阴症。

川芎（二钱半）	当归（六钱）
炙草（五分）	桃仁（十五粒）
麻仁（二钱，炒）	肉苁蓉（酒洗去甲，一钱）

Yǎng Zhèng Tōng Yōu Tāng (养正通幽汤, Healthy Qi Reinforcing and Constipation Relieving Decoction): treats postpartum constipation belonging to the quasi-cold damage syndromes of the three yin meridians.

chuān xiōng (Sichuan lovage root), *2.5 qian*

dāng guī (Chinese angelica), 6 *qian*

zhì cǎo (prepared licorice root), 5 *fen*

táo rén (peach kernel), 15 pieces

má rén (hemp seed), 2 *qian* (dry-fried)

ròu cōng róng (desert cistanche), 1 *qian* (washed with millet wine and scaled)

汗多便实,加黄芪一钱,麻黄根一钱,人参二钱;口燥渴,加人参、麦冬各一钱;腹满溢便实,加麦冬一钱,枳壳六分,人参二钱,苁蓉一钱;汗出谵语便实,乃气血虚竭,精神失守,宜养荣安神,加茯神、远志、苁蓉各一钱,人参、白术各二钱,黄芪、白芷各一钱,柏子仁一钱。

Formula Variations:

If there is profuse sweating and solid stools, add 1 *qian má huáng* gēn (麻黄根, ephedra root) and 2 *qian* Ginseng.

If there is dry mouth and thirst, add Ginseng and *mài dōng* (麦冬, dwarf lilyturf tuber), each 1 *qian*.

If there is an over-full abdomen and solid stools, add 1 *qian mài dōng* (麦冬, dwarf lilyturf tuber), 6 *fen zhǐ qiào* (枳壳, bitter orange), 2 *qian* Ginseng, 1 *qian ròu cōng róng* (肉苁蓉, desert cistanche).

Suppose there is sweating, incoherent speech, and solid stools caused by qi and blood deficiency and exhaustion, as well as spirit failing to keep to its abode, in that case, it is proper to nourish and quiet the spirit by adding *fú shén* (茯神, Indian bread with hostwood), *yuǎn zhì* (远志, thin-leaf milkwort root), *ròu cōng róng* (肉苁蓉, desert cistanche) each 1 *qian*, Ginseng, *bái zhú* (白术, white atractylodes rhizome) each 2 *qian*, *huáng qí* (黄芪, astragalus root), *bái zhǐ* (白芷, angelica root), each 1 *qian*, and *bǎi zǐ rén* (柏子仁, oriental arborvitael) 1 *qian*.

以上数等大便燥结症,非用当归,人参至斤数,难取功效。大抵产后虚中伤寒,口伤食物,外症虽见头痛发热,或胁痛腰痛,是外感宜汗,犹当重产亡血禁汗。惟宜生化汤,量为加减,调理无失。又如大便秘结,犹当重产亡血禁下,宜养正助血通滞,则稳当矣。

又润肠粥:治产后日久,大便不通。

芝麻一升,研末,和米二合,煮粥食。肠润即通。

The above several categories of dry, bound stools hardly show improvement before the patient consumes as much as *dāng guī* (当归, Chinese angelica) 1 *jin* and Ginseng. Generally speaking, even though postpartum deficiency with cold and food damage shows external signs of headache and fever, or lateral costal and lumbar pain, these external-contraction signs seem like they should be treated with a sweating treatment. The priority should, nevertheless, be given to the postpartum condition. A sweating treatment is prohibited for postpartum blood collapse. The only appropriate choice is *Shēng Huà Tāng* (生化汤, Engendering and Transforming Decoction) which can be modified according to the specific syndromes. It will achieve coordination and rectification without fail.

If there is constipation, it typically cannot be treated with a sweating method, and priority should be given to a postpartum blood collapse syndrome. It is proper to nurture the healthy qi and assist blood circulation to free stagnation. This is the safe way.

Additionally, *Rùn Cháng zhōu* (润肠粥, Intestine Moistening Gruel) treats postpartum constipation for days.

zhī ma (sesame seed), 1 *Sheng* (about 200 ml.), ground, mixed with 2 *He* (about 40 ml.) millets, boil them into a gruel, and take it. When the intestines are moistened, the stool is freed.

[1] The three *Chéng Qì Tāng*: refers to the *Dà Chéng Qì Tāng* (Major Purgative Decoction), *Xiǎo Chéng Qì Tāng* (Minor Purgative Decoction), and *Tiáo Wèi Chéng Qì Tāng* (Stomach Balancing Purgative Decoction). They are all purgative formulas.

[2] *Fù Rén Liáng Fāng* (妇人良方, *Fine Formulas for Women*): This is a famous compendium of gynecological formulas compiled by Chen Ziming and published in 1337 CE. It is also referred to as *Fù Rén Dà Quán Liáng Fāng* (妇人大全良方, *The Complete Compendium of Fine Formulas for Women*). It was the first systematic work specializing in gynecology in Chinese medicine.

Chapter Eighty-five

Treatment Methods for Various Postpartum Symptoms XII

产后诸症治法 十二

类中风
Quasi-Windstroke

产后气血暴虚，百骸少血濡养，忽然口噤牙紧，手足筋脉拘搐等症，类中风痫痉。虽虚火泛上有痰，皆当以末治之。勿执偏门，而用治风消痰之方，以重虚产妇也。治法当先服生化汤，以生旺新血。如见危症，三服后，即用加参，益气以救血脱也。如有痰火，少佐橘红、炒芩之类，竹沥、姜汁亦可加之。黄柏、黄连切不可并用，慎之。

After delivery, qi and blood become abruptly deficient, and bones are short of blood to moisten and nourish them. The patient may suddenly show the manifestations such as clenched jaws and teeth, contraction of muscles and tendons of hands and feet. These are quasi-wind stroke, convulsive diseases, and epilepsy. Even if deficient fire flames upward with phlegm, these should be treated as the branch, not the root. Interns should not adhere to a one-sided view and use wind treating and phlegm dispersing formulas, making the birthing woman more deficient. First of all, the proper treatment is to administrate *Shēng Huà Tāng* (生化汤, Engendering and Transforming Decoction) to engender and make effulgent new blood.

In critical cases, after 3 *ji Shēng Huà Tāng* (生化汤, Engendering and Transforming Decoction) is taken, it is necessary to change to *Jiā Shēn Shēng Huà Tāng* (加参生化汤, Engendering and Transforming Decoction Plus Ginseng) to boost qi to save blood collapse. If the patient has phlegm fire, add a small amount of *jú hóng* (橘红, red tangerine peel), dry-fried *huáng qín* (黄芩, scutellaria root), *zhú lì* (竹沥, bamboo sap), and ginger juice can also be added. However, *huáng bǎi* (黄柏, amur cork-tree bark) and *huáng lián* (黄连, coptis rhizome) should not be used together. Be cautious!

滋荣活络汤：治产后血少，口噤项强，筋搐类风症。

川芎（一钱半）	当归（二钱）
熟地（二钱）	人参（二钱）
黄芪（一钱）	茯神（一钱）
天麻（一钱）	炙草（一钱）
陈皮（四分）	荆芥穗（四分）
防风（四分）	羌活（四分）

黄连（八分，姜汁炒）

Zī Róng Huó Luò Tāng (滋荣活络汤，Construction Nourishing and Collaterals Invigorating Decoction): treats quasi-windstroke caused by postpartum blood deficiency, which manifests as clenched jaws, contraction of muscles and tendons.

chuān xiōng (Sichuan lovage root), 1 *qian* and 5 *fen*

dāng guī (Chinese angelica), 2 *qian*

shú dì (prepared rehmannia root), 2 *qian*

rén shēn (ginseng), 2 *qian*

huáng qí (astragalus root), 1 *qian*

fú shén (Indian bread with hostwood), 1 *qian tiān má* (tall gastrodis tuber), 1 *qian*

zhì cǎo (prepared licorice root), 4 *fen*

chén pí (aged tangerine peel), 4 *fen*

jīng jiè suì (fineleaf schizonepeta spike), 4 *fen*

fáng fēng (saposhnikovia root) , 4 *fen*

qiāng huó (notoptetygium root), 4 *fen*

huáng lián (coptis rhizome), 8 *fen* (dry-fried with ginger juice)

有痰，加竹沥、姜汁、半夏，渴加麦冬、葛根。有食，加山楂、砂仁以消肉食，神曲、麦芽以消饭食。大便闭加肉从蓉一钱半，汗多，加麻黄根一钱，惊悸加枣仁一钱。

Formula Variations:

If there is phlegm, add *zhú lì* (竹沥，bamboo sap), Ginger Juice, and *bàn xià* (半夏，pinellia rhizome).

In case there is thirst, add *mài dōng* (麦冬，dwarf lilyturf tuber), *gé gēn* (葛根，kudzuvine root).

I case there is food damage (indigestion), add *shān zhā* (山楂，Chinese hawthorn fruit), *shā rén* (砂仁, villous amomum fruit) to digest meat, or *shén qū* (神曲, medicated leaven), and *mài yá* (麦芽, germinated barley) to disperse grains.

In case there is the retention of feces, add 1 *qian* and 5 *fen ròu cōng róng* (肉苁蓉, desert cistanche).

In case there is profuse sweating, add *má huáng gēn* (麻黄根, ephedra root) 1 *qian*.

In case there is fright palpitation, add *zǎo rén* (枣仁, spiney date seed) 1 *qian*.

天麻丸：治产后中风，恍惚语涩，四肢不利。

天麻（一钱）	防风（一钱）
川芎（七分）	羌活（七分）
人参（一钱）	远志（一钱）
柏子仁（一钱）	山药（一钱）
麦冬（一钱）	枣仁（一两）
细辛（一钱）	南星曲（八分）
石菖蒲（一钱）	

研细末，炼蜜为丸，辰砂为衣，清汤下六七十丸。

（一本枣仁用一钱，细辛用四分，存参。）

Tiān Má Wán (天麻丸, Tall Gastrodis Tuber Pill): treats postpartum wind stroke manifests abstraction of the spirit, difficult speech, and inhibition of four limbs.

tiān má (tall gastrodis tuber), 1 *qian*

fáng fēng (saposhnikovia root) , 4 *fen*, 1 *qian*

chuān xiōng, (Sichuan lovage root), 7 *fen*

qiāng huó (notoptetygium root), 7 *fen*

rén shēn (ginseng), 1 *qian*

yuǎn zhì (thin-leaf milkwort root), 1 *qian*

bǎi zǐ rén (oriental arborvitael), 1 *qian*

shān yào (common yam rhizome), 1 *qian mài dōng* (dwarf lilyturf tuber), 1 *qian*

zǎo rén (spiney date seed), 1 *liang*

xì xīn (asarum), 1 *qian*

nán xīng qū (fermented jackinthepulpit tuber) , 8 *fen*

shí chāng pú (grassleaf sweetflag rhizome), 1 *qian*

Grind above medicines into a fine powder, mix with honey and make into pills coated with *chén shā* (辰砂 cinnabar). Take 60-70 pills with water.

(In a variant edition, *zǎo rén* (枣仁, spiney date seed) is 1 *qian*, *xì xīn* (细辛, asarum) is 4 *fen,* and Ginseng is kept.)

产后诸症治法 十三

类痉
Quasi-Tetany

产后汗多，即变痉者，项强而身反，气息如绝，宜速服加减生化汤。加减生化汤专治有汗变痉者。

川芎（一钱）	麻黄根（一钱）
当归（四钱）	桂枝（五分）
人参（一钱）	炙草（五分）
羌活（五分）	天麻（八分）
附子（一片）	羚羊角（八分）

如无汗类痉者中风，用川芎三钱，当归一两酒洗，枣仁、防风俱无分量。

（一本引用生姜一片，枣一枚。）

After delivery, if there is profuse sweating, followed by tetany or rigidity of the neck and arched back, with feeble breathing, it is necessary to take *Jiā Jiǎn Shēng Huà Tāng* (加减生化汤 Modified Engendering and Transforming Decoction) immediately.

Jiā Jiǎn Shēng Huà Tāng (加减生化汤, Engendering and Transforming Variant Decoction): especially treats sweating accompanied by tetany.

chuān xiōng (Sichuan lovage root), 1 *qian*

Mahuanggen (ephedra root), 1 *qian*

dāng guī (Chinese angelica), 4 *qian*

Guizhi, Cassia Twig, 5 *fen*

rén shēn (ginseng), 1 *qian*

zhì cǎo (prepared licorice root), 5 *fen*

qiāng huó (notoptetygium root), and Root, 5 *fen*

tiān má (tall gastrodis tuber), 8 *fen*

fù zǐ (prepared aconite root), 1 *slice*

líng yáng jiǎo (antelope horn), 8 *fen*

In case there is quasi-tetanic wind stroke without sweating, use *chuān Xiōng* (川芎, Sichuan lovage root) 3 *qian*, *dāng guī* (当归, Chinese angelica) (washed with millet wine) 1 *liang*, in addition to *zǎo rén* (枣仁, spiney date seed) and *fáng fēng* (防风, saposhnikovia root), both in indefinite amounts.

(A variant edition has a slice of Ginger and a piece of *zǎo* (枣, Chinese date).

产后诸症治法 十四

出汗
Sweating

凡分娩时汗出，由劳伤脾，惊伤心，恐伤肝也。产妇多兼三者而汗出，不可即用敛汗之剂，神定而汗自止。若血块作痛，芪、术未可遽加，宜服生化汤二三帖，以消块痛，随继服加参生化汤，以止虚汗。若分娩后倦甚，濈濈然汗出，形色又脱，乃亡阳脱汗也。汗本亡阳，阳亡则阴随之，故又当从权，速灌加参生化汤，倍参以救危，毋拘块痛。妇人产多汗，当健脾以敛水液之精，益荣卫以嘘血归源，灌溉四肢，不使妄行。杂症虽有自汗、盗汗之分，然当归六黄汤不可治产后之盗汗也，并宜服加参生化汤及加味补中益气二方。若服参、芪而汗多不止，及头出汗而不至腰足，必难疗矣。如汗出而手拭不及者，不治。产后汗出气喘等症，虚之极也，不受补者，不治。

Without exception, sweating in the course of delivery is caused by taxation damage of the spleen, fright damage of the heart, and fear damage of the liver. Most birthing women have all three symptoms simultaneously, and it results in sweating. It is improper to administer sweat-constraining formulas at that time. When the spirit becomes tranquil, perspiration will stop by itself.

If there are blood clots causing pain, *huáng qí* (黄芪, astragalus root) and *bái zhú* (白术, white atractylodes rhizome) may not be used for the time being. It is appropriate to administer 2~3 *ji* of *Shēng Huà Tāng* (生化汤, Engendering and Transforming Decoction) to relieve the lump pain and then later take *Jiā Shēn Shēng Huà Tāng* (加参生化汤, Engendering and Transforming Decoction Plus Ginseng) to stop deficient sweating.

If the patient, after delivery, has incessant sweating, feels very fatigued, and shows body and complexion prostration, it is sweating due to yang collapse (exhaustion). Sweating can lead to yang's collapse. When there is yang collapse, yin follows. Therefore, a measure of expediency should be taken. Immediately administer *Jiā Shēn Shēng Huà Tāng* (加参生化汤, Engendering and Transforming Decoction Plus Ginseng) with a double amount of Ginseng to rescue yang without any regard to clots or lump pain. In case of profuse sweating in the birthing woman, it is imperative to invigorate the spleen to preserve the essence of water and fluid and strengthen ying (nutrient) qi and zheng qi (defensive qi) in order to urge the blood to return to its source. Thus, the blood may irrigate the four limbs and does not flow chaotically. In some miscellaneous syndromes, sweating is classified as spontaneous sweating or night sweating.

Dāng Guī Liù Huáng Tāng (当归六黄汤, Chinese Angelica Six Yellow Decoction) is not an appropriate formula for treating postpartum night sweating. The two formulas which are appropriate to administer are *Jiā Shēn Shēng Huà Tāng* (加参生化汤, Engendering and Transforming Decoction Plus Ginseng) and *Jiā Wèi Bǔ Zhōng Yì Qì Tāng* (加味补中益气汤, Supplemented Center-Supplementing and Qi-Boosting Decoction).

If sweating is still profuse and unstoppable after taking *rén shēn* (人参, ginseng) and *huáng qí* (黄芪, astragalus root), or sweat appears only on the head but is absent from the lumbar region down to the feet, these are complex cases. If sweat pours so quickly that the hand does not have enough time to wipe it off, the case is incurable. Postpartum sweating, wheezing, and the symptoms indicate extreme deficiency. If the patient is incompatible with supplementation, the case is incurable.

麻黄根汤：治产后虚汗不止。

人参（二钱）	当归（二钱）
黄芪（一钱半，炙）	白术（一钱，炒）
桂枝（五分）	麻黄根（一钱）
粉草（五分，炒）	牡蛎（研，少许）
浮麦（一大撮）	

Má Huáng Gēn Tāng (麻黄根汤, Ephedra Root Decoction): treats incessant postpartum deficient sweating.

rén shēn (ginseng), 2 *qian*

dāng guī (Chinese angelica), 2 *qian*

huáng qí (astragalus root), 1 *qian* and 5 *fen* (honey-fried) *bái zhú* (white atractylodes rhizome), 1 *liang* (dry-fried)

guì zhī (cinnamon twig), 5 *fen*

má huáng gēn (ephedra root), 1 *qian*

fén cǎo (licorice root), 5 *fen* (dry-fried)

mǔ lì (oyster shell), a tiny amount, (ground)

Fú mài (blighted wheat), a big handful

虚脱汗多，手足冷，加黑姜四分，熟附子一片；渴加麦冬一钱，五味十粒。肥白人产后多汗，加竹沥一盏，姜汁一小匙，以清痰火。恶风寒加防风、桂枝各五分，血块不落加熟地三钱，晚服八味地黄丸。

山茱萸（八钱）	山药（八钱）
丹皮（八钱）	云苓（八钱）
泽泻（五钱）	熟地（八钱）
五味子（五钱）	炙黄芪（一两）

炼蜜为丸。阳加于阴则汗，因而遇风，变为瘛疭者有之，尤难治。故汗多，宜谨避风寒。汗多小便不通，乃亡津液故也，勿用利水药。

Formula Variations:

If there is a deficient collapse with profuse sweating and cold hands and feet, add 4 *fen* prepared dried ginger and a slice of *fù zǐ* (附子, prepared aconite root).

If there is thirst, add 1 *qian mài dōng* (麦冬, dwarf lilyturf tuber) and *wǔ wèi zǐ* (五味子, Chinese magnolivine fruit) 10 pieces.

For an obese woman with a pale complexion and profuse sweating, add 1 cup of *zhú lì* (竹沥, bamboo sap) and a spoonful of ginger juice to clear phlegm fire.

If there is an aversion to wind and cold, add *fáng fēng* (防风, saposhnikovia root) and *guì zhī* (桂枝, cinnamon twig) 5 *fen* each.

In case there is a retention of blood clots, add 3 *qian shú dì* (熟地, prepared rehmannia root) and take *Bā Wèi Dì Huáng Wán* (八味地黄丸, Eight-Ingredient Rehmannia Pill) at night.

shān zhū yú (Asiatic cornelian cherry fruit), 8 *qian*

shān yào (common yam rhizome), 8 *qian*

dān pí (cortex moutan), 8 *qian*

yún líng (poria), 8 *qian*

zé xiè (water plantain rhizome), 5 *qian*

shú dì (prepared rehmannia root), 8 *qian*

wǔ wèi zǐ (Chinese magnolivine fruit), 5 *qian*

huáng qí (astragalus root), 1 *liang* (honey-fried)

Mix the above medicine powder with heated honey and make it into pills. Sweating occurs when yang qi join yin fluid.

If encountered by wind, convulsion and slackening will occur. These are difficult to treat. Therefore, the patient with profuse sweating should carefully keep away from wind and cold. Profuse sweating with urinary stoppage is the reason of fluid exhaustion. Water disinhibiting medicinals are prohibited.

Chapter Eighty-eight

Treatment Methods for Various Postpartum Symptoms XV

产后诸症治法 十五

盗汗
Night Sweating

产后睡中汗出，醒来即止，犹盗瞰入睡，而谓之盗汗，非汗自至之比。《杂症论》云：自汗阳亏，盗汗阴虚。然当归六黄汤又非产后盗汗方也，惟兼气血而调治之，乃为得耳。

止汗散：治产后盗汗。

人参（二钱）	当归（二钱）
熟地（一钱半）	麻黄根（五分）
黄连（五分，酒炒）	浮小麦（一大撮）
枣（一枚）	

又方：牡蛎（段细末，五分）、小麦面（炒黄，研末）。

（一本牡蛎、小麦炒黄，各五分，空心调服。）

After delivery, perspiring happens during sleep but stops when the patient is awake. This is called *daohan* or thief sweating (night sweating) since it is like a thief peeping in at a sleeping person. It is different from perspiration that comes spontaneously. "*Zazheng Lun* (杂症论, *The Treatise on Miscellaneous Syndromes*)"*: "Spontaneous sweating is due to yang deficiency; while night sweating is due to yin deficiency." But *Dāng Guī Liù Huáng Tāng* (当归六黄汤, Chinese Angelica Six Yellow Decoction) again is not the appropriate formula to treat postpartum night sweating. Only that which can regulate qi and blood to stop sweating is appropriate.

Zhǐ Hàn Sǎn (止汗散, Sweat Stopping Powder): treats postpartum night sweating.

rén shēn (ginseng), 2 *qian*

dāng guī (Chinese angelica), 2 *qian*

shú dì (prepared rehmannia root), 1 *qian* and 5 *fen*

má huáng gēn (ephedra root), 5 *fen*

huáng lián (coptis rhizome), 5 *fen* (dry-fried with millet wine)

fú xiǎo mài (blighted wheat), a big handful

zǎo (枣, Chinese date), 1 piece

Another formula:

mǔ lì (牡蛎, oyster shell), 5 *fen,* calcined, and ground into fine powder

wheat, dry-fried until yellow in color, ground into fine powder

(Anther edition gives oyster shell and wheat, fried until yellow in color, each 5 *fen*, to be taken on an empty stomach.)

*

Zazheng Lun (杂症论, The Treatise on Miscellaneous Syndromes): This is a part of Zhang Jingyue's complete writings, called in Chinese, *Jingyue Quanshu*. Zhang Jingyue is also known as Zhang Jiebin and lived from 1563A.D.~1640A.D.

Treatment Methods for Various Postpartum Symptoms XVI

产后诸症治法 十六

口渴兼小便不利
Thirsty with Inhibited Urination

产后烦躁，咽干而渴，兼小便不利，由失血汗多所致。治当助脾益肺，升举气血，则阳升阴降，水入经而为血为液，谷入胃而气长脉行，自然津液生而便调利矣。若认口渴为火，而用芩、连、栀、柏以降之；认小便不利为水滞，而用五苓散以通之，皆失治也。必因其劳损而温之益之，因其留滞而濡之行之，则庶几矣。

生津止渴益水饮

人参（三钱）	麦冬（三钱）
当归（三钱）	生地（三钱）
黄芪（一钱）	葛根（一钱）
升麻（四分）	炙草（四分）
茯苓（八分）	五味子（十五粒）

汗多，加麻黄根一钱、浮小麦一大撮，大便燥，加肉苁蓉一钱五分，渴甚，加生脉散，不可疑而不用。

Postpartum agitation, dry throat, and thirst with inhibited urination result from blood loss and profuse sweating.

Treatment should be to assist the spleen, benefit the lungs, and lift qi and blood. This will cause the yang to ascend while causing yin to descend. Water enters the meridians and transforms into blood and fluids; grains enter the stomach so that qi grows and the pulse becomes smooth. Naturally, fluids are engendered, and urination is regulated and disinhibited.

Thirst being diagnosed as a fire syndrome, with the use of *huáng qín* (黄芩,

scutellaria root), *huáng lián* (黄连, coptis rhizome), *zhī zǐ* (栀子, gardenia), and *huáng bǎi* (黄柏, amur cork-tree bark) to downbear it, is erroneous.

Equally erroneous would be inhibited urination diagnosed as stagnated water, using *Wǔ Líng Sǎn* (五苓散, Five Substances Powder with Poria) in order to free it.

If it is warmed, supplemented, moistened, and moved given fatigue, the fluid retention and stagnation, then success is not far off.

The proper treatment is the use of *Shēng Jīn Zhǐ Kě Yì Shuǐ Yǐn* (生津止渴益水饮, Fluid Engendering to Quench Thirst and Water Boosting Decoction)

rén shēn (ginseng), 3 *qian*

mài dōng (dwarf lilyturf tuber), 3 *qian*

dāng guī (Chinese angelica), 3 *qian*

shēng dì (rehmannia root)

huáng qí (astragalus root), 1 *qian*

shēng má (black cohosh rhizome), 4 *fen*

zhì gān cǎo (prepared licorice root), 4 *fen*

fú líng (poria), 8 *fen*

wǔ wèi zǐ (Chinese magnolivine fruit), 15 pieces

Formula Variations:

If there is profuse sweating, add 1 *qian má huáng gēn* (麻黄根, ephedra root) and a big handful of *fú xiǎo mài* (浮小麦, blighted wheat).

If there is constipation, add *ròu cōng róng* (肉苁蓉, desert cistanche) 1 *qian* and 5 *fen*.

If there is severe thirst, add *Shēng Mài Sǎn* (生脉散, Pulse Engendering Powder). Do not doubt this and not use it.

Chapter Ninety

Treatment Methods for Various Postpartum Symptoms XVII

产后诸症治法 十七

遗尿
Enuresis

气血太虚，不能约束，宜八珍汤加升麻、柴胡，甚者加熟附子一片。

This is due to extreme qi and blood deficiency failing to retain (water). It is appropriate to administer *Bā Zhēn Tāng* (八珍汤，Eight-Gem Decoction), add *shēng má* (升麻，black cohosh rhizome), *chái hú* (柴胡，thotowax root). In severe cases, add one slice of *shú fù zǐ* (prepared aconite root).

Volume Ten

Postpartum Disorders Ⅱ

产后篇 下卷

Chapter Ninety-one

Treatment Methods for Various Postpartum Symptoms XVIII

产后诸症治法 十八

患淋
Dribbling Urination

由产后虚弱，热客于脬中，内虚频数，热则小便淋涩作痛，曰淋。

茅根汤：凡产后冷热淋并治之。

石膏（一两）	白茅根（一两）
瞿麦（五钱）	白茯苓（五钱）
葵子（一钱）	人参（一钱）
桃胶（一钱）	滑石（一钱）

石首鱼头（四个）

灯心水煎，入齿末，空心服。

一本小注载：症由内虚，方用石膏一两，无此治法，不可拘执陈方以致误人。一本石膏作一钱，无滑石。一作各等分。

This is due to postpartum deficiency and weakness, with heat settling in the bladder. Internal deficiency makes urination frequent. Heat makes urination dribbling, inhibited, and painful. This is called Lin (dribbling, strangury).

Máo Gēn Tāng (茅根汤，Woolly Grass Decoction): treats postpartum strangury, either cold or heat syndrome.

shí gāo (gypsum), 1 *liang*

bái máo gēn (woolly grass), 1 *liang*

qú mài (lilac pink), 5 *qian*

bái fú líng (poria), 5 *qian*

kuí zǐ (cluster mallow seed), 1 *qian*

rén shēn (ginseng), 1 *qian*

táo jiāo (peach gum), 1 *qian*

huá shí (talcum powder), 1 *qian*

shí shǒu yú tóu (head of pseudosciaena crocea (richardson）or little yellow croaker), 4

Decoct the formula in the decoction of *dēng xīn* (灯心, Juncus), add fish teeth powder in, and take it before meals.

An annotation says the syndrome is caused by internal deficiency, so using *shí gāo* (石膏, gypsum) 1 *liang* is unreasonable. Doctors should not adhere to the formula and try to avoid mistreatment. In another version, *shí gāo* (石膏, gypsum) is 1 *qian*, and *huá shí* (滑石, talcum powder) is not used. There is also another version where *shí gāo* (石膏, gypsum) and *huá shí* (滑石, talcum powder) are used at the same dosage.

又方：治产后小便痛淋血。

白茅根	翟麦
葵子	车前子
通草	鲤鱼齿（一百个）

水煎服。亦入齿末。

Another Formula Varitation: treats postpartum strangury and hematuria:

bái máo gēn (woolly grass)

qú mài (lilac pink)

kuí zǐ (cluster mallow seed)

chē qián zǐ (plantago seed)

tōng cǎo (rice paper plant pith)

lǐ yú chǐ (carp teeth), 100 pieces (ground)

Decoct the formula in water and take it orally. Carp teeth may be ground.

Chapter Ninety-two

Treatment Methods for Various Postpartum Symptoms XIX

产后诸症治法 十九

便数
Frequent Urination

由脬内素有冷气，因产发动，冷气入脬故也。用赤石脂二两为末，空心服。
又方：治小便数及遗尿，用益智仁二十八枚为末，米饮送下二钱。

又：桑螵蛸散

桑螵蛸（三十个）	人参（三钱）
黄芪（三钱）	鹿茸（三钱）
牡蛎（三钱）	赤石脂（三钱）

空心服二钱，米饮送下。

This is due to cold qi having stayed in the bladder during pregnancy. Delivery sets it in motion. The cold qi then enters into the bladder tissue. Take 2 *liang chì shí zhī* (赤石脂, halloysite) powder on an empty stomach to treat this condition.

Two other formula variations treat frequent urination and enuresis:

1) Use 28 pieces of *yì zhì rén* (益智仁, sharp leaf glangal fruit), ground up. Take 2 *qian* of the powder with millet soup.

2) *Sāng Piāo Xiāo Sǎn* (桑螵蛸散, Mantis Egg Shell Powder):

sāng piāo xiāo, (桑螵蛸, mantis egg-case), 30 pieces

rén shēn (ginseng), 3 *qian,*

huáng qí (astragalus root), 3 *qian*

lù róng (deer velvet), 3 *qian*

mǔ lì, (oyster shell), 3 *qian*

chì shí zhī (halloysite), 3 *qian*

Ground above medicinals into powder, and take 2 *qian* of the powder with millet soup on an empty stomach.

Chapter Ninety-three

Treatment Methods for Various Postpartum Symptoms XX

产后诸症治法 二十

泻
Diarrhea

　　产后泄泻，非杂症有食泄、湿泄、水谷注下之论，大率气虚食积与湿也。气虚宜补、食积宜消、湿则宜燥。然恶露未净，遽难骤燥，当先服生化汤二三帖，化旧生新，加茯苓以利水道。俟血生，然后补气以消食，燥湿以分利水道，使无滞涩虚虚之失。若产旬日外，方论杂症，尤当论虚实而治也。如痛下清水，腹鸣，米饮不化者，以寒泄治；如粪水黄赤，肛门作痛，以热泄治之。有因饮食过多，伤脾成泄，气臭如败卵，以食积治之。又有脾气久虚少食，食下即鸣，急尽下所食之物方觉快者，以虚寒泄治之。治法寒则温之，热则清之，脾伤食积，分利健脾，兼消补虚，善为调治，无失也。产后虚泻，眠昏人不识，弱甚形脱危症，必用人参二钱，白术、茯苓各二钱，附子一钱，方能回生。若脉浮弦，按之不鼓，即为中寒，此盖阴先亡而阳欲去，速宜大补气血，加附子、黑姜以回元阳，万勿忽视。

　　Unlike in various diseases, postpartum diarrhea is not classified into food diarrhea, watery diarrhea, and downpouring of water and grains diarrhea. Generally, it is due to either food accumulation caused by qi deficiency or dampness. qi deficiency requires supplementation; food accumulation requires dispersion; dampness requires drying. However, when there is still lochia inside, it is hard to dry dampness right away. Therefore, it is appropriate first to administer 2~3 *ji Shēng Huà Tāng* (生化汤, Engendering and Transforming Decoction) to transform the stale and engender the new.

　　Fú líng (茯苓, poria) is added to regulate the waterways. When blood has been engendered, supplementing qi to digest food and drying dampness to regulate the waterways can be used. This can prevent the trouble of stagnating the inhibited and weakening what is already deficient. Only ten days after delivery can diarrhea be regarded as a miscellaneous disease. The treatment must still first differentiate the deficiency and excess. Watery stools with pain, abdominal rumbling, and inability to digest even porridge should be treated as cold diarrhea. Reddish yellow watery stools with pain around the anus should be treated as heat diarrhea. If the stools smell like rotten eggs due to injury of the spleen by overeating, it should be treated as food accumulation. Patients taking less food with enduring spleen qi deficiency, rumbling upon taking food, with relieved feeling only after diarrhea of what has just been taken in should be treated as a deficient cold syndrome.

The treatments are to warm the cold syndrome, clear the heat syndrome, promote urination, remove dampness and strengthen the spleen if the spleen is injured and there is food accumulation. If one combines dispersing with the supplementing of deficiency and coordinates the treatment, there will be no failure.

Postpartum deficient diarrhea with lethargic sleep and loss of consciousness is an acute syndrome due to extreme weakness and body collapse. To rescue life, it must be treated with *rén shēn* (人参, ginseng), *bái zhú* (白术, white atractylodes rhizome), and *fú líng* (茯苓, poria) each 2 *qian*, and *fù zǐ* (附子, repared aconite root) 1 *qian*.

If the pulse is floating and wiry and does not beat with force when pressed, this is a cold attack. This is a case of yin collapsing first and yang being on the verge of departure. It is proper then to supplement qi and blood greatly and immediately. Add *fù zǐ* (附子, prepared aconite root) and *hēi jiāng* (黑姜, prepared dried ginger) to recover yang. It does not allow any hesitation.

加减生化汤: 治产后块未消患泻症。

川芎（二钱）	茯苓（二钱）
当归（四钱）	黑姜（五分）
炙草（五分）	桃仁（十粒）
莲子（八枚）	

水煎, 温服。

Jiā Jiǎn Shēng Huà Tāng (加减生化汤, Engendering and Transforming Variant Decoction): Treats postpartum diarrhea with clots not yet eliminated.

chuān xiōng (Sichuan lovage rhizome), 2 *qian*

fú líng (poria), 2 *qian*

dāng guī (Chinese angelica), 4 *qian*

hēi jiāng (prepared dried ginger), 5 *fen*

zhì cǎo (prepared licorice root), 5 *fen*

táo rén (peach kernel), 10 pieces

lián zǐ (lotus seed), 8 pieces

Decoct the formula in water and take it when it is warm.

健脾利水生化汤：治产后块已除，患泻症。

川芎（一钱）	茯苓（一钱半）
归身（二钱）	黑姜（四分）
陈皮（五分）	炙草（五分）
人参（三钱）	肉果（一个，制）
白术（一钱，土炒）	泽泻（八分）

Jiàn Pí Lì Shuǐ Shēng Huà Tāng (Spleen Strengthening and Water Disinhibiting, Engendering and Transforming Decoction): treats postpartum diarrhea with clots eliminated.

chuān xiōng (Sichuan lovage root), 1 *qian*

fú líng (poria), 1 *qian* and 5 *fen*

guī shēn [Chinese Angelica (body part)], 2 *qian*

hēi jiāng (prepared dried ginger), 4 *fen*

chén pí (aged tangerine peel), 5 *fen*

zhì cǎo (prepared licorice root), 5 fen

rén shēn (ginseng), 3 qian

ròu guǒ (nutmeg), 1 piece (prepared)

bái zhú (white atractylodes rhizome), 1 *qian* (dry-fried with earth)

zé xiè (water plantain rhizome), 8 *fen*

寒泻，加干姜八分；寒痛，加砂仁、炮姜各八分；热泻，加炒黄连八分；泻水腹痛，米饮不化，加砂仁八分，麦芽、山楂各一钱；泻有酸嗳臭气，加神曲、砂仁各八分。脾气久虚，泻出所食物方快，以虚寒论；泻水者，加苍术一钱以燥湿；脾气弱，元气虚，必须大补，佐消食清热却寒药。弱甚形色脱，必须第一方，参、术、苓、附，必用之药也。诸泻俱加升麻酒炒，莲子十粒。

Formula Variations

If there is cold diarrhea, add *gān jiāng* (干姜, dried ginger rhizome) 8 *fen.*

If there is cold pain, add *shā rén* (砂仁, villous amomum fruit), *páo jiāng* (炮

姜, Rhizoma Zingiberis Preparata) each eight *fen*.

If there is heat diarrhea, add dry-fried *huáng lián* (黄连, coptis rhizome) 8 *fen*.

If there is watery diarrhea with abdominal pain and indigestion (even when eating thin porridge), add *shā rén* (砂仁, villous amomum fruit) 8 *fen*, *mài yá* (麦芽, germinated barley), *shān zhā* (山楂, Chinese hawthorn fruit) each 1 *qian*.

If there is diarrhea with an acidic, putrid smell, add *shén qū* (神曲, medicated leaven) and *shā rén* (砂仁, villous amomum fruit) each 8 *fen*.

Enduring spleen qi deficiency with relieved feeling only after diarrhea of what has just been taken in should be treated as deficient cold syndrome.

In case of watery diarrhea, add *cāng zhú* (苍术, atractylodes rhizome) 1 *qian* to dry dampness.

If there is spleen qi weakness and original qi deficiency, substantial supplementation is necessary. Food dispersing, heat-clearing, and cold dispersing medicinals should be used as assistants.

Suppose there is a severe weakness as well as body and complexion collapse. In that case, the first formula (Jiajian Shenghua Tang) is the only choice. *Rén shēn* (人参, ginseng), *bái zhú* (白术, white atractylodes rhizome), *fú líng* (茯苓, poria), and *fù zǐ* (附子, prepared aconite root) are necessary.

For all types of diarrhea, add wine-fried *shēng má* (升麻, black cohosh rhizome) and ten pieces of *lián zǐ* (莲子, lotus seed).

Chapter Ninety-four

Treatment Methods for Various Postpartum Symptoms XXI

产后诸症治法 二十一

完谷不化
Whole Grains Not Transformed (i.e., Undigested Grains in Stool)

因产后劳倦伤脾，而运转稽迟也，名飧泄。又饮食太过，脾胃受伤，亦然，俗呼水谷痢是也。然产方三日内，块未消化，此脾胃衰弱，参、芪、术未可遽加，且服生化汤加益智、香、砂，少温脾气，俟块消后，加参、芪、术补气，肉果、木香、砂仁、益智温胃，升麻、柴胡清胃气，泽泻、茯苓、陈皮以利水，为上策也。

加味生化汤：治产后三日内完谷不化，块未消者。

川芎（一钱）	益智（一钱）
当归（四钱）	黑姜（四分）
炙草（四分）	桃仁（十粒）
茯苓（一钱半）	

（一本当归作三钱，有枣一枚。）

This is caused by retarded transportation and transformation due to postpartum overexertion and fatigue damaging the spleen. It is called sunxie (lienteric diarrhea). Besides, damage of the spleen and stomach due to overeating can cause the same problem. This is what is known as water and grain diarrhea. However, if this occurs within three days after the delivery when lumps are not yet cleared or transformed, it is due to asthenia and weakness of the Spleen and Stomach.

Ginseng, *huáng qí* (黄芪, asastragalus root), and *bái zhú* (白术, white atractylodes rhizome) should not be used in a hurry. Administer *Shēng Huà Tāng* (生化汤, Engendering and Transforming Decoction) added with *yì zhì rén* (益智仁, sharp leaf glangal fruit), *mù xiāng* (木香, common aucklandia root), and *shā rén* (砂

仁, villous amomum fruit) to warm the spleen qi gradually. After the clots or lumps are cleared, add ginseng, *huáng qí* (黄芪, asastragalus root) and *bái zhú* (白术, white atractylodes rhizome) to supplement qi; add *ròu guì* (肉桂, cinnamon bark), *mù xiāng* (木香, common aucklandia root), *shā rén* (砂仁, villous amomum fruit), and *yì zhì rén* (益智仁, sharp leaf glangal fruit) to warm the stomach. Additionally, add *shēng má* (升麻, black cohosh rhizome) and *chái hú* (柴胡, thotowax root) to clean the stomach qi. Add *zé xiè* (泽泻, water plantain rhizome), *fú líng* (茯苓, poria), *chén pí* (陈皮, aged tangerine peel) to disinhibit water. This is the best strategy.

Jiā Wèi Shēng Huà Tāng (加味生化汤, Supplemented Engendering and Transforming Decoction): treats undigested food in stools less than three days after the delivery when clots are not yet cleared.

> *chuān xiōng* (Sichuan lovage root), 1 *qian*
>
> *yì zhì* (sharp leaf glangal fruit), 1 *qian*
>
> *dāng guī* (Chinese angelica), 4 *qian*
>
> *hēi jiāng* (prepared dried ginger), 4 *fen*
>
> *zhì cǎo* (prepared licorice root), 4 *fen*
>
> *táo rén* (peach kernel), 10 Pieces
>
> *fú líng* (poria), 1 *qian* and 5 *fen*

In anther version, *dāng guī* (当归, Chinese angelica) is 3 *qian,* with 1 piece of *zǎo* (枣, Chinese date).

参苓生化汤: 治产后三日内块已消, 谷不化, 胎前素弱患此症者。

川芎(一钱)	当归(二钱)
黑姜(四分)	炙草(五分)
人参(二钱)	茯苓(一钱)
白芍(一钱, 炒)	益智(一钱, 炒)
白术(二钱, 土炒)	肉果(一个, 制)

泻水多, 加泽泻、木通各八分; 腹痛, 加砂仁八分; 渴, 加麦冬、五味子; 寒泻, 加黑姜一钱, 木香四分; 食积, 加神曲、麦芽消饭面, 砂仁、山楂消肉食。产后泻痢日久, 胃气虚弱, 完谷不化, 宜温助胃气, 六君子汤加木香四分, 肉果一个(制)。

（一本有莲子八枚, 去心, 枣三枚。）

Shēn Líng Shēng Huà Tāng (参苓生化汤, Ginseng & Poria Engendering and Transforming Decoction): treats the inability to digest food within three days after the delivery when clots are already cleared, with diarrhea existing before pregnancy due to a weak constitution.

chuān xiōng (Sichuan lovage root), 1 *qian*

dāng guī (Chinese angelica), 2 *qian*

hēi jiāng (prepared dried ginger), 4 *fen*

zhì cǎo (prepared licorice root), 5 *fen*

rén shēn (ginseng), 2 *qian*

fú líng (poria), 1 *qian*

bái sháo (white peony root), 1 *qian*

yì zhì (sharp leaf glangal fruit), 1 *qian*

bái zhú (white atractylodes rhizome), 2 *qian*

ròu guì (cinnamon bark), 1 Piece

Formula Variations:

If there is diarrhea with much water, add *zé xiè* (泽泻, water plantain rhizome) and *mù tōng* (木通, akebia stem), each 8 *fen*.

If there is abdominal pain, add *shā rén* (砂仁, villous amomum fruit) 8 *fen*.

If there is thirst, add *mài dōng* (麦冬, dwarf lilyturf tuber) and *wǔ wèi zǐ* (五味子, Chinese magnolivine fruit).

If there is diarrhea due to cold, add *hēi jiāng* (黑姜, prepared dried ginger) 1 *qian* and *mù xiāng* (木香, common aucklandia root) 4 *fen*.

If there is food accumulation, add *shén qū* (神曲, medicated leaven) and *mài yá* (麦芽, germinated barley) to disperse grain-based food or *shā rén* (砂仁, villous amomum fruit) and *shān zhā* (山楂, Chinese hawthorn fruit) to digest meat-based food.

Suppose there is long-term postpartum diarrhea with weak and deficient stomach qi as well as inability to transform food. In that case, it is proper to warm and assist stomach qi using *Liù Jūn Zǐ Tāng* (六君子汤, Six Gentlemen Decoction) with *mù xiāng* (木香, common aucklandia root) 4 *fen*, and 1 piece of prepared *ròu guǒ* (肉果, nutmeg) added.

(Another edition added with eight pieces of *lián zǐ* (莲子, lotus seed, hearts removed) and three pieces of *zǎo* (枣, Chinese date)

Chapter Ninety-five
Treatment Methods for Various Postpartum Symptoms XXII

产后诸症治法 二十二

痢
Dysentery

产后七日内外，患赤白痢，里急后重频并，最为难治。欲调气行血，而推荡痢邪，犹患产后元气虚弱；欲滋荣益气，而大补虚弱，又助痢之邪，惟生化汤减干姜，而代以木香、茯苓，则善消恶露，而兼治痢疾，并行而不相悖也。再服香连丸，以俟一、二日后，病势如减，可保无虞。若产七日外，有患褐花色后重，频并虚痢，即当加补无疑。若产妇禀厚，产期已经二十余日，宜服生化汤加连、芩、厚朴、芍药行积之剂。

Red and white dysentery with frequent abdominal pain and tenesmus around the seventh day after delivery is very difficult to treat. Suppose the treatment methods of qi regulating and blood moving are used to wipe out dysenteric pathogenic factors. In that case, there is a concern that postpartum original qi is still deficient and weak. If the method of enriching and qi benefiting is used to supplement deficiency and weakness significantly, the concern is that it will assist the pathogenic factors. The only appropriate way is using *Shēng Huà Tāng* (生化汤, Engendering and Transforming Decoction), but substitute *mù xiāng* (木香, common aucklandia root) and *fú líng* (茯苓, poria) for *gān jiāng* (干姜, dried ginger rhizome). The formula is good at dispersing lochia and can treat dysentery at the same time. So the two functions are going in a similar and compatible way. Afterward, administer *Xiāng Lián Wán* (香连丸, Common Aucklandia Root and Coptis Rhizome Pill). If the condition gets better in 1 to 2 days, safety will be ensured.

Supplementation is undoubtedly needed if there is frequent deficient dysentery with brown flower-like stools and tenesmus more than seven days after delivery. On the other hand, suppose the birthing woman is of strong constitution, and more than 20 days have passed since delivery. In that case, it is appropriate to take *Shēng Huà Tāng* (生化汤, Engendering and Transforming Decoction) added with accumulation moving medicines such as *huáng lián* (黄连, coptis rhizome), *huáng qín* (黄芩, scutellaria root), *hòu pò* (厚朴, magnolia bark), and *sháo yào* (芍药, peony root).

加减生化汤：治产后七日内患痢。

川芎（二钱）　　　　　　　当归（五钱）

炙草（五分）　　　　　　　桃仁（十二粒）

茯苓（一钱）　　　　　　　陈皮（四分）

木香（磨，三分）

红痢腹痛，加砂仁八分。

Jiā Jiǎn Shēng Huà Tāng (加减生化汤, Engendering and Transforming Variant Decoction): Treats dysentery occuring within 7 days after delivery.

chuān xiōng (Sichuan lovage root), 2 *qian*

dāng guī (Chinese angelica), 5 *qian*

zhì gān cǎo (prepared licorice root), 5 *fen*

táo rén (peach kernel), 12 pieces

fú líng (poria), 1 *qian*

chén pí (aged tangerine peel), 4 *fen*

mù xiāng (common aucklandia root), 3 *fen,* ground

If there is red dysentery, add *shā rén* (砂仁, villous amomum fruit) 8 *fen*.

青血丸：治噤口痢。

香连为末，加莲肉粉，各一两半，和匀为丸，酒送下四钱。凡产三，四日后，块散，痢疾少减，共十症，开后依治：

一产后久泻：元气下陷，大便不禁，肛门如脱，宜服六君子汤，加木香四分，肉果一个（制），姜汁（五分）；

二产后泻痢：色黄，乃脾土真气虚损，宜服补中益气汤，加木香、肉果；

三产后伤面食：泻痢，宜服生化汤，加神曲、麦芽（一本神曲，麦芽下有各一钱）；

四产后伤肉食：泻痢，宜服生化汤，加山楂、砂仁；

五产后胃气虚弱：泻痢，完谷不化，当温助胃气，宜服六君子汤，加木香四分，肉果一个（制）；

六产后脾胃虚弱：四肢浮肿，宜服六君子汤，加五皮散（见后水肿）；

七产后泻痢：无后重，但久不止，宜服六君子汤，加木香、肉果；

八产后赤白痢：脐下痛，当归、厚朴、黄连、肉果、甘草，桃仁、川芎；

九产后久痢：色赤，属血虚，宜四物汤，加荆芥、人参；

十产后久痢：色白，属气虚，宜六君子汤，加木香、肉果。

Qīng Xuè Wán (青血丸, Green-Blue Blood Pills): treats food-denying dysentery.

Make powder of *mù xiāng* (木香, common aucklandia root) and *huáng lián* (黄连, coptis rhizome) and mix with lotus root powder, each 1.5 *liang*. The three kinds of powder should be mixed evenly and made into pills. Take 4 *qian* with millet wine.

Three or four days after delivery, with clots cleared, ten symptoms may arise when dysentery has been ameliorated a little. They are listed below and can be treated as instructed:

1. Postpartum persisting diarrhea: If the original qi has fallen with incontinent defecation and the anus has seemingly prolapsed, it is appropriate to take *Liù Jūn Zǐ Tāng* (六君子汤, Six Gentlemen Decoction), with *mù xiāng* (木香, common aucklandia root) 4 *fen*, *ròu guǒ* (肉果, nutmeg) 1 Piece and Ginger juice 5 *fen* added.

2. Postpartum diarrhea and dysentery: If the patient has yellow stools, it indicates deficiency and damage of the true qi of spleen earth. It is proper to take *Bǔ Zhōng Yì Qì Tāng* (补中益气汤, Center-Supplementing and Qi-Boosting Decoction), with *mù xiāng* (木香, common aucklandia root) and *ròu guǒ* (肉果, nutmeg) added.

3. If there is diarrhea and dysentery due to postpartum cereal (grain) based food damage: take *Shēng Huà Tāng* (生化汤, Engendering and Transforming Decoction), adding *shén qū* (神曲, medicated leaven) and *mài yá* (麦芽, germinated barley).

4. If there is diarrhea and dysentery due to postpartum meat-based food damage: It is proper to take *Shēng Huà Tāng* (生化汤, Engendering and Transforming Decoction) while adding *shān zhā* (山楂, Chinese hawthorn fruit) and *shā rén* (砂仁, villous amomum fruit).

5. If there is diarrhea and dysentery with undigested food in stools due to postpartum deficiency and weakness of stomach qi: It is proper to warm and assist stomach qi with *Liù Jūn Zǐ Tāng* (六君子汤, Six Gentlemen Decoction), adding *mù xiāng* (木香, common aucklandia root) 4 *fen* and a piece of *ròu guǒ* (肉果, nutmeg).

6. If there is edema of four limbs due to postpartum deficiency and weakness

of spleen and stomach: It is proper to administer *Liù Jūn Zǐ Tāng* (六君子汤, Six Gentlemen Decoction), add *Wǔ Pí Sǎn* (五皮散, Five-Peel Powder) (See edema in a later section).

7. Suppose there is postpartum diarrhea and dysentery: (presents as no pressure in the rectum but diarrhea continues for a long time and no signs of it stopping). In that case, it is appropriate to take *Liù Jūn Zǐ Tāng* (六君子汤, Six Gentlemen Decoction), adding *mù xiāng* (木香, common aucklandia root) and *ròu guǒ* (肉果, nutmeg).

8. If there is postpartum red and white dysentery: (presents as pain below the navel), take *dāng guī* (当归, Chinese angelica), *hòu pò* (厚朴, magnolia bark), *huáng lián* (黄连, coptis rhizome), *ròu guǒ* (肉果, nutmeg), *gān cǎo* (甘草, licorice root), *táo rén* (桃仁, *peach kernel*) and *chuān xiōng* (川芎, Sichuan lovage root).

9. If there is postpartum chronic dysentery: red stools indicate blood deficiency. It is proper to take *Sì Wù Tāng* (四物汤, Four Substances Decoction), adding *jīng jiè* (荆芥, schizonepeta), and *rén shēn* (人参, ginseng).

10. If there is enduring postpartum dysentery: (presents as white stools), which is ascribed to qi deficiency, it is proper to administer *Liù Jūn Zǐ Tāng* (六君子汤, Six Gentlemen Decoction), with *mù xiāng* (木香, common aucklandia root) and *ròu guǒ* (肉果, nutmeg) added.

Chapter Ninety-six

Treatment Methods for Various Postpartum Symptoms XXIII

产后诸症治法 二十三

霍乱
Sudden Turmoil Disorder (i.e., Cholera-like Disease)

由劳伤气血，脏腑空虚，不能运化食物，及感冷风所致，阴阳升降不顺，清浊乱于脾胃，冷热不调，邪正相搏，上下为霍乱。

生化六和汤：治产后血块痛未除，患霍乱。

川芎（二钱）	当归（四钱）
黑姜（四分）	炙草（四分）
陈皮（四分）	藿香（四分）
砂仁（六分）	茯苓（一钱）

姜三片，煎。

If qi and blood are damaged by overexertion, the zang and fu organs are empty, deficient, and unable to transport and transform food. When attacked by the cold wind, ascending and descending of yin and yang become abnormal, the clear and turbid are disordered in the spleen and stomach, cold and heat are in disharmony, pathogenic factors and healthy qi are struggling with each other. Therefore, the clear can not go upward, and the turbid cannot go downward, resulting in sudden turmoil disorder.

Shēng Huà Liù Hé Tāng (生化六和汤, Engendering, Transforming and Six Harmony Decoction): treats postpartum cholera-like disease with clots and pain not eliminated yet.

chuān xiōng (Sichuan lovage root), 2 *qian*

dāng guī (Chinese angelica), 4 *qian*

hēi jiāng (prepared dried ginger), 4 *fen*

zhì cǎo (prepared licorice root), 4 *fen*

chén pí (aged tangerine peel), 4 *fen*

huò xiāng, (agastache), 4 *fen*

shā rén (villous amomum fruit), 6 *fen*

fú líng (poria), 1 *qian*

jiāng (ginger), 3 slices

Decoct the medicinals in water.

附子散：治产后霍乱吐泻，手足逆冷，须无块痛方可服。

白术（一钱）	当归（二钱）
陈皮（四分）	黑姜（四分）
丁香（四分）	甘草（四分）
附子（五分）	

共为末，粥饮送下二钱。

fù zǐ Sǎn (附子散，Prepared Aconite Root Powder): treats postpartum cholera-like disease with vomiting, diarrhea, counterflow cold of the extremities. It can be taken only when a clot or lump pain has disappeared.

bái zhú (white atractylodes rhizome), 1 *qian*

dāng guī (Chinese angelica), 2 *qian*

chén pí (aged tangerine peel), 4 *fen*

hēi jiāng (prepared dried ginger), 4 *fen*

dīng xiāng (clove flower), 4 *fen*

gān cǎo (licorice root), 4 *fen*

fù zǐ (prepared aconite root), 5 *fen*

Grind above medicines into a powder. Take 2 *qian* with porridge.

温中汤：治产后霍乱吐泻不止，无块痛者可服。

人参（一钱）	白术（一钱半）
当归（二钱）	厚朴（八分）
黑姜（四分）	茯苓（一钱）
草豆蔻（六分）	姜三片，水煎服

Wēn Zhōng Tāng (温中汤，Center Warming Decoction): Treats postpartum cholera-like disease with endless vomiting and diarrhea. It can be taken only when a clot or lump pain has disappeared.

rén shēn (ginseng), 1 *qian*

bái zhú (white atractylodes rhizome), 1 *qian* and 5 *fen*

dāng guī (Chinese angelica), 2 *qian*

hòu pò (magnolia bark), 8 *fen*

hēi jiāng (prepared dried ginger), 4 *fen*

fú líng (poria), 1 *qian*

cǎo dòu kòu (katsumada's galangal seed), 6 *fen*

jiāng (ginger), 3 slices

Decoct above medicines in water and take orally.

Chapter Ninety-seven

Treatment Methods for Various Postpartum Symptoms XXIV

产后诸症治法 二十四

呕逆不食
Vomiting and Inability to Eat

产后劳伤脏腑，寒邪易乘于肠胃，则气逆呕吐而不下食也。又有瘀血未净而呕者，亦有痰气入胃，胃口不清而呕者，当随症调之。

加减生化汤：治产妇呕逆不食。

川芎（一钱）	当归（三钱）
黑姜（五分）	砂仁（五分）
藿香（五分）	淡竹叶（七片）

水煎，和姜汁二匙服。

After delivery, if the zang (viscera) and fu (bowels) organs are damaged by over-fatigue, the pathogenic cold will find its way to exploit the intestine and spleen, resulting in qi counterflow, retching, and vomiting with an inability to eat. There are also cases of vomiting due to uncleared static blood or cases of vomiting due to unclear stomach caused by phlegm qi entering the stomach. These should be balanced according to the syndrome.

Jiā Jiǎn Shēng Huà Tāng (加减生化汤, Engendering and Transforming Variant Decoction): treats postpartum counterflow, retching with an inability to eat.

chuān xiōng (Sichuan lovage root), 1 *qian*

dāng guī (Chinese angelica), 5 *fen*

hēi jiāng (prepared dried ginger), 5 *fen*

shā rén (villous amomum fruit), 5 *fen*

huò xiāng (agastache), 5 *fen*

dàn zhú yè (salvia root), 7 pieces

Decoct above medicines in water, and mix the decoction with 2 spoons of ginger juice and take it orally.

温胃丁香散: 治产后七日外, 呕逆不食。

当归（三钱）　　　　　　　白术（二钱）

黑姜（四分）　　　　　　　丁香（四分）

人参（一钱）　　　　　　　陈皮（五分）

炙草（五分）　　　　　　　前胡（五分）

藿香（五分）　　　　　　　姜三片, 水煎服。

Wēn Wèi Dīng Xiāng Sǎn (温胃丁香散, Stomach Warming Clove Powder): Treats vomiting and inability to eat more than seven days after delivery.

dāng guī (Chinese angelica), 3 *qian*

bái zhú (white atractylodes rhizome), 2 *qian*

hēi jiāng (prepared dried ginger), 4 *fen*

dīng xiāng (clove), 4 *fen*

rén shēn (ginseng), 1 *qian*

chén pí (aged tangerine peel), 5 *fen*

zhì cǎo (prepared licorice root), 5 *fen*

qián hú (hogfennel root), 5 *fen*

huò xiāng (agastache), 5 *fen*

jiāng (ginger), 3 *slices*.

Decoct the formula with water and take it orally.

石莲散: 治产妇呕吐, 心冲目弦。

石莲子（去壳, 去心, 一两半）　　　白茯苓（一两）

丁香（五分）

共为细末, 米饮送下。

一本有白术, 无白茯苓, 丁香作五钱, 用者酌之。

Shí Lián Sǎn (石莲散, Nelumbinis Seed Powder): Treats vomiting, (qi) surging up into the heart and visual dizziness in the birthing woman.

shí lián zǐ (nelumbinis seed), hulled, pith discarded, 1.5 *liang*

bái fú líng (poria), 1 *liang*

dīng xiāng (clove), 5 *fen*

Mix above medicines and grind into a fine powder; take it with millet soup.

In a variant edition, there is *bái zhú* (白术, white atractylodes rhizome) instead of *bái fú líng* (白茯苓, poria). *Dīng xiāng* (丁香, clove) is 5 *qian*. Physicians can use it according to their consideration.

生津益液汤：治产妇虚弱，口渴气少，由产后血少多汗内烦不生津液。

人参（一两）	麦冬（一两，去心）
茯苓（一两）	大枣
竹叶	浮小麦
炙草	栝蒌根

大渴不止，加芦根。

（一本人参一钱，麦冬、茯苓三钱，存参。）

Shēng Jīn Yì Yè Tāng (生津益液汤, Fluids Engendering and Humor Boosting Decoction): treats thirst with shortness of breath in weak and deficient birthing women. These are due to insufficiency of blood and profuse sweating and interior vexation failing to engender fluids and humor (spirit).

rén shēn (ginseng), 1 *liang*

mài dōng (dwarf lilyturf tuber), 1 *liang* (pith discarded)

fú líng (poria), 1 *liang*

dà zǎo (Chinese date)

zhú yè (henon bamboo leaf)

fú xiǎo mài (blighted wheat)

zhì cǎo (prepared licorice root)

guā lóu gēn (snakegourd root)

In case of constant severe thirst, add *lú gēn* (芦根, reed rhizome).

(In another edition, Ginseng is given at 1 *qian*; *mài dōng* (麦冬, dwarf lilyturf tuber) and *fú líng* (茯苓, poria), each 3 *qian*. This cloud be used as reference)

Chapter Ninety-eight

Treatment Methods for Various Postpartum Symptoms XXV

产后诸症治法 二十五

咳嗽
Coughing

治产后七日内，外感风寒，咳嗽鼻塞，声重恶寒，勿用麻黄以动汗；嗽而胁痛，勿用柴胡汤；嗽而有声，痰少面赤，勿用凉药。凡产有火嗽，有痰嗽，必须调理半月后，方可用凉药，半月前不当用。

加味生化汤：治产后外感风寒、咳嗽及鼻塞声重。

川芎（一钱）　　　　　　当归（二钱）

杏仁（十粒）　　　　　　桔梗（四分）

知母（八分）

有痰，加半夏曲；虚弱有汗咳嗽，加人参。总之产后不可发汗。

【知母一本作（四分）。】

In treating external wind-cold invasion within seven days after delivery with cough, nasal congestion, heavy voice, and aversion to cold, do not use *Má Huáng Tāng* (麻黄汤, Ephedra Decoction) to promote perspiration.

In treating coughing with lateral costal pain, do not use *Chái Hú Tāng* (柴胡汤, Thotowax Root Decoction).

In treating coughing with lung rales, little phlegm, and red facial complexion, do not use cold-natured herbs.

For postpartum coughing caused either by fire or phlegm, no cold-natured herbs should be used until after half a month of regulating and rectifying. In no case should they be used earlier.

Jiā Wèi Shēng Huà Tāng (加味生化汤, Supplemented Engendering and Transforming Decoction): treats postpartum external wind-cold invasion with coughing, nasal congestion, and heavy nasal tone.

chuān xiōng (Sichuan lovage root), 1 *qian*

dāng guī (Chinese angelica), 2 *qian*

xìng rén (apricot kernel), 10 pieces

jié gěng (platycodon root), 4 *fen*

zhī mǔ (common anemarrhena rhizome), 8 *fen*

If there is phlegm, add *bàn xià qū* (半夏曲, fermented pinellia rhizome).

If there is deficient, weak sweating and coughing, add Ginseng. In a word, diaphoresis is prohibited after delivery.

[In a variant edition, *zhī mǔ* (知母, common anemarrhena rhizome) is given at 4 *fen*.]

加参安肺生化汤：治产后虚弱，旬日内外感风寒，咳嗽声重有痰，或身热头痛及汗多者。

川芎（一钱）	人参（一钱）
知母（一钱）	桑白皮（一钱）
当归（二钱）	杏仁（十粒，去皮尖）
甘草（四分）	桔梗（四分）
半夏（七分）	橘红（三分）

虚人多痰，加竹沥一杯，姜汁半匙。

按：咳嗽论中，明示纵有火嗽，在半月前，犹不得轻用凉药，垂戒綦严。而第一与第二方中，均有知母，小注均有"外感风寒"云云。此必于既感之后，将蕴而为燥热，不得已而用之，小注未及申明。如谓不然，苟初感即用此凉品，岂不与前论显为枘凿。读者须会前人微意，庶不致用古方而自少权衡耳。

Jiā Shēn Ān Fèi Shēng Huà Tāng (加参安肺生化汤, Lung Calming, Engendering and Transforming Decoction Plus Ginseng): treats postpartum deficiency and weakness with external wind-cold invasion within ten days after delivery, presenting as cough, heavy nasal voice, and phlegm or fever, headache, and profuse sweating.

chuān xiōng (Sichuan lovage root), 1 *qian*

rén shēn (ginseng), 1 *qian*

zhī mǔ (common anemarrhena rhizome), 1 *qian*

sāng bái pí (white mulberry root-bark), 1 *qian*

dāng guī (Chinese angelica), 2 *qian*

xìng rén (apricot kernel), peeled, ten pieces

gān cǎo (licorice root), 4 *fen*

jié gěng (platycodon root), 4 *fen*

bàn xià qū (pinellia rhizome), 7 *fen*

jú hóng (red tangerine peel), 3 *fen*

For patients with a deficient syndrome with profuse phlegm, add a cup of Zhuli (Henon Bamboo Juice) and a half spoonful of Ginger juice.

Note: In the discussion on coughing given above, it is clearly stated that even in the case of fire coughing, cold-natured herbs should not be used inadvertently any earlier than two weeks after delivery. This is a stringent rule which should be followed rigidly. However, in both the first and the second formulas that are given above, there is *zhī mǔ* (知母, common anemarrhena rhizome). There are minor characters inserted as a note reading, "external wind-cold invasion." These must imply that after such invasion, dryness and heat are already brewed. *Zhī mǔ* (知母, common anemarrhena rhizome) is used because there is no alternative. However, this implication is not mentioned in that note. If this were not the case and such a cool medicine was meant to be used immediately following the external invasion, these formulas and this discussion would differ.

Readers should try to understand the subtle meaning between the lines and avoid using old formulas without being circumspect.

加味四物汤: 治半月后干嗽有声, 痰少者。

川芎（一钱）	白芍（一钱）
知母（一钱）	瓜蒌仁（一钱）
生地（二钱）	当归（二钱）
诃子（二钱）	冬花（六分）
桔梗（四分）	甘草（四分）
兜铃（四分）	生姜（一大片）

Jiā Wèi Sì Wù Tāng (加味四物汤, Supplemented Four Substances Decoction): treats dry cough with lung rales and little phlegm occurring more than two weeks after delivery.

chuān xiōng (Sichuan lovage root), 1 *qian*

bái sháo (white peony root), 1 *qian*

zhī mǔ (common anemarrhena rhizome), 1 *qian*

guā lóu rén (snakegourd seed), 1 *qian*

shēng dì (rehmannia root), 2 *qian*

dāng guī (Chinese angelica), 2 *qian*

hē zǐ (medicine terminalia fruit), 2 *qian*

dōng huā (common coltsfoot flower), 6 *fen*

jié gěng (platycodon root), 4 *fen*

gān cǎo (licorice root), 4 *fen*

dōu líng (birthwort fruit), 4 *fen*

Shengjiang (ginger), 1 big slice

Chapter Ninety-nine

Treatment Methods for Various Postpartum Symptoms XXVI

产后诸症治法 二十六

水肿
Edema

产后水气，手足浮肿，皮肤见光荣色，乃脾虚不能制水，肾虚不能行水也。必以大补气血为先，佐以苍术、白术、茯苓补脾；壅满，用陈皮、半夏、香附消之；虚火，加人参、木通；有热，加黄芩、麦冬以清肺金。健脾利水，补中益气汤；七日外，用人参、白术各二钱，茯苓、白芍各一钱，陈皮五分，木瓜八分，紫苏、木通、大腹皮、苍术、厚朴各四分；大便不通，加郁李仁、麻仁各一钱。如因寒邪湿气伤脾，无汗而肿，宜姜皮、半夏，苏叶加于补气方，以表汗。

五皮散：治产后风湿客伤脾经，气血凝滞，以致面目浮虚，四肢肿胀气喘。

五加皮（一钱）	地骨皮（一钱）
大腹皮（一钱）	茯苓皮（一钱）
姜皮（一钱）	枣一枚，水煎服。

Postpartum water qi manifesting itself as edema of the hands and feet with a bright, shiny complexion is due to deficiency of the spleen failing to restrain water and deficiency of the Kidneys failing to move Water.

The first thing to do in order to treat this syndrome should be to supplement qi and blood significantly and use *cāng zhú* (苍术, atractylodes rhizome), *bái zhú* (白术, white atractylodes rhizome), and *fú líng* (茯苓, poria) as assistants to supplement the spleen.

If there is a feeling of congestion and fullness, use *chén pí* (陈皮, aged tangerine peel), *bàn xià* (半夏, pinellia rhizome), and *xiāng fù* (香附, cyperus) to disperse them.

For patients with deficient fire, use *rén shēn* (人参, ginseng) and *mù tōng* (木

通, akebia stem).

For patients with heat, add *huáng qín* (黃芩, scutellaria root), *mài dōng* (麦冬, dwarf lilyturf tuber) to clear the lung (metal), and use *Bǔ Zhōng Yì Qì Tāng* (补中益气汤, Center-Supplementing and Qi-Boosting Decoction) to strengthen the spleen and disinhibit water.

If edema is still presenting seven days after delivery, add *rén shēn* (人参, ginseng) and *bái zhú* (白术, white atractylodes rhizome), each 2 *qian*. Additionally, add *fú líng* (茯苓, poria) and *bái sháo* (白芍, white peony root), each 1 *qian, chén pí* (陈皮, aged tangerine peel) 5 *fen*, *mù guā* (木瓜, Chinese quince fruit) 8 *fen*, *zǐ sū* (紫苏, perilla leaf), *mù tōng* (木通, akebia stem), *dà fù pí* (大腹皮, areca peel), *cāng zhú* (苍术, atractylodes rhizome), and *hòu pò* (厚朴, magnolia bark), each 4 *fen*.

For patients with constipation, add *yù lǐ rén* (郁李仁, Chinese dwarf cherry seed), *má rén* (麻仁, hemp seed), each 1 *qian*.

Suppose there is edema with no sweating due to the spleen's damage by pathogenic cold and damp qi. In that case, it is appropriate to add *jiāng pí* (姜皮, ginger peel), *bàn xià qū* (半夏曲, pinellia rhizome), *sū yè* (苏叶, perilla leaf) to a qi supplementing formula to effuse sweat.

Wǔ Pí Sǎn (五皮散, Five-Peel Powder): treats postpartum edema of the face and eyes, swelling and distention of four limbs, and asthma due to wind dampness invading and damaging the Spleen.

wǔ jiā pí (acanthopanax root bark), 1 *qian*

dì gǔ pí (Chinese wolfberry root-bark), 1 *qian*

dà fù pí (areca peel), 1 *qian*

fú líng pí (poria exodermis), 1 *qian*

jiāng pí (ginger peel), 1 *qian*

dà zǎo (Chinese date), 1 piece.

Decoct above medicines with water and take it orally.

又云，产后恶露不净，停留胞络，致令浮肿，若以水气治之，投以甘遂等药，误矣！但服调经散，则血行而肿消矣。

调经散：

没药（另研，一钱）　　　　　琥珀（另研，一钱）

肉桂（一钱）　　　　　　　　赤芍（一钱）

当归（一钱）

上为细末，每服五分，姜汁、酒各少许，调服。

（此方能调经治腹痛。）

In addition, after delivery, if the lochia is not cleared up, it will be retained in the uterus vessels, which results in edema. It is wrong to treat it as water qi and use *gān suì* (甘遂, gansui root) or similar medicines. Administer *Tiáo Jīng Sǎn* (调经散, Menstruation Regulating Powder), and blood will be moved and edema dispersed.

Tiáo Jīng Sǎn (调经散, Menstruation Regulating Powder):

mò yào (myrrh), 1 *qian* (ground separately)

hǔ pò (amber), 1 *qian* (ground separately)

ròu guì (cinnamon bark), 1 *qian*

chì sháo (red peony root) 1 *qian*

dāng guī (Chinese angelica), 1 *qian*

Grind above medicines into a fine powder. Take 5 *fen* each time. Take it with a small amount of Ginger juice mixed with millet wine.

(This formula can regulate menstruation and treat abdominal pain.)

Treatment Methods for Various Postpartum Symptoms XXVII

产后诸症治法 二十七

流注
Streaming Sore (Multiple Abscess)

产后恶露流于腰臂足关节之处，或漫肿、或结块，久则肿起作痛，肢体倦怠，急宜用葱熨法以治外肿；内服参归生化汤以消血滞，无缓也。未成者消，已成者溃。

葱熨法：用葱一握，炙热，捣烂作饼，敷痛处，用厚布二、三层，以熨斗火熨之。

参归生化汤：

川芎（一钱半）	当归（二钱）
炙草（五分）	人参（二钱）
黄芪（一钱半）	肉桂（五分）
马蹄香（二钱）	

After delivery, the lochia may flow into the joints of the waist, arms, and feet, resulting in diffuse swelling or lumps. If this lingers long, the swelling will grow, causing pain and fatigue of the body and limbs. It is necessary to immediately perform the green onion ironing method to treat the swelling externally. Internally, administer *Shēn Guī Shēng Huà Tāng* (参归生化汤, Engendering and Transforming Decoction Plus Ginseng and Chinese Angelica) to disperse blood stagnation. The immature swelling will be dispersed, and the mature swelling will break up.

Scallion ironing method:

Heat a handful of scallion, smash, and make it into a cake. Apply the cake to the painful area. Cover with 2~3 layers of cloth and iron it.

Shēn Guī Shēng Huà Tāng (参归生化汤, Engendering and Transforming

Decoction Plus Ginseng and Chinese Angelica):

chuān xiōng (Sichuan lovage root), 1 *qian* and 5 *fen*

dāng guī (Chinese angelica), 2 *qian*

zhì cǎo (prepared licorice root), 5 *fen*

rén shēn (ginseng), 2 *qian*

huáng qí (astragalus root), 1 *qian* and 5 *fen*

ròu guì cinnamon bark, 5 *fen*

mǎ tí xiāng (saruma henryi), 2 *qian*

此症若不补气血，节饮食，慎起居，未有得生者。如肿起作痛，起居饮食如常，是病气未深，形气未损，易治；若漫肿微痛，起居倦怠，饮食不足，最难治。或未成脓，未溃，气血虚也，宜服八珍汤；憎寒恶寒，阳气虚也，宜服十全大补汤；补后大热，阴血虚也，宜服四物汤加参、术、丹皮；呕逆，胃气虚也，宜服六君子汤加炮姜、干姜；食少体倦，脾气虚也，宜服补中益气汤；四肢冷逆，小便频数，肾气虚也，补中益气汤加益智仁一钱。神仙回洞散治产后流注恶露，日久成肿，用此宜导其脓，若未补气血旺，不可服此方。

No patients with this syndrome can survive unless qi and blood are supplemented, temperance in eating and drinking is practiced, and care is taken about daily life. If the swelling has become enlarged and painful, but daily life is not affected, the pathogenic qi has not yet penetrated deep, and the body and qi have not yet been damaged. Therefore it is easy to recover. It is challenging to treat diffuse swelling with slight pain, fatigue, and insufficient food intake. If there is no pus or failure of the pus to ulcerate due to qi and blood deficiency, it is proper to take *Bā Zhēn Tāng* (八珍汤，Eight-Gem Decoction).

Abhorrence of and aversion to cold is due to yang qi deficiency and should be treated with *Shí Quán Dà Bǔ Tāng* (十全大补汤，Perfect Major Supplementation Decoction).

Suppose the patient presents with great heat after supplementing (due to yin and blood deficiency). In that case, the patient should be treated with *Sì Wù Tāng* (四物汤，Four Agents Decoction), added with *rén shēn* (人参，ginseng), *bái zhú* (白术，white atractylodes rhizome), and *dān pí* (丹皮，tree peony bark).

In case there is vomiting and belching due to stomach qi deficiency, take *Liù Jūn Zǐ Tāng* (六君子汤，Six Gentlemen Decoction), and add *páo jiāng* (炮姜，prepared dried ginger) and *gān jiāng* (干姜，dried ginger rhizome).

Poor appetite and fatigue are due to spleen deficiency. It is, therefore, proper to administer *Bǔ Zhōng Yì Qì Tāng* (补中益气汤, Center-Supplementing and Qi-Boosting Decoction).

Coldness of extremities and frequent urination is due to kidney qi deficiency. It is, therefore, proper to take *Bǔ Zhōng Yì Qì Tāng* (补中益气汤, Center-Supplementing and Qi-Boosting Decoction), added with *yì zhì rén* (益智仁, sharp leaf glangal fruit) 1 *qian*.

Shēn Xiān Huí dòng Sǎn (神仙回洞散, Acute Mastitis Powder) is used to treat postpartum streaming sore (multiple abscesses), which has been retained long enough to result in swelling. The powder is used to conduct pus, but it should not be used before qi and blood are supplemented and made effulgent.

注：

乳痈方（即神仙回洞散）：

蒲公英、天花粉、金银花、连翘、白芷、甘草若是吹乳，加防风。久破烂，加人参、黄芪。

Note: *Shén Xiān Huí dòng Sǎn* (神仙回洞散, Acute Mastitis Powder):

pú gōng yīng (蒲公英, dandelion), *tiān huā fěn* (天花粉, snakegourd root), *jīn yín huā* (金银花, honeysuckle flower), *lián qiào* (连翘, weeping forsythia capsule), *bái zhǐ* (白芷, angelica root), *gān cǎo* (甘草, licorice root).

Variations:

In case of breast blowing (mammary with swelling abscess), add *fáng fēng* (防风, saposhnikovia root).

In case of long-time ulceration, add *rén shēn* (人参, ginseng) and *huáng qí* (黄芪, astragalus root).

Treatment Methods for Various Postpartum Symptoms XXVIII

产后诸症治法 二十八

膨胀
Distention

妇人素弱，临产又劳，中气不足，胸膈不利，而转运稽迟。若产后即服生化汤以消块止痛，又服加参生化汤以健脾胃，自无中满之症。其膨胀，因伤食而误消，因气郁而误散，多食冷物而停留恶露，又因血虚大便燥结，误下而愈胀。殊不知气血两虚，血块消后，当大补气血，以补中虚。治者若但知伤食宜消，气郁宜散，恶露当攻，便结可下，则胃气反损，满闷益增，气不升降，湿热积久，遂成膨胀。岂知消导坐于补中，则脾胃强，而所伤食气消散，助血兼行，大便自通，恶露自行。

Suppose the patient has a weak constitution and has been exhausted in the course of labor. *Zhong* (Central) qi is insufficient, and the chest and diaphragm are inhibited. As a result, transformation and transportation are retarded. If *Shēng Huà Tāng* (生化汤, Engendering and Transforming Decoction) is administered immediately after delivery to disperse clots and relieve pain, and *Jiā Shēn Shēng Huà Tāng* (加参生化汤, Engendering and Transforming Decoction Plus Ginseng) is taken in addition to strengthen the spleen and stomach, the symptom of fullness in the center will not arise.

Distention is caused by misapplication of dispersing in the case of food damage (indigestion), dissipating in the case of qi depression, and retention of lochia due to overeating cold food. This symptom can be further aggravated by inappropriate precipitation in the case of dry, bound stools due to blood deficiency. Interns hardly know that when qi and blood are both deficient, they should be significantly supplemented as soon as the clots are dispersed in order to supplement the central deficiency. Suppose the doctor knows no more than the fact that dispersing is appropriate for food damage, or that dissipating is appropriate for qi depression, or that lochia should be attacked, and that constipation requires precipitation. Therefore, the stomach qi will be damaged. The feeling of fullness and oppression will worsen, and the qi will stop ascending and descending. When damp-heat accumulates for a long time, distention comes into being. Doctors should understand that, in postpartum cases, if abduction of dispersing is realized through central supplementation, the spleen and stomach will be strong, and the food qi causing damage will be dispersed and dissipated. If blood is assisted and simultaneously moved, defecation will automatically be freed, and the lochia naturally moved.

如产后中风，气不足，微满，误服耗气药而胀者，服补中益气汤。

人参（五分）	当归（五分）
白术（五分）	白茯苓（一钱）
川芎（四分）	白芍（四分）
萝卜子（四分）	木香（三分）

（一本人参、白术俱作一钱，当归作二钱，有姜一片。）

In the case of a postpartum wind attack with qi insufficiency and minor fullness that has developed into distention as a result of the misapplication of qi-consuming medicines; take *Bǔ Zhōng Yì Qì Tāng* (补中益气汤，Center-Supplementing and Qi-Boosting Decoction):

rén shēn (ginseng), 5 *fen*

dāng guī (Chinese angelica), 5 *fen*

bái zhú (white atractylodes rhizome), 5 *fen*

bái fú líng (poria), 1 *qian*

chuān xiōng (Sichuan lovage root), 4 *fen*

bái sháo (white peony root), 4 *fen*

luó bo zǐ, (radish seed), 4 *fen*

mù xiāng (common aucklandia root), 3 *fen*

(In a variant edition, *rén shēn* (人参，ginseng) and *bái zhú* (白术，white atractylodes rhizome) are both 1 *qian*, *dāng guī* (当归，Chinese angelica) is 2 *qian*. Moreover, there is a piece of ginger.)

如伤食，误服消导药成胀，或胁下积块，宜服健脾汤

人参（三钱）	白术（三钱）

当归（三钱）　　　　　白茯苓（一钱）

白芍（一钱）　　　　　神曲（一钱）

吴萸（一钱）　　　　　大腹皮（四分）

陈皮（四分）　　　　　砂仁（五分）

麦芽（五分）

（一本人参、白术作二钱。）

In case there is food damage developing into distention or accumulation of lumps in the lateral costal region due to misapplication of food stagnation-removing medicines, administering *Jiàn Pí Tāng* (健脾汤，Spleen-Fortifying Decoction) will be beneficial:

rén shēn (ginseng), 3 *qian*

bái zhú (white atractylodes rhizome), 3 *qian*

dāng guī (Chinese angelica), 3 *qian*

bái fú líng (poria), 1 *qian*

bái sháo (white peony root), 1 *qian*

shén qū (medicated leaven), 1 *qian*

wú yú (medicinal veodia fruit), 1 *qian*

dà fù pí (areca peel), 4 *fen*

chén pí (aged tangerine peel), 4 *fen*

shā rén (villous amomum fruit), 5 *fen*

mài yá (germinated barley), 5 *fen*

In a variant edition *rén shēn* (人参，ginseng) and *bái zhú* (白术，white atractylodes rhizome) are given at 2 *qian*.

如大便不通，误服下药成胀，及腹中作痛，宜服养荣生化汤。

当归（四钱）　　　　　白芍（一钱）

白茯苓（一钱）　　　　人参（一钱）

白术（二钱）　　　　　陈皮（五分）

大腹皮（五分）　　　　香附（五分）

苁蓉（一钱）　　　　　桃仁（十粒，制）

块痛，将药送四消丸。屡误下，须用参、归半斤，大便方通，膨胀方退。凡误用消食耗气药，以致绝谷，长生活命丹屡效。方见伤食条。

（一本无桃仁。）

In case there is constipation that has developed into distention with abdominal pain resulting from misapplication of precipitation medicines, it is proper to take *Yǎng Róng Shēng Huà Tāng* (养荣生化汤, Engendering and Transforming Decoction for Nourishing):

    dāng guī (Chinese angelica), 4 *qian*

    bái sháo (white peony root), 1 *qian*

    bái fú líng (poria), 1 *qian*

    rén shēn (ginseng), 1 *qian*

    bái zhú (white atractylodes rhizome), 2 *qian*

    chén pí (aged tangerine peel), 5 *fen*

    dà fù pí (areca peel), 5 *fen*

    xiāng fù (cyperus), 5 *fen*

    cōng róng (desert cistanche), 1 *qian*

    táo rén (peach kernel), 10 pieces, prepared

In case there is lump pain, take *Sì Xiāo Wán* (四消丸, Four Dispersing Pill) with the above decoction.

In case there is repeated inappropriate precipitation, it is proper to administer half a *jin* (250g) of Ginseng and *dāng guī* (当归, Chinese angelica). Doing so will relieve constipation and distention.

If there is lump pain, take *Sì Xiāo Wán* (四消丸, Four Dispersing Pill) with the above decoction.

If there is repeated inappropriate precipitation, it is proper to administer half a *jin* (250g) of ginseng and *dāng guī* (当归, Chinese angelica). Doing so will relieve constipation and distention.

If there is any circumstance where the patient mistakenly takes digestive medicines, qi-consuming medicines, or the patient is made not to take in food, administer *Cháng Shēng Huó Mìng Dān* (长生活命丹, Life-Saving Pill). The formula can be seen in the previous chapter of Food Damage.

In a variant edition, there is no *táo rén* (桃仁, peach kernel).

Treatment Methods for Various Postpartum Symptoms XXIX

产后诸症治法 二十九

怔忡惊悸
Palpitation and Heart-throb with Fear

由产忧惊劳倦，去血过多，则心中跳动不安，谓之怔忡。若惕然震惊，心中怯怯，如人将捕之状，谓之惊悸。治此二症，惟调和脾胃，志定神清而病愈矣。如分娩后血块未消，宜服生化汤，且补血行块，血旺则怔定惊平，不必加安神定志剂。如块消痛止后患此，宜服加减养荣汤。

当归（二钱）	川芎（二钱）
茯神（一钱）	人参（一钱）
枣仁（一钱，炒）	麦冬（一钱）
远志（一钱）	白术（一钱）
黄芪（一钱，炙）	元肉（八枚）
陈皮（四分）	炙草（四分），姜煎。

虚烦加竹沥、姜汁，去川芎、麦冬，再加竹茹一团。加木香即归脾汤。

If the heart jumps and beats irregularly and is uneasy, it is usually because of worry, fright, taxation, fatigue, and blood loss during delivery. This is called palpitation.

Being hypersensitive, easy to be shocked and frightened, being timid or fainthearted (as if fearing being arrested) is called Heart-throb with Fear.

There is no other choice to treat either of the two symptoms but to harmonize the spleen and stomach. When the mind is stabilized, and the spirit is quiet and clear the patient recovers. If blood clots are not eliminated after delivery, it is proper to administer *Shēng Huà Tāng* (生化汤, Engendering and Transforming Decoction) to supplement blood and move the clots. When the blood is made effulgent, the palpitations will become stabilized, and heart-throb with fear will become peaceful. There is no need to use spirit calming or mind stabilizing formulas.

If these disorders arise after clots are eliminated, and pain is relieved, it is advisable to administer *Jiā Jiǎn Yǎng Róng Tāng* (加减养荣汤, Variant Nourishing Decoction):

dāng guī (Chinese angelica), 2 *qian*

chuān xiōng (Sichuan lovage root), 2 *qian*

fú shén (Indian bread with hostwood), 1 *qian*

rén shēn (ginseng), 1 *qian*

zǎo rén (spiney date seed), 1 *qian*

mài dōng (dwarf lilyturf tuber), 1 *qian*

yuǎn zhì (thin-leaf milkwort root), 1 *qian*

bái zhú (white atractylodes rhizome), 1 *qian*

huáng qí (astragalus root), 1 *qian* (honey-fried)

yuán ròu (longan aril), 8 pieces

chén pí (aged tangerine peel), 4 *fen*

zhì cǎo (prepared licorice root), 4 *fen*

jiāng (ginger)

Decoct the formula.

If there is deficient vexation, add *zhú lì* (竹沥, bamboo sap), ginger juice, subtract *chuān xiōng* (川芎, Sichuan lovage root) and *mài dōng* (麦冬, dwarf lilyturf tuber), and then add a ball of *zhú rú* (竹茹, bamboo shavings).

The formula becomes *Guī Pí Tāng* (归脾汤, Spleen-Restoring Decoction) if *mù xiāng* (木香, common aucklandia root) is added.

养心汤: 治产后心血不定, 心神不安。

炙黄芪（一钱）	茯神（八分）
川芎（八分）	当归（二钱）
麦冬（一钱八分）	远志（八分）
柏子仁（一钱）	人参（一钱半）
炙草（四分）	五味（十粒）

姜, 水煎服。

（一本有元肉六枚。）

Yǎng Xīn Tāng (养心汤, Heart Nourishing Decoction): treats unsteady heart blood and restless heart spirit:

huáng qí (astragalus root), 1 *qian* (honey-fried)

fú shén (Indian bread with hostwood)

chuān xiōng (Sichuan lovage root)

dāng guī (Chinese angelica)

mài dōng (dwarf lilyturf tuber)

yuǎn zhì (thin-leaf milkwort root),

bǎi zǐ rén (oriental arborvitael)

rén shēn (ginseng)

zhì cǎo (prepared licorice root)

wǔ wèi zǐ (Chinese magnolivine fruit)

jiāng (ginger)

Decoct the formula in water and take orally.

[In a variant edition there are 6 pieces of *yuán ròu* (元肉，longan aril).]

Treatment Methods for Various Postpartum Symptoms XXX

产后诸症治法 三十

心痛
Heart Pain

此即胃脘痛。因胃脘在心之下，劳伤风寒及食冷物而作痛，俗呼为心痛。心可痛乎？血不足，则怔仲惊悸不安耳。若真心痛，手足青黑色，且夕死矣。治当散胃中之寒气，消胃中之冷物。必用生化汤，佐消寒食之药，无有不安。若绵绵而痛，可按止之，问无血块，则当论虚而加补也。产后心痛腹痛二症相似，因寒食与气上攻于心则心痛，下攻于腹则腹痛，均用生化汤加肉桂、吴萸等温散之药也。

In fact, this is stomach ache or epigastric pain. Because the site of the pain is below the heart, the pain is due to taxation damage, wind-cold, or eating cold food. This pain is popularly known as "heart" pain. How can the heart be painful? When blood is insufficient, the patient feels severe palpitation, fearful throbbing, and is disquieted. If it is really the heart feels very painful, the hands and feet look green-blue, and the patient is at death's door.

The treatment is to dissipate the cold qi and disperse the cold substance in the stomach. *Shēng Huà Tāng* (生化汤, Engendering and Transforming Decoction) is indispensable, assisted with medicinals for dispersing cold food accumulation. Then, recovery is ensured without fail. If the pain is dull and relivable by pressure, it should be diagnosed as a deficient syndrome and treated with supplementation. Postpartum heart pain and abdominal pain are similar. When cold food and qi go up and attack the "heart," there occurs "heart" pain. If they go down and attack the abdomen, there occurs abdominal pain. In either case, administer *Shēng Huà Tāng* (生化汤, Engendering and Transforming Decoction) added with warming and dissipating medicinals such as *ròu guì* (肉桂, cinnamon bark) and *wú yú* (吴萸, medicinal evodia fruit), and the like.

加味生化汤：

川芎（一钱）	当归（三钱）
黑姜（五分）	肉桂（八分）
吴萸（八分）	砂仁（八分）
炙草（五分）	

伤寒食加肉桂、吴萸，伤面食加神曲、麦芽，伤肉食加山楂、砂仁，大便不通加肉苁蓉。

Jiā Wèi Shēng Huà Tāng (加味生化汤, Supplemented Engendering and Transforming Decoction):

chuān xiōng (Sichuan lovage root), 1 *qian*

dāng guī (Chinese angelica), 3 *qian*

hēi jiāng (prepared dried ginger), 5 *fen*

ròu guì (cinnamon bark), 8 *fen*

wú yú (medicinal evodia fruit) 8 *fen*

shā rén (villous amomum fruit), 8 *fen*

zhì cǎo (prepared licorice root), 5 *fen*

Formula Variations:

If there is cold food damage, add additional *ròu guì* (肉桂, cinnamon bark), and *wú yú* (吴萸, medicinal evodia fruit).

If there is cereal (grain) food damage (stagnation), add *shén qū* (神曲, medicated leaven) and *mài yá* (麦芽, germinated barley).

If there is meat food damage (stagnation), add *shān zhā* (山楂, Chinese hawthorn fruit), *shā rén* (砂仁, villous amomum fruit).

In case of constipation, add *ròu cōng róng* (肉苁蓉, desert cistanche).

Treatment Methods for Various Postpartum Symptoms XXXI

产后诸症治法 三十一

腹痛
Abdominal Pain

先问有块无块。块痛只服生化汤，调失笑散二钱，加元胡一钱；无块则是遇风冷作痛，宜服加减生化汤。

川芎（一钱）	当归（四钱）
黑姜（四分）	炙草（四分）
防风（七分）	吴萸（六分）
白蔻（五分）	桂枝（七分）

痛止去之。随伤食物，所加如前。

First of all, enquire about the presence or absence of clots. If there is clot or lump pain, take *Shēng Huà Tāng* (生化汤, Engendering and Transforming Decoction) plus 2 *qian* of *Shī Xiào Sǎn* (失笑散, Sudden Smile Powder) and 1 *qian yuán hú* (元胡, corydalis tuber).

If there are no clots, and the pain occurs when exposed to wind and cold, it is proper to take *Jiā Wèi Shēng Huà Tāng* (加味生化汤, Supplemented Engendering and Transforming Decoction).

chuān xiōng (Sichuan lovage root), 1 *qian*

dāng guī (Chinese angelica), 4 *qian*

hēi jiāng (prepared dried ginger), 4 *fen*

zhì cǎo (prepared licorice root), 4 *fen*

fáng fēng (saposhnikovia root) 7 *fen*

wú yú (medicinal evodia fruit), 6 *fen*

bái kòu (round cardamon kernel), 5 *fen*

guì zhī (cinnamon twig), 7 *fen*

After the pain stops, delete what has been added. Modify the formula as instructed previously, following the type of food damage.

Treatment Methods for Various Postpartum Symptoms XXXII

产后诸症治法 三十二

小腹痛
Lower abdominal Pain

产后虚中，感寒饮冷，其寒下攻小腹作痛，又有血块作痛者，又产后血虚脐下痛者，并治之以加减生化汤。

川芎（一钱）	当归（三钱）
黑姜（四分）	炙草（四分）
桃仁（十粒）	

有块痛者，本方中送前胡散，亦治寒痛。若无块，但小腹痛，亦可按而少止者，属血虚，加熟地三钱，前胡、肉桂各一钱，为末，名前胡散。

After delivery, the patient will be deficient in her spleen and stomach. If there is an invasion of cold or if drinking cold drinks, the cold may attack the lower abdomen and cause pain. Blood clots or lumps can also cause such pain. Also, postpartum blood deficiency can result in pain below the navel. All these types of pain should be treated with *Jiā Jiǎn Shēng Huà Tāng* (加减生化汤, Engendering and Transforming Variant Decoction):

chuān xiōng (Sichuan lovage root), 1 *qian*

dāng guī (Chinese angelica), 3 *qian*

hēi jiāng (prepared dried ginger), 4 *fen*

zhì cǎo (prepared licorice root), 4 *fen*

táo rén (peach kernel), 10 pieces

If there is lump pain, the formula should be administered with *Qián Hú Sǎn* (前胡散, Hogfennel Root Powder). This method can also treat cold pain. Lower abdominal pain without clots and can be slightly relieved with pressure is due to blood deficiency. For this, add *shú dì* (熟地, prepared rehmannia root) 3 *qian*, q*ián hú* (前胡, hogfennel root), and *ròu guì* (肉桂, cinnamon bark) each 1 *qian*, ground into powder, called *Qián Hú Săn* (前胡散, Hogfennel Root Powder).

产后诸症治法 三十三

遍身疼痛
Generalized Pain

产后百节开张，血脉流散。气弱则经络间血多阻滞，累日不散，则筋牵脉引，骨节不利，故腰背不能转侧，手足不能动履，或身热头痛。若误作伤寒，发表出汗，则筋脉动荡，手足发冷，变症出焉。宜服趁痛散。

当归（一钱）　　　　　甘草（八分）

黄芪（八分）　　　　　白术（八分）

独活（八分）　　　　　肉桂（八分）

桑寄生（一钱）　　　　牛膝（八分）

薤白（五根）　　　　　姜三片，水煎服。

（一本无桑寄生。）

During delivery, the joints of the whole body are opened and extended. The blood in the vessels flows in scattered way. As qi is weak, the blood becomes stagnated around the channels and collaterals. If it does not disperse for days, the tendons will contract and the vessels will be tugged. The bone joints will then become inhibited. As a result, the lower and upper back are unable to turn and the hands and feet are unable to move. The patient may have generalized fever and headache. If this is mistakenly diagnosed as cold damage (exogenous cold disease), and treated with exterior-releasing herbs that promote perspiration, the tendons and vessels will become restless and the hands and feet will be cold. Transmutation will occur. It is therefore proper to administer *Chèn Tòng Sǎn* (Pain Expelling Powder).

dāng guī (Chinese angelica), 1 *qian*

gān cǎo (licorice root), 8 *fen*

huáng qí (astragalus root), 8 *fen*

bái zhú (white atractylodes rhizome), 8 *fen*

dú huó (double teeth pubescent angelica root), 8 *fen*

ròu guì (cinnamon bark), 8 *fen*

sāng jì shēng (Chinese taxillus), 1 *qian*

niú xī (two-toothed achyranthes root), 8 *fen*

xiè bái (long stamen onion bulb), 5 pieces

jiāng (ginger), 3 slices

[In a variant edition, there's no *sāng jì shēng* (Chinese taxillus)]

产后诸症治法 三十四

腰痛
Lumbar Pain

由女人肾位系胞，腰为肾府，产后劳伤肾气，损动胞络，或虚未复而风乘之也。

养荣壮肾汤：治产后感风寒，腰痛不可转。

当归（二钱）	防风（四分）
独活（八分）	桂心（八分）
杜仲（八分）	续断（八分）
桑寄生（八分）	生姜（三片）

水煎服。两帖后痛未止，属肾虚，加熟地三钱。

（一本川芎八分。）

The Kidneys are tied to the uterus for women, and the lumbar is where the kidneys are located. Therefore, lumbar pain may occur after delivery by taxation (deficiency or overwork), damage of the kidney qi, damage of the network vessels of the uterus, or wind overwhelming the patient before recovery from deficiency.

The formula to use is *Yǎng Róng Zhuàng Shèn Tāng* (养荣壮肾汤, Body Nourishing and Kidney Invigorating Decoction): treats postpartum wind-cold invasion and lumbar pain with inability to turn.

dāng guī (Chinese angelica), 2 *qian*

fáng fēng (saposhnikovia root),4 *fen*

dú huó (double teeth pubescent angelica root), 8 *fen*

guì xīn (cinnamon bark, rough skin peeled) 8 *fen*

dù zhòng (eucommia bark), 8 *fen*

xù duàn (himalayan teasel root), 8 *fen*

sāng jì shēng (Chinese taxillus), 8 *fen*

shēng jiāng (fresh ginger), 3 slices

Decoct the formula in water and take it orally. If, after taking 2 *ji*, the pain has not been relieved, it is a kidney deficiency syndrome. Add *shú dì* (熟地, prepared rehmannia root) 3 *qian*.

In a variant edition, use *chuān xiōng* (川芎, Sichuan lovage root) 8 *qian*.

◎加味大造丸：治产后日久，气血两虚，腰痛肾弱，方见骨蒸条。

◎青娥丸：

胡桃（十二个）　　　　　　　　破故纸（八两，酒浸，炒）

杜仲（一斤，姜汁炒，去丝）

为细末，炼蜜丸，淡醋汤送六十丸。

（胡桃一本作二十个。）

Jiā Wèi Dà Zào Wán (加味大造丸, Supplemented Great Building Pills): treats postpartum qi and blood deficiency that has lasted for an extended period and manifests as lumbar pain and weak kidneys. For the formula, see the chapter about steaming bones.

Qīng é Wán (青娥丸, Young Maid Pill)

hé táo (核桃, walnut), 12 pieces

pò gù zhǐ (破故纸, oroxylum seed), 8 *liang,* soaked in millet wine and then stir fried.

dù zhòng (杜仲, eucommia bark), 1 *jin*, stir fried with ginger juice, stripped of fibers.

Grind the medicinals into a fine powder, mix it with honey, and shape it into pills. Take 60 pills with boiled, dilute vinegar and water.

(In a variant edition, Walnut is 20 pieces.)

产后诸症治法 三十五

胁痛
Rib-side Pain

乃肝经血虚气滞之故。气滞，用四君子汤加青皮、柴胡，血虚用四物汤加柴胡、人参、白术。若概用香燥之药，则反伤清和之气，无所生矣。

补肺散：治胁痛。

山萸	当归
五味	山药
黄芪	川芎
熟地	木瓜
白术	独活
枣仁	

各等分。水煎服。

（一本山萸二钱，当归二钱，五味十粒，黄芪八分，川芎六分，熟地钱半，木瓜、白术各一钱，独活八分，枣仁一钱，姜一片，无山药，存参。）

This pain is due to blood deficiency and qi stagnation. If it is qi stagnation, use *Sì Jūn Zǐ Tāng* (四君子汤, Four Gentlemen Decoction) plus *qīng pí* (青皮, green tangerine peel), *chái hú* (柴胡, thotowax root).

For blood deficiency, use *Sì Wù Tāng* (Four Substances Decoction) plus *chái hú* (柴胡, thotowax root), *rén shēn* (人参, ginseng), and *bái zhú* (白术, white atractylodes rhizome).

Using dry and aromatic medicinals without exception will damage clear and harmonious qi, and nothing can be engendered.

Generally, the formula to use is *Bǔ Fèi Sǎn* (补肺散, Lung Supplementing

Powder): treats rib-side pain.

shān yú (fructus corni)

dāng guī (Chinese angelica)

wǔ wèi (Chinese magnolivine fruit)

shān yào (common yam rhizome)

huáng qí (astragalus root)

chuān xiōng (sichuan lovage root)

shú dì (prepared rehmannia root)

mù guā (Chinese quince fruit)

bái zhú (white atractylodes rhizome)

dú huó (double teeth pubescent angelica root)

zǎo rén (spiney date seed)

Take the same amount of each medicine above and decoct in water.

In a variant edition, *shān yú* (山萸, fructus corni) is 2 *qian*, *dāng guī* (当 归, Chinese angelica) is 2 *qian*; *wǔ wèi* (五味, Chinese magnolivine fruit), 10 pieces; *huáng qí* (黄芪, astragalus root) 8 *fen*, *chuān xiōng* (川芎, sichuan lovage root) 6 *fen*, *shú dì* (熟地, prepared rehmannia root) 1 *qian* and 5 *fen*, *mù guā* (木 瓜, Chinese quince fruit) and *bái zhú* (白术, white atractylodes rhizome) each 1 *qian*, *dú huó* (独活, double teeth pubescent angelica root) 8 *fen*, *zǎo rén* (枣仁, spiney date seed) 1 *qian*, ginger 1 *slice*. There is no *shān yào* (山药, common yam rhizome).

Treatment Methods for Various Postpartum Symptoms XXXVI

产后诸症治法 三十六

阴痛
Vaginal Pain

产后起居太早，产门感风作痛，衣被难近身体，宜用祛风定痛汤。

川芎（一钱）	当归（三钱）
独活（五分，炒黑）	防风（五分，炒黑）
肉桂（五分，炒黑）	荆芥（五分，炒黑）
茯苓（一钱）	地黄（二钱）

Suppose after delivery, the patient starts out-of-bed activity too soon. At this time, the birth gate is invaded by wind and can cause such pain that the body can not touch clothes or quilt.

It is proper to take *Qù fēng Dìng Tòng Tāng* (祛风定痛汤, Wind Dispelling and Pain Settling Decoction).

chuān xiōng (Sichuan lovage root), 1 *qian*

dāng guī (Chinese angelica), 1 *qian*

dú huó (double teeth pubescent angelica root), 5 *fen*

fáng fēng (saposhnikovia root), 5 *fen*

ròu guì (cinnamon bark), 5 *fen*

jīng jiè (schizonepeta), 5 *fen* (charred)

fú líng (poria), 1 *qian*

dì huáng (rehmannia root), 2 *qian*

zǎo (Chinese date), 2 pieces

Decoct the formula in water and take it.

又附阴疮阴蚀。阴中疮曰匿疮，或痛或痒，如虫行状，浓汁淋漓。阴蚀几尽者，由心肾烦郁，胃气虚弱，致气血流滞。经云：诸疮痛痒，皆属于心。治当补心养肾，外以药熏洗。宜用十全阴疮散。

川芎	当归
白芍	地榆
甘草	

各等分。水五碗，煎二碗，去渣熏。日三夜四，先熏后洗。

Note on vaginal sores and ulcers: Sores in the vaginal area are called private sores. They may be painful or itching like worms crawling and thick discharge dripping wet. In nearly all these cases, vaginal sores and ulcers are due to stagnated qi and blood caused by vexed and depressed heart, kidney, and stomach qi deficiency. The classic states, "All types of sores with pain and itching are ascribed to the heart." The proper treatment should be supplementing the heart and nourishing the kidneys. Externally, the patient should steam and wash the sore with medicinals.

The appropriate formula is *Shí Quán Yīn Gān Sǎn* (十全阴疮散，Perfect Vaginal Sore Powder):

chuān xiōng (Sichuan lovage root)

dāng guī (Chinese angelica)

bái sháo (white peony root)

dì yú, (garden burnet root)

gān cǎo (licorice root)

Boil the formula (same amount) in 5 bowls of water down to 2 bowls. Remove the dregs and steam the affected area with the decoction, then wash the sores and ulcers with the same decoction, three times in the day and four times at night.

产后诸症治法 三十七

恶露
Lochia

　　即系裹儿污血。产时恶露随下，则腹不痛而产自安。若腹欠温暖，或伤冷物，以致恶露凝块，日久不散，则虚症百出。或身热骨蒸，食少羸瘦，或五心烦热，月水不行，其块在两胁，动则雷鸣，嘈杂晕眩，发热似疟，时作时止。如此数症，治者欲泄其邪，先补其虚，必用补中益气汤送三消丸，则元气不损，恶露可消。

If the lochia is discharged with delivery, there will be no abdominal pain, and the delivery will go smoothly. If the abdomen is not warm enough or is affected by cold substances (i.e., food), the lochia will coagulate into clots and be retained for a long time. Various deficient symptoms will then arise. For instance, generalized fever, steaming bone, less food intake, marasmus, vexing heat in the chest, palms, and soles, or menstrual stoppage (amenorrhea). If the clots are scattered around the ribs, then there may be thunderous rumbling upon movement, gastric upset, dizziness, and malaria-like fever with fitful attacks.

To treat these various symptoms, physicians should first supplement the deficiency to drain the pathogenic factors. Additionally, to protect the original qi from damage and disperse the lochia, the indispensable formula choice is to take *Bǔ Zhōng Yì Qì Tāng* (补中益气汤, Center-Supplementing and Qi-Boosting Decoction) with *Sān Xiāo Wán* (三消丸, Three Dispersing Pills).

　　加味补中益气汤：
　　人参（一钱）　　　　　　　　　白术（二钱）

当归（三钱）　　　　　黄芪（一钱，炙）

白芍（一钱）　　　　　广皮（四分）

甘草（四分）　　　　　姜、枣煎服

Variation:

Jiā Wèi Bǔ Zhōng Yì Qì Tāng (加味补中益气汤，Supplemented Center-Supplementing and Qi-Boosting Decoction):

rén shēn (ginseng), 1 *qian*

bái zhú (white atractylodes rhizome), 2 *qian*

dāng guī (Chinese angelica), 3 *qian*

huáng qí (astragalus root), 1 *qian*

bái sháo (white peony root), 1 *qian*

guǎng pí, (pericarpium citri reticulatae chachiensis), 4 *fen*

gān cǎo (licorice root), 4 *fen*

Decoct the formula with Ginger and *zǎo* (枣，Chinese date) in water and take orally.

三消丸：治妇人死血、食积、痰三等症。

黄连（一两，一半用吴萸煎汁去渣浸炒，　　　川芎（五钱）

一半用益智仁炒，去益智仁不用）

莱菔子（一两五钱，炒）　　　　　桃仁（十粒）

山栀（五钱，醋炒）　　　　　　　青皮（五钱，醋炒）

三棱（五钱，醋炒）　　　　　　　莪术（五钱，醋炒）

山楂（一两）　　　　　　　　　　香附（一两，童便浸炒）

上为末，蒸饼为丸。食远服，用补中益气汤送下五六十丸；或用白术三钱，陈皮五钱，水一盅，煎五分送下亦可。

此方治产后伤食，恶露不尽。若初产恶露不下，宜服生化汤加楂炭三钱。每日一帖，连服四剂，妙。

Sān Xiāo Wán (三消丸，Three Dispersing Pills): Treats the three symptoms of stagnated blood, food accumulation and phlegm in women.

huáng lián (黄连，coptis rhizome) 1 *liang*, half soaked and dry-fried in decocted *wú yú* (吴萸，medicinal evodia fruit) with dregs removed; half dry-fried with *yì zhì rén* (益智仁，Semen Amomi Amari) which is removed afterwards.

chuān xiōng (Sichuan lovage root), 5 *qian*

lái fú zǐ (radish seed), 1 liang and 5 *qian*

táo rén (peach kernel), 10 pieces

shān zhī (cape jasmine fruit), 5 *qian*

qīng pí (green tangerine peel), 5 *qian*

sān léng (common burr reed tuber), 5 *qian*

é zhú (curcumae rhizome), 5 *qian*

shān zhā (Chinese hawthorn fruit), 1 *liang*

xiāng fù (cyperus), 1 *liang*

Grind the above medicinals into powder, steam it and make it into pills. Administer between meals. Take 50-60 pills with *Bǔ Zhōng Yì Qì Tāng* (补中益气 汤, Center-Supplementing and Qi-Boosting Decoction) or with 3 *qian* of *bái zhú* (白 术, white atractylodes rhizome) and 5 *qian* of *chén pí* (陈皮, aged tangerine peel), which are boiled in a cup of water down to half.

This formula treats postpartum food damage and retention of the lochia.

For retention of the lochia shortly after delivery, it is advisable to take *Shēng Huà Tāng* (生化汤, Engendering and Transforming Decoction) with 3 *qian* of charred *shān zhā* (山楂, Chinese hawthorn fruit). 1 *ji* per day. If the patient takes 4 *ji* in succession, a magic effect will be seen.

Chapter One Hundred and Eleven
Treatment Methods for Various Postpartum Symptoms XXXVIII

产后诸症治法 三十八

乳痈
Mammary Yong (Acute Mastitis)

乳头属足厥阴肝经,乳房属足阳明胃经。若乳房臃肿,结核色红,数日外肿痛溃稠脓,脓尽而愈,此属胆胃热毒,气血壅滞,名曰乳痈,易治。若初起内结小核,不红不肿不痛,积之岁月,渐大如巉岩山,破如熟榴,难治。治法:痛肿寒热宜发表散邪,痛甚宜疏肝清胃,脓成不溃用托里。肌肉不生,脓水清稀,宜补脾胃;脓出及溃,恶寒发热,宜补血气;饮食不进,或作呕吐,宜补胃气。乳岩初起,用益气养荣汤加归脾汤,间可内消。若用行气破血之剂,速亡甚矣。

The nipples belong to the foot *jueyin* liver meridian, while the breasts belong to the foot *yangming* stomach meridian. If swelling of the breast with red nodules occurs several days after delivery, the nodules become painful ulcers with sticky pus that discharges, which then heal with the elimination of pus; it is due to toxic heat in the gallbladder and stomach as well as stagnation of qi and blood. This condition is called "mammary yong" (acute mastitis), and it is easy to treat.

If initially, inside the breasts, there are small nodules which do not show a red color and are not swollen or painful, but last for years and grow larger until they are like precipitous rocky mountains, and then become like ripe pomegranate fruits when breaking, this is called "mammary rock" (breast cancer), and it is difficult to treat.

Treatment methods:

If there is pain, swelling, and alternating cold and fever, effuse the exterior and disperse pathogenic factors.

If there is severe pain, soothe the liver and clear the stomach.

If there is the development of pus that does not discharge, expel the pus by strengthening vital qi.

If the wounds do not mend and the skin does not come together, and there is a thin, clear pus discharge, supplement the spleen and stomach.

It is appropriate to supplement qi and blood for discharging of pus and aversion to cold with fever.

It is advisable to supplement stomach qi for inability to eat or retching and vomiting.

At the initial stage of mammary rock (breast cancer), use *Yì Qì Yǎng Róng Tāng* (益气养荣汤, Qi Boosting and Construction Nourishing Decoction) plus *Guī Pí Tāng* (归脾汤, Spleen-Restoring Decoction). Occasionally, it may be possible to melt away.

Using qi-removing and blood cracking formulas will only hasten death.

瓜蒌散：治一切痈疽，并治乳痈。痈者，六腑不和之气，阳滞于阴则生之。

瓜蒌（一个，连皮捣烂）	生甘草（五分）
当归（三钱）	乳香（五分，灯心炒）
金银花（三钱）	白芷（一钱）
没药（五分，灯心炒）	青皮（五分）

水煎，温服。

Guā Lóu Sǎn (瓜蒌散, Snakegourd Fruit Powder): treats all types of swelling abscess and flat abscess, including acute mastitis. A swelling abscess is due to disharmony of the qi of the six bowels.

If yang stagnates within yin, yong (swelling abscess) may be generated.

guā lóu (snakegourd fruit), 1 piece (smashed with its pericarpium)

shēng gān cǎo (fresh licorice root), 5 *fen*

dāng guī (Chinese angelica), 3 *qian*

rǔ xiāng (frankincense), 5 *fen* [dry-fried with *dēng xīn* (灯心, juncus)]

jīn yín huā (honeysuckle flower), 3 *qian*

bái zhǐ (angelica root), 1 *qian*

mò yào (myrrh), 5 *fen* [dry-fried with *dēng xīn* (灯心, juncus)]

qīng pí (green tangerine peel), 5 *fen*

Decoct the formula in water and take orally.

回脉散：乳痈未溃时服此，毒从大便出，虚人不用。

大黄（三钱半）　　　　　　白芷（八分）

乳香（五分）　　　　　　　木香（五分）

没药（五分）　　　　　　　穿山甲（五分，蛤粉拌炒）

共为末，人参二钱煎汤，调药末服。

（一本大黄作三钱，有人参三钱。）

（穿山甲现为国家一级保护动物，捕猎穿山甲是违法的。穿山甲不准入药。）

Huí Mài Săn (回脉散, Pulse Retrieving Powder): This powder should be used before the mammary yong breaks, the pus is not yet discharged, and the toxins are discharged through defecation. It should not be used in patients with a deficient syndrome.

dà huáng (rhubarb root and rhizome), 3.5 *qian*

bái zhĭ (angelica root), 8 *fen*

rŭ xiāng (frankincense), 5 *fen*

mù xiāng (common aucklandia root), 5 *fen*

mò yào (myrrh), 5 *fen*

chuān shān jiǎ (pangolin scales), 5 *fen*, dry-fried with *gé fĕn* (蛤粉, clam shell powder)

(The pangolin is now one of the Class I State Protected Animals. It is illegal to catch and hunt Pangolins. They can no longer be used for medicinal purposes.)

Grind above medicinals into powder. Decoct 2 *qian* of *rén shēn* (人参, ginseng), mix *rén shēn* (人参, ginseng) docotion in the powdered medicinals and take.

(In a variant edition, *dà huáng* (大黄, rhubarb root and rhizome) is 3 *qian* and *rén shēn* (人参, ginseng) is also 3 *qian*)

十全大补汤：

人参（三钱）　　　　　　　白术（三钱）

黄芪（三钱）　　　　　　　熟地（三钱）

茯苓（八分）　　　　　　　甘草（五分）

川芎（八分）　　　　　　　金银花（三钱）

泻加黄连、肉果，渴，加麦冬、五味，寒热往来用马蹄香捣散。凡乳痈服薏苡仁粥好。又方，用乌药软白香辣者五钱，研，水一碗，牛皮胶一片，同煎七分，温服。如孕妇腹内痛，此二方可通用。

一本人参四味各二钱。

又有乳吹，乃小儿饮乳，口气所吹，乳汁不通，壅结作痛。不急治则成痈，宜速服瓜蒌散，更以手揉散之。

Shí Quán Dà Bǔ Tāng (十全大补汤, Perfect Major Supplementation Decoction):

rén shēn (ginseng), 3 qian

bái zhú (white atractylodes rhizome), 3 qian

huáng qí (astragalus root), 3 qian

shú dì (prepared rehmannia root), 3 qian

fú líng (poria), 8 fen

gān cǎo (licorice root), 5 fen

chuān xiōng (Sichuan lovage root), 8 fen

jīn yín huā (honeysuckle flower), 3 qian

Formula Variations:

If there is diarrhea, add huáng lián (黄连, coptis rhizome), ròu guǒ (肉果, nutmeg).

If there is thirst, add mài dōng (麦冬, dwarf lilyturf tuber) and wǔ wèi (五味, Chinese magnolivine fruit).

If there is alternating fever and chills, add pounded mǎ tí xiāng (马蹄香, saruma henryi).

For any mammary yong, it is beneficial to take yì yǐ rén (薏苡仁, coix seed) gruel.

Alternative Formula:

Use 5 qian wū yào (乌药, combined spicebush root), which is soft, white, smells fragrant, and tastes spicy, ground and boiled with one slice of ox-hide glue in a bowl of water down to 7/10. Take it warm. For abdominal pain in pregnant women, either of these two formulas may be used.

(In a variant edition, rén shēn (人参, ginseng) and the other three medicinals are each 2 qian.)

In addition, there is ru chui (suckling breast abscess), a condition caused by the stoppage of milk due to congestion and binding. If not treated immediately, it will develop into yong. It is appropriate in this case to administrate *Guā Lóu Sǎn* (瓜蒌散, Snakegourd Fruit Powder) without delay and rub the breast with hands to free the congestion.

Treatment Methods for Various Postpartum Symptoms XXXIX

产后诸症治法 三十九

风甚
Severe Wind

用山羊血取色新者，于新瓦上焙干，研末，老酒冲下五六分为度。重者用至八分，其效如神。

又用抱不出壳鸡子，瓦上焙干，酒调服。

如治虚寒危症，用蓝须子根刮皮，新瓦上焙干，研末，温服一钱为度。虽危可保万全。

Take fresh goat's blood, bake it dry on a new clay tile, and grind it. Administer 5~6 *fen* per dose with old millet wine. In serious cases, use as much as 8 *fen*. It has a magical effect.

Another method: bake eggs with chicken not hatched yet on a clay tile till dry. Mix with millet wine and take.

To treat critical conditions such as a deficient cold syndrome, use the root bark of *lanxuzi**, bake it on a new tile till dry, and grind it into powder. Take warm, 1 *qian* per dose. No matter how dangerous, this is a trusted remedy.

*

lanxuzi: Unidentifiable. Possibly *yuán hú suǒ* (corydalis rhizome).

Treatment Methods for Various Postpartum Symptoms XL

产后诸症治法 四十

不语
Aphasia

乃恶血停蓄于心，故心气闭塞，舌强不语，用七珍散。

人参（一两）	石菖蒲（一两）
川芎（一两）	生地（一两）
辰砂（五分，研）	防风（五钱）
细辛（一钱）	

共为细末，用薄荷汤下一钱。因痰气郁结，闭口不语者，用好明矾一钱，水飞过，沸汤送下。

一方治产后不语。

人参	石莲子（去心）
石菖蒲	

各等分。水煎服。

《妇人良方》云：产后喑，心肾虚不能发声，七珍散。脾气郁结，归脾汤，脾伤食少，四君子汤。气血俱虚，八珍汤，不应，独参汤，更不效急加附子，盖补其血气以生血。若单用佛手散等破血药，误矣。

Loss of voice (aphasia), is due to malign blood stagnating and accumulating in the heart. The heart qi is blocked and the tongue becomes stiff and results in loss of speech.

Use *Qī Zhēn Sǎn* (七珍散, Seven Gem Powder) for this condition.

rén shēn (ginseng), 1 *liang*

shí chāng pú (grassleaf sweetflag rhizome), 1 *liang*

chuān xiōng (Sichuan lovage root), 1 *liang*

shēng dì (rehmannia root), 1 *liang*

chén shā (cinnabar), 5 *fen*

fáng fēng (saposhnikovia root), 5 *qian*

xì xīn (asarum), 1 *qian*

Grind the above medicinals into a fine powder. Take 1 *qian* the powder and wash it down with *Bò He Tāng* (薄荷汤，Wild Mint Herb Decoction).

For aphasia due to accumulating and binding of phlegm, use 1 *qian* high quality *míng fán* (明矾，alum), and grind it with water. Take it down with hot water.

Another alternative formula for postpartum loss of speech:

rén shēn (ginseng)

shí lián zǐ (nelumbinis seed) (plumules removed)

shí chāng pú (grassleaf sweetflag rhizome)

All in equal amounts. Decoct in water and take it orally.

Furen Liangfang (《妇人良方》，*Complete Book of Effective Prescriptions for Women*) says:

If there is postpartum loss of voice, or inability of the voice due to heart and kidney deficiency, use *Qī Zhēn Sǎn* (七珍散，Seven Gem Powder). If it is due to spleen qi stagnation, use *Guī Pí Tāng* (归脾汤，Spleen-Restoring Decoction). If there is loss of appetite due to damage of the spleen, use *Sì Jūn Zǐ Tāng* (四君子 汤，Four Gentlmen Decoction). For dual deficiency of qi and blood, use *Bā Zhēn Tāng* (八珍汤，Eight-Gem Decoction). If it fails to respond, *Dú Shēn Tāng* (独参 汤，Pure Ginseng Decoction) is advisable. Add *fù zǐ* (附子，prepared aconite root) immediately when use of *Dú Shēn Tāng* (独参汤，Pure Ginseng Decoction) has no effect, since blood is generated through supplementing qi. It is a serious mistake if only formulas for breaking blood stasis such as *Fó Shǒu Sǎn* (佛手散，Finger Citron Powder) are used.

Addendum

补集

产后大便不通

　　用生化汤内减黑姜，加麻仁。胀满加陈皮，血块痛加肉桂、元胡。如燥结十日以上，肛门必有燥粪，用蜜枣导之。

　　炼蜜枣法：

　　用好蜜二三两，火炼滚，至茶褐色，先用湿桌，倾蜜在桌上，用手作如枣样。插肛门，待欲大便，去蜜枣，方便。

　　又方，用麻油，口含竹管入肛门内，吹油四五口，腹内粪和即通。或猪胆亦可。

　　To treat postpartum constipation, use *Shēng Huà Tāng* (生化汤，Engendering and Transforming Decoction), and substitute *má rén* (麻仁，Hemp Seed) for *hēi jiāng* (黑姜，prepared dried ginger).

　　If there is fullness and distention, add *chén pí* (陈皮，aged tangerine peel).

　　If there is blood clot pain, add *ròu guì* (肉桂，cinnamon bark), *yuán hú* (元胡，corydalis tuber).

　　If the accumulation of dry feces lasts more than ten days, there must be dry feces in the anus. Therefore, use the honey date to conduct it out.

　　Method for processing honey date:

　　Take 2~3 *liang* high-quality honey. Heat it to be boiling and do not stop till it turns to tea-brown color. Pour the honey onto a moist table and shape it by hand into a "date" (a suppository in date shape). Put the "date" into the anus and retain it till a desire appears to defecate. Then, remove the date and defecate.

　　Another method:

　　Insert a bamboo tube into the anus, hold sesame oil in the mouth, and then blow 4~5 mouthfuls of oil into the anus. When the oil has mixed with the feces in the intestine, the bowels will relax. Pig bile can substitute for oil.

Chapter One Hundred and Fifteen
Postpartum Chicken's Claw Wind

治产后鸡爪风

桑柴灰（三钱，存性）　　　　　鱼胶（三钱，炒）
手指甲（十二个，炒）
共为末，黄酒送下，取汗即愈。

Chicken's claw wind is a syndrome of hypertonicity of the sinews with body trembling, handshaking, and difficulty moving. In addition, spasms make the hands look like a chicken's claw. This results from the over-effulgent liver fire drying up the blood.

sāng chái huī (mulberry twig burned into ash, without destroying nature), 3 *qian*,

yú jiāo, (fish gelatin), 3 *qian*

shǒu zhǐ jiǎ (fingernail), 12, dry-fried

Grind the above materials into a powder, take it with millet wine. When the patient begins to sweat, recovery is achieved.

Bǎo Chǎn Wú Yōu Sǎn (Safe Pregnancy Without Worry Powder)

保产无忧散

当归（钱半，酒洗）　　　　炒黑芥穗（八分）

川芎（钱半）　　　　　　　艾叶（七分，炒）

面炒枳壳（六分）　　　　　炙黄芪（八分）

菟丝子（钱四分，酒炒）　　厚朴（七分，姜炒）

羌活（五分）　　　　　　　川贝母（一钱，去心）

白芍（钱二分，酒炒）　　　甘草（五分）

姜三片，温服。

上方保胎，每月三五服。临产热服，催生如神。

dāng guī (Chinese angelica), 1 *qian* and 5 *fen* (washed with millet wine)

hēi jiè suì (charred schizonepeta), 8 *fen*

chuān xiōng (Sichuan lovage root), 1 *qian* and 5 *fen*

ài yè (mugwort leaf), 7 *fen*

zhǐ qiào (bitter orange), 6 *fen*, (dry-fried with wheat flour)

huáng qí (astragalus root), 5 *fen* (honey fried)

tù sī zǐ (dodder seed), 1 *qian* and 4 *fen* (dry-fried with millet wine)

hòu pò (magnolia bark), 7 *fen*

qiāng huó (notoptetygium root), 5 *fen*

chuān bèi mǔ (Sichuan fritillaria bulb) , 1 *qian* (pith removed)

bái sháo (white peony root), 1 *qian* and 2 *fen* (dry-fried with millet wine)

gān cǎo (licorice root), 5 *fen*

jiāng (ginger), 3 *slices*

Take the decoction warm.

The above formula protects the fetus. Take 3~5 times per month. Towards delivery, take warm. The formula hastens delivery magically.

治遍体浮肿

是脾虚水溢之过。凡浮肿者可通用，俱神效。

真缩砂仁四两，莱菔子二两四钱，研末，水浸浓取汁，浸砂仁，候汁尽，晒干，研极细末。每服一钱，渐加至二钱为度，淡姜汤送下。

Generalized edema is caused by water overflow/spillage due to spleen deficiency. The following formula is advisable for any water edema, and it can always result in a miraculous effect.

Shā rén (砂仁, villous amomum fruit) 4 *liang, lái fú zǐ* (莱菔子, radish seed) 2 *liang* and 4 *qian,* grind and dip *lái fú zǐ* (莱菔子, radish seed) in water, when it is thoroughly soaked, put *shā rén* (砂仁, villous amomum fruit) in this juice till all the juice has been absorbed. Dry *shā rén* (砂仁, villous amomum fruit) in the sun and finally grind it very fine. Administer 1 *qian* at a time. Increase the dosage gradually to 2 *qian* at the most. Swallow it with dilute boiled ginger water.

Bǎo Chǎn Shén Xiào Fāng (Child-birth Protecting Magic Formula)

保产神效方

未产能安，临产能催。偶伤胎气，腰疼腹痛，甚至见红不止，势欲小产，危急之际，一服即愈，再服全安。临产时交骨不开，横生逆下，或子死腹中，命在垂危，服之奇效。

全当归（一钱五分，酒洗）　　　紫厚朴（七分，姜汁炒）

真川芎（一钱五分）　　　　　　菟丝子（一钱五分，酒泡）

川贝母（二钱，去心）　　　　　枳壳（六分，面炒）

川羌活（六分）　　　　　　　　荆芥穗（八分）

黄芪（八分，蜜炙）　　　　　　蕲艾（五分，醋炒）

炙草（五分）　　　　　　　　　白芍（一钱二分，冬用二钱，酒炒）

生姜（三片）

水二盅，煎八分，渣水一盅，煎六分，产前空心预服二剂，临产随时热服。此方仙传奇方，慎勿以庸医轻加减其分两。

This formula can ensure safety before delivery and hasten parturition in the preliminary stage of labor.

In the case of accidentally hurting the fetal qi with lumbar and abdominal pain (also in the case of a critical condition of incessant bleeding bordering on abortion), taking the following formula one time can stop the bleeding.

Taking the following formula a second time will make the delivery go smoothly. If there is a failure of the pubic bones to move in the course of labor, transverse or inverted presentation, or fetus's death in the abdomen with the mother's life in danger, take it, and a magical effect will be seen.

dāng guī (Chinese angelica), 1 *qian* and 5 *fen* (washed with millet wine)

hòu pò (magnolia bark), 7 *fen* (fried with ginger juice)

chuān xiōng (Sichuan lovage root), 1 *qian* and 5 *fen*

tù sī zǐ (dodder seed), 1 *qian* and 5 *fen* (dipped in millet wine)

chuān bèi mǔ (Sichuan fritillaria bulb) , 2 *qian* (pith removed)

zhǐ qiào (bitter orange), 6 *fen* (dry-fried with flour)

qiāng huó (notoptetygium root), 6 *fen* (honey-fried)

jīng jiè suì (fineleaf schizonepeta spike), 8 *fen*

huáng qí (astragalus root), 8 *fen*

qí ài (mugwort leaf), 5 *fen*

zhì cǎo (prepared licorice root), 5 *fen*

bái sháo (white peony root), 1 *qian* and 2 *fen* (dry-fried with millet wine, use only 2 *fen* in winter)

shēng jiāng (ginger), 3 slices

Decoct the formula in 2 bowls of water, take 8/10 of decoction, then decoct the dregs in 1 bowl of water and take 6/10 decoction. Take 2 *ji* on an empty stomach before delivery. Take it warm any time near the time of labor. Do not modify the dosage of the formula casually.

Herbal Formulas and Variations for Various Symptoms Steaming Bone

骨蒸

宜服保真汤。先服清骨散。

柴胡梅连汤：即清骨散作汤，速效。

柴胡（二两）	前胡（二两）
黄连（二两）	乌梅（二两，去核）

共为末听用。再将猪脊骨一条，猪苦胆一个，韭菜白十根，各一寸，同捣成泥，入童便一酒盏，搅如稀糊，入药末，再捣为丸，如绿豆大，每服三四十丸，清汤送下。如上膈热多，食后服。此方凡男女骨蒸皆可用之，不专治产妇。

It is advisable to take *Bǎo Zhēn Tāng* (保真汤, True Safeguarding Decoction). However, before that, take *Qīng Gǔ Sǎn* (清骨散, Bones Clearing Powder) first.

Chái Hú Méi Lián Tāng (柴胡梅连汤, Bupleurum, Smoked Plum, and Coptis Rhizome Decoction): also known as *Qīng Gǔ Sǎn* (清骨散, Bones Clearing Powder). A rapid effect can be seen if decocted.

chái hú (bupleurum),

qián hú (hogfennel root)

huáng lián (coptis rhizome)

wū méi (smoked plum)

Each 2 *liang*, powdered for use.

Next, get one pig spine, one pig gallbladder, and ten white sections of Chinese chive stalk, 1 *cun* each (about 3.3cm). Crush these materials together, mix with a tiny cup of little boy's urine, and stir into a thin paste. Add the medicine powder into the paste and pound again. Make pills the size of mung beans. Take 30~40 pills each time with water.

If there is heat above the diaphragm, take the pills after meals. This formula can be used for steaming bones in both males and females and is not just specific to birthing women.

保真汤：

黄芪（六分）	人参（二钱）
白术（二钱，炒）	炙草（四分）
川芎（六分）	当归（二钱）
天冬（一钱）	麦冬（二钱）
白芍（二钱）	枸杞（二钱）
黄连（六分，炒）	黄柏（六分，炒）
知母（二钱）	生地（二钱）
五味（十粒）	地骨皮（六分）

枣（三枚，去核）

水煎服。（一本无麦冬、黄连。）

Bǎo Zhēn Tāng (保真汤，True Safeguarding Decoction):

huáng qí (astragalus root), 6 *fen*

rén shēn (ginseng), 2 *qian*

bái zhú (white atractylodes rhizome), 2 *qian*

zhì gān cǎo (prepared licorice root), 4 *fen*

chuān xiōng (Sichuan lovage root), 6 *fen*

dāng guī (Chinese angelica), 2 *qian*

tiān dōng (asparagus tuber), 1 *qian*

mài dōng (dwarf lilyturf tuber), 2 *qian*

bái sháo (white peony root), 2 *qian*

gǒu qǐ (Chinese wolfberry fruit), 2 *qian*

huáng lián (coptis rhizome), 6 *fen*

huáng bǎi (amur cork-tree bark), 6 *fen*

zhī mǔ (common anemarrhena rhizome), 2 *qian*

shēng dì (rehmannia root), 2 *qian*

wǔ wèi (Chinese magnolivine fruit), 10 pieces

dì gǔ pí (Chinese wolfberry root-bark), 6 *fen*

zǎo (Chinese date), 3 pieces (pitted)

Decoct the above formula in water and take orally.

[In a variant edition there is no *mài dōng* (麦冬，dwarf lilyturf tuber) and *huáng lián* (黄连，coptis rhizome).]

加味大造汤: 治骨蒸劳热。若服清骨散、梅连丸不效服此方。

人参（一两）	当归（一两）
麦冬（八分）	石斛（八分，酒蒸）
柴胡（六钱）	生地（二两）
胡连（五钱）	山药（一两）
枸杞（一两）	黄柏（七分，炒）

先将麦冬、地黄捣烂，后入诸药同捣为丸，加蒸紫河车另捣，焙干为末，炼蜜丸。

（一本麦冬、石斛仅作八钱，柴胡五钱，黄柏四分，酒炒。）

Jiā Wèi Dà Zào Wán (加味大造汤, Supplemented Great Building Pills): Treats steaming bone deficiency fever. Take this formula if *Qīng Gǔ Sǎn* (清骨散, Bones Clearing Powder) or *Chái Hú Méi Lián Wán* (柴胡梅连丸, Bupleurum, Smoked Plum, and Coptis Rhizome Pill) failed to bring effect:

rén shēn (ginseng), 1 *liang*

dāng guī (Chinese angelica), 1 *liang*

mài dōng (dwarf lilyturf tuber), 8 *fen*

shí hú (dendrobium), 8 *fen* (steamed with millet wine)

chái hú (bupleurum), 6 *qian*

shēng dì (rehmannia root), 2 *liang*

hú lián (figwort flower), 5 *qian*

shān yào (common yam rhizome), 1 *liang*

gǒu qǐ (Chinese wolfberry fruit), 1 *liang*

huáng bǎi (amur cork-tree bark), 7 *fen* (dry-fried)

First, smash *mài dōng* (麦冬, dwarf lilyturf tuber) and *shēng dì* (生地, rehmannia root). Then mix it with the rest of the medicinals and pound together. Make the mixture into pills. Next, steam and then pound *zǐ hé chē* (紫河车, human placenta). Bake and powder it. Then mix it with heated honey and make it into pills.

[In a variant edition, *mài dōng* (麦冬, dwarf lilyturf tuber) and *shí hú* (石斛, dendrobium) are given at 8 *qian*. *Chái hú* (柴胡, bupleurum) is given at 5 *qian*, *huáng bǎi* (黄柏, amur cork-tree bark) is dry-fried with millet wine at 4 *fen*.]

虚劳

指节冷痛，头汗不止。

人参（三钱）　　　　　　当归（三钱）

黄芪（二钱）　　　　　　淡豆豉（十粒）

生姜（三片）　　　　　　韭白（十寸）

猪肾（二个）

先将猪肾煮熟，取汁煎药八分，温服。

（一本有或用猪胃一个。先将胃略煮后，再煎汤煮药。）

Symptoms: The joints of fingers are cold and painful with incessant sweating on the head.

rén shēn (ginseng), 3 *qian*

dāng guī (Chinese angelica), 3 *qian*

huáng qí (astragalus root), 2 *qian*

dàn dòu chǐ (prepared soybean), 10 pieces

shēng jiāng (ginger), 3 *slices*

jiǔ bái (white part of Chinese chives), 10 *cùn* (about 33 cm)

zhū shèn (pig's kidney), 2

First, cook the kidney well and then decoct the medicinals in the soup down to 8/10. Take it warm.

(A variant edition uses 1 pig's stomach instead of kidneys. The stomach is boiled for a while and then the medicinals are decocted in the soup.)

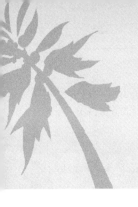

附录1

· 中药汇总表 ·

阿胶	donkey-hide gelatin	赤石脂	Halloysite
艾叶	Argy Wormwood Leaf	川贝	Sichuan Fritillaria (Bulb)
巴戟天	Morinda Root	川贝母	Tendrilleaf Fritillaria Bulb
白扁豆	Hyacinth Bean	川芎	Sichuan Lovage Rhizome
白矾、明矾	Alum	葱白	Fistular Onion Stalk
白果	ginkgo nut	大葱	Green Chinese Onion
白芨	Hyacinth Bletilla	大腹皮	Areca Peel
白蔻	Cardamon Fruit	大黄	rhubarb root and rhizome
白茅根	Cogon Grass Rhizome	大枣、红枣、枣	Fructus Ziziphi Jujubae
白芍、白芍药	white peony root	丹皮、粉丹皮	cortex moutan
白术	white atractylodes rhizome	胆星曲	Bile Arisaema Leaven
白芷	Dahurian Angelica Root	淡豆豉	Fermented Soybean
柏子仁	Chinese Arborvitae Kernel		Decoction
半夏	Pinellia Tuber	淡豆豉	Fermented Soybean
半夏曲	Fermented Pinellia	淡竹叶	Lophatherum Herb
薄荷	Wild Mint Herb	当归	Chinese angelica
荸荠	Chinese Water-chestnut	党参	Tangshen
蓖麻子	Castor Seed	灯心草	Common Rush
扁豆	Dolichos Lablab	地骨皮	Chinese Wolfberry Root-bark
槟榔	Areca Seed	地榆	Garden Burnet Root
补骨脂	Malaytea Scurfpea Fruit	丁香	Clove
苍术	atractylodes rhizome	冬葵子	Cluster Mallow Fruit
草豆蔻	Katsumada Galangal Seed	独活	Doubleteeth Pubescent
草果	Fruit of Caoguo		Angelica Root
柴胡	thotowax root	杜仲	Eucommia Bark
常山	Antifeverile Dichroa Root	莪术	curcumae rhizome
车前子	plantago seed	发灰、血余炭	Crinis Carbonisatus
陈皮	aged tangerine peel	防风	Divaricate Saposhnikovia
赤芍	Peony Root		Root

中药汇总表

粉草	Chinese Mesona	黄芩	scutellaria root
佛手	Finger Citron	藿香	Cablin Patchouli Herb
茯苓	poria	姜黄	Turmeric
茯神	Poria with Hostwood	僵蚕	Stiff Silkworm
浮小麦	Immature Wheat	金银花	Honeysuckle Bud and Flower
附子	prepared aconite root	荆芥	Fineleaf Schizonepeta Herb
覆盆子	Palmleaf Raspberry Fruit	荆芥穗	Spica Schizonepetae
甘草	licorice root	桔梗	Platycodon Root
甘遂	Gansui Root	橘红	Red Tangerine Peel
干姜	Dried Ginger	款冬花	Common Coltsfoot Flowe
葛根	Kudzuvine Root	莱菔子	Radish Seed
枸杞	Chinese Wolfberry Fruit	连翘	Weeping Forsythia Capsule
瓜蒌	Snakegourd Fruit	莲子	Lotus Seed
瓜蒌根	Snakegourd Root	灵芝	Glossy Ganoderma
贯众炭	charred cyrtomii rhizome	羚羊角	Antelope Horn
归尾	Angelicae Sinensis Radicis Extremita	刘寄奴	artemisia
		硫磺	Sulfur
龟板	Tortoise Carapace and Plastron	芦根	Reed Rhizome
桂心	cinnamon bark (Rough Skin Peeled)	鹿角	Deer Horn
		鹿角灰	ash of Deer Horn
桂圆肉	Longan Aril	鹿角霜	Degelatined Deer Horn Powder
桂枝	Cassia Twig		
蛤粉、蛤蜊粉	Concha Cyclinae Powder	鹿茸	Pilose Antler
蛤蚧	Tokay Gecko	萝卜籽	Radish Seed
诃子	Medicine Terminalia Fruit	麻黄	Ephedra
荷叶	Lotus Leaf	麻黄根	Ephedra Root
黑姜	prepared dried ginger	麻仁	Hemp Seed
黑芥穗	charred schizonepeta	马蹄香	Saruma Henryi
红花	Safflower	马蹄香	Saruma Henryi
厚朴	magnolia bark	麦冬	dwarf lilyturf tuber
胡黄连	Figwortflower Picrorhiza Rhizome	麦芽	Germinated Barley
		芒硝	Crystallized Sodium Sulfate
琥珀	Amber	没药	Myrrh
花椒	Pricklyash Peel	母丁香	Fructus Caryophylli（Mother of Clove）
滑石粉	Talcum Powder		
黄柏	amur cork-tree bark	牡蛎	Oyster Shell
黄连	coptis rhizome	木耳	Edible Tree Fungus
连须	scallion with fibrous root	木瓜	Common Floweringqince Fruit
黄芪	astragalus root		

木通	Akebia Stem	生地、地黄	rehmannia root
木香	Common Aucklandia Root	石菖蒲	Grassleaf Sweetflag Rhizome
牛膝、怀牛膝	two-toothed achyranthes root	石膏	gypsum
炮姜	Dry-fried Ginger	石斛	Dendrobium
莆草	Stem or Leaf of Cattail	熟地	prepared rehmannia root
蒲公英	Dandelion	苏木	Sappan Wood
蒲黄	Cattail Pollen	苏叶	Common Perilla Leaf
前胡	Hogfennel Root	苏子	Perilla Fruit
芡实	euryale seed	桃胶	Peach Gum
羌活	Incised Notopterygium Rhizome and Root	桃仁	*peach kernel*
		天冬	Cochinchinese Asparagus Root
青蒿	Sweet Wormwood Herb	天花粉	Snakegourd Root
青皮	green tangerine peel	天麻	Tall Gastrodia Tuber
瞿麦	Lilac Pink Herb	通草	Ricepaperplant Pith
人参	ginseng	菟丝子	Dodder Seed
肉苁蓉	Herba Cistanches	王不留行	cowherb seed
肉豆蔻、肉果	Nutmeg	乌梅	Smoked Plum
肉桂	cinnamon bark	乌药	Combined Spicebush Root
乳香	Frankincense	吴茱萸	Medicinal Evodia Fruit
三棱	*common burr reed tuber*	五倍子	Gold Thread
三七	Sanqi	五加皮	Acanthopanax Root Bark
桑白皮	White Mulberry Root-bark	五灵脂	Flying Squirrel's Droppings
桑寄生	Chinese Taxillus Herb	五味子	Chinese Magnoliavine Fruit
桑螵蛸	Mantis Egg-case	细辛	Asarum sieboldi Mig.
桑叶	Mulberry Leaf	香附	cyperus
沙参	Adenophora Stricta	薤白	Longstamen Onion Bulb
砂仁	Villous Amomum Fruit	杏仁	Bitter Apricot Seed
芍药	peony root	雄黄	Realgar
山药	common yam rhizome	续断	Himalayan Teasel Root
山萸肉	Fructus Corni	益母草	Motherwort Herb
山楂	Hawthorn Fruit	益智仁	Semen Amomi Amari
山茱萸	Asiatic Cornelian Cherry Fruit	益智仁	Semen Amomi Amari
		薏苡仁	Coix Seed
蛇床子	Common Cnidium Fruit	茵陈	virgate wormwood herb
蛇蜕	Snake Slough	鱼胶	Fish Gelatin
麝香	Musk	郁金	Turmeric Root Tuber
神曲	Medicated Leaven	郁李仁	Chinese Dwarf Cherry Seed
升麻	Largetrifoliolious Bugbane rhizome	元参	Kakuda Figwort Root
		元胡	corydalis tuber

中药汇总表

远志	Milkwort Root	炙甘草	Prepared Radix Glycyrrhizae
枣仁	Spine Date Seed	炙黄芪	Milkvetch Root (Honey-fried)
泽泻	Oriental Waterplantain Rhizome	朱砂、辰砂	Cinnabar
		竹沥	Henon Bamboo Juice
知母	common anemarrhena rhizome	竹茹	Bamboo Shavings
		竹叶	Folia Bambosae
栀子	gardenia	紫河车	Human Placenta
枳壳	Fructus Aurantii	紫苏	Purple Perilla
枳实	Immature Orange Fruit	棕榈	Fortune Windmillpalm Petiole

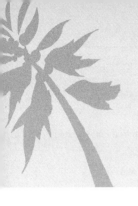

附录2

方剂汇总表

中文名称	英译	
安奠二天汤	Innate and Postnatal Tocolysis Decoction	Chapter Thirty-nine
安老汤	The Decoction for Calming the Aged	Chapter Seventeen
安神生化汤	Spirit Quieting, Engendering and Transforming Decoction	Chapter Seventy-nine
安神丸	Mind Tranquilizing Pills	Chapter Sixty-eight
安心汤	Heart Calming Decoction	Chapter Fifty-six
八味地黄丸	Eight Flavors Rehmannia Pills	Chapter Eighty-seven
八珍汤	Eight Precious Ingredients Decoction	Chapter Sixty-nine/Seventy/Ninety
保产神效方	Child-birth Protecting Magic Formula	Chapter One Hundred and Eighteen
保产无忧散	Carefree Pregnancy Powder	Chapter One Hundred and Eighteen
保真汤	True Safeguarding Decoction	Chapter One Hundred and Nineteen
并提汤	Double Lifting Decoction	Chapter Twenty-eight
补肺散	Lung Supplementing Powder	Chapter One Hundred and Eight
补气解晕汤	Qi Supplementing and Fainting Relieving Decoction	Chapter Fifty-four
补气解晕汤	Qi Supplementing and Fainting Relieving Decoction	Chapter Fifty-four
补气升肠饮	Qi Supplementing and Intestine Lifting Decoction	Chapter Fifty-seven
补气养荣汤	Qi Supplementing and Nutrient Nourishing Decoction	Chapter Seventy-eight
补血汤	Blood Supplementing Decoction	Chapter Twenty-five
补中益气汤	Middle Tonifying and qi Benefiting Decoction	Chapter One Hundred and One
参归生化汤	Engendering and Transforming Decoction with Ginseng and Chinese Angelica	Chapter One Hundred
参苓生化汤	Ginseng & Poria Engendering and Transforming Decoction	Chapter Ninety-four

方剂汇总表

参术膏	Ginseng and Largehead Atractylodes Rhizome Orally Taken Paste	Chapter Eighty-two
柴胡梅连汤	Chinese Thorowax, Smoked Plum and Gold Thread Decoction	Chapter One Hundred and Nineteen
柴胡清肝饮	Chinese Thorowax Root Liver Clearing Decoction	Chapter Eighty-two
肠宁汤	Intestine-quieting Decoction	Chapter Fifty-eight
趁痛散	Pain Expelling Powder	Chapter One Hundred and Six
承气汤	Purgative Decoction	Chapter Seventy-three
催生兔脑丸	Birth Hastening Rabbit Brain Pills	Chapter Seventy-one
当归补血汤	Chinese Angelica Blood-Supplementing Decoction	Chapter Fifty-five
当归六黄汤	Chinese Angelica Six Yellow Decoction	Chapter Eighty-seven/Eighty-eight
定经汤	Menstruation Regulating Decoction	Chapter Fifteen
独参汤	Pure Ginseng Decoction	Chapter Fifty-five/Sixty-two/One Hundred and Thirteen
独活汤	Doubleteeth Pubescent Angelica Decoction	Chapter Sixty-nine
夺命丹	Life Clutching Elixir	Chapter Seventy-one
佛手散	Finger Citron Powder	Chapter One Hundred and Thirteen
扶气止啼汤	Qi supporting and Cry Stopping Decoction	Chapter Forty-five
附子散	prepared aconite root Powder	Chapter Ninety-six
固本止崩汤	Constitution Strengthening and Bleeding Stopping Decoction	Chapter Six
固气汤	Qi Consolidating Decoction	Chapter Eight
固气填精汤	Qi Securing and Essence Replenishing Decoction	Chapter Forty-eight
瓜蒌散	Snakegourd Fruit Powder	Chapter One Hundred and Eleven
归脾汤	Spleen Invigorating Decoction	Chapter One Hundred and Two/One Hundred and Three
河车丸	Human Placenta Pills	Chapter Eighty-two
化水种子汤	Water Transforming and Conception Promoting Decoction	Chapter Thirty-six
黄芪补气汤	Milkvetch Root qi Supplementing Decoction	Chapter Fifty-one
黄芪补气汤	Milkvetch Root qi Supplementing Decoction	Chapter Fifty-two
回脉散	Pulse Retrieving Powder	Chapter One Hundred and Eleven
加参安肺生化汤	Lungs Calming, Engendering and Transforming Decoction Added with Ginseng	Chapter Ninety-eight

加参生化汤	Engendering and Transforming Decoction Added with Ginseng	Chapter Seven-six/Seventy-eight
加减补中益气汤	Modified Middle Tonifying and qi Benefiting Decoction	Chapter Thirty-eight
加减当归补血汤	Chinese Angelica Blood-Supplementing Variant Decoction	Chapter Seven
加减生化汤	Modified Engendering and Transforming Decoction	Chapter Eighty-six/Ninety-three/Ninety-five/Chapter Ninety-seven/One Hundred and Four/One Hundred and Five
加减四物汤	Modified Four Agents Decoction	Chapter Twenty-three/Chapter Fifty
加减养荣汤	Modified Construction Nourishing Decoction	Chapter One Hundred and Two
加减养胃汤	Modified Stomach Nourishing Decoction	Chapter Eighty-two
加味补中益气汤	Supplemented Middle Tonifying and qi Benefiting Decoction	Chapter Thirty-three/One Hundred and Ten
加味大造丸	Supplemented Great Creation Pills	Chapter One Hundred and Seven
加味生化汤	Supplemented Engendering and Transforming Decoction	Chapter Fifty-six/Sixty-one/Seventy-four/Eighty/Eighty-three/Chapter Ninety-four/Ninety-eight/One Hundred and three
加味四物汤	Supplemented Four Agents Decoction	Chapter Eighteen/Ninety-eight
加味逍遥散	Supplemented Free Wanderer Powder	Chapter Fifteen
加味芎归汤	Supplemented Sichuan Lovage Rhizome and Chinese Angelica Decoction	Chapter Seventy/Seventy-one
健固汤	Strengthening and Consolidating Decoction	Chapter Twenty-four
健脾化食散气汤	Spleen Strengthening, Food Transforming and qi Dispersing Decoction	Chapter Eighty-one
健脾利水生化汤	Spleen Strengthening and Water Disinhibiting, Engendering and Transforming Decoction	Chapter Ninety-three
健脾汤	Spleen Strengthening Decoction	Chapter One Hundred and One
健脾消食生化汤	Spleen Strengthening, Food Dispersing, Engendering and Transforming Decoction	Chapter Eighty
解郁汤	Depression Relieving Decoction	Chapter Forty-two
救败求生汤	Collapse Rescuing and Life Rekindling Decoction	Chapter Sixty-two
救损安胎汤	Injury Rescuing and Fetus Calming Decoction	Chapter Forty-three
救脱活母汤	Collapse Rescuing and Mother Saving Decoction	Chapter Fifty-nine

方剂汇总表

开郁种玉汤	Stagnation Relieving and Fertilization Improving Decoction	Chapter Thirty-two
宽带汤	*Dai mai* Releasing Decoction	Chapter Thirty-one
理气散瘀汤	Qi Regulating and Stasis Dissipating Decoction	Chapter Forty-nine
利火汤	Fire Discharging Decoction	Chapter Four
利气泄火汤	Qi Soothing and Fire Purging Decoction	Chapter Forty-seven
两地汤	Shengdi and Digupi Decoction	Chapter Thirteen
两收汤	Dual Withdrawing Decoction	Chapter Sixty-five
流气引子	Qi Flowing Drink	Chapter Eighty-one
六君子汤	Six Gentlemen Decoction	Chapter Ninety-five
麻黄根汤	Ephedra Root Decoction	Chapter Eighty-seven
茅根汤	Cogon Grass Rhizome Decoction	Chapter Ninety-one
木香槟榔丸	Common Aucklandia and Areca Seeds Pill	Chapter Eighty-one
木香生化汤	Common Aucklandia Root Engendering and Transforming Decoction	Chapter Eighty-one
平肝开郁止血汤	Liver Soothing, Depression Relieving, and Blood Stopping Decoction	Chapter Ten
平胃散	Stomach Harmonizing Powder	Chapter Seventy-one
七珍散	Seven Gem Powder	Chapter One Hundred and Thirteen
羌活养荣汤	Incised Notopterygium Nutrient-Nourishing Decoction	Chapter Sixty-eight
青娥丸	Young Maid Pills	Chapter One Hundred and Seven
青血丸	Green-Blue Blood Pills	Chapter Ninety-five
清骨滋肾汤	Bone Clearing and Kidney Nourishing Decoction	Chapter Thirty-four
清肝止淋汤	Liver Clearing and Liver-Clearing and Discharge Stopping Decoction	Chapter Five
清骨散	Bones Clearing Powder	Chapter One Hundred and Nineteen
清海丸	Sea of Blood Clearing Bolus	Chapter Twelve
清经散	Meridians Clearing Powder	Chapter Thirteen
祛风定痛汤	Wind Dispelling and Pain Settling Decoction	Chapter One Hundred and Nine
润肠粥	Intestine Moistening Gruel	Chapter Eighty-four
润燥安胎汤	Dryness Moistening and Fetus Calming Decoction	Chapter Fourth
三消丸	Three Dispersing Pills	Chapter One Hundred and Ten
散结定疼汤	Mass Dissipating and Pain Relieving Decoction	Chapter Fifty-eight
桑螵蛸散	Mantis Egg-case Powder	Chapter Ninety-two

升带汤	*Dai mai* Raising Decoction	Chapter Thirty-five
升举大补汤	Upraising and Greatly Tonifying Decoction	Chapter Seventy-seven
生化六和汤	Engendering, Transforming and Six Harmoniaztions Decoction	Chapter Ninety-six
生化汤	Engendering and Transforming Decoction	Chapter Seventy-one/Seventy-four
生津益液汤	Fluids Engendering and Humor Boosting Decoction	Chapter Ninety-seven
生津止渴益水饮	Fluid Engendering to Quench Thirst and Water Boosting Decoction	Chapter Eighty-nine
生脉散	Pulse Engendering Powder	Chapter Seventy-three/Seventy-six/Eighty-nine
生乳丹	Milk Producing Pills	Chapter Sixty-six
生血止崩汤	Blood Engendering and Bleeding Stopping Decoction	Chapter Seventy-seven
失笑散	Sudden Smile Powder	Chapter Seventy-one
十全大补汤	Perfect Major Supplementation Decoction	Chapter Sixty/One Hundred and Eleven
十全阴疳散	Perfect Vaginal Malnutrition Powder	Chapter One Hundred and Nine
石莲子散	Fructus Nelumbinis Powder	Chapter Ninety-seven
疏肝化滞汤	Liver Soothing and Stagnation Transforming Decoction	Chapter Thirty-seven
顺肝益气汤	Liver Soothing and qi Benefiting Decoction	Chapter Thirty-seven
顺经两安汤	Menstruation Normalizing and Heart and Kidneys Calming Decoction	Chapter Twenty-five
顺经汤	Menses Normalizing Decoction	Chapter Twenty-one
四君子汤	Four Gentlmen Decoction	Chapter One Hundred and Eight
四物汤	Four Agents Decoction	Chapter Ninety-five
四消丸	Four Dispersing Pills	Chapter One Hundred and One
送胞汤	Placenta Delivering Decoction	Chapter Fifty-three
送胞汤	Placenta Delivering Decoction	Chapter Fifty-three
天麻丸	Tall Gastrodia Tuber Pills	Chapter Eighty-five
调肝汤	Liver Regulating Decoction	Chapter Twenty
调经散	Menstruation Regulating Powder	Chapter Ninety-nine
通肝生乳汤	Liver Freeing and Milk Producing Decoction	Chapter Sixty-seven
通乳丹	Lactation Promoting Pills	Chapter Sixty-six
完胞饮	Uterus Renewing Decoction	Chapter Sixty-three
完带汤	Discharge-Ceasing Decoction	Chapter One
温胞饮	Uterus Warming Decoction	Chapter Twenty-nine

方剂汇总表

温经摄血汤	Meridians Warming and Blood Controlling Decoction	Chapter Fourteen
温脐化湿汤	Navel Warming and Dampness Dispelling Decoction	Chapter Twenty-two
温肾止呕汤	Kidney Warming and Vomit Stopping Decoction	Chapter Sixty-one
温土毓麟汤	Spleen-Earth Warming and Uterus Nourishing Decoction	Chapter Thirty
温胃丁香散	Stomach Warming Clove Powder	Chapter Ninety-seven
温中汤	Center Warming Decoction	Chapter Ninety-six
五苓散	Powder of Five Ingredients with Poria	Chapter Seventy-five
五皮散	Five-Peel Powder	Chapter Ninety-nine
息焚安胎汤	Flames Quenching and Fetus Calming Decoction	Chapter Forty-six
逍遥散	Free Wanderer Powder	Chapter Two
消块汤	Lumps Resolving Decoction	Chapter Seventy-four
宣郁通经汤	Depression Relieving and Menstruation Promoting Decoction	Chapter Nineteen
养精种玉汤	Essence Nourishing and Fertilization Improving Decoction	Chapter Twenty-seven
养荣生化汤	Engendering and Transforming Decoction for Construction Nourishing	Chapter One Hundred and One
养荣壮肾汤	Constructive Nourishing and Kidney Invigorating Decoction	Chapter One Hundred and Seven
养心汤	Heart Nourishing Decoction	Chapter One Hundred and Two
养正通幽汤	Healthy qi Reinforcing and Constipation Relieving Decoction	Chapter Eighty-four
易黄汤	Yellow-Transforming Decoction	Chapter Three
益经汤	Menses Nourishing Decoction	Chapter Twenty-six
	Qi Boosting and Construction Nourishing Decoction	Chapter One Hundred and Eleven
引精止血汤	Semen Drawing and Bleeding Stopping Decoction	Chapter Nine
引气归血汤	Qi Conducting and Blood Returning Decoction	Chapter Fifty-two
引气归血汤	Qi Conducting and Blood Returning Decoction	Chapter Fifty-two
援土固胎汤	Earth Supporting and Fetus Securing Decoction	Chapter Forty-one

长生活命丹	Life Saving and Prolonging Pill	Chapter Eighty/One Hundred and One
止汗散	Sweat Stopping Powder	Chapter Eighty-eight
逐瘀止血汤	Blood Stasis Removing and Bleeding Stopping Decoction	Chapter Eleven
助气补漏汤	qi Assisting and Bleeding Stopping Decoction	Chapter Forty-four
助仙丹	Immortal Assisting Pill	Chapter Sixteen
转气汤	Qi Changing Decoction	Chapter Sixty-four
滋荣活络汤	Construction Nourishing and Collaterals Invigorating Decoction	Chapter Eighty-five
滋荣养气扶正汤	Construction Nourishing, qi Boosting and Healthy-Qi Reinforcing Decoction	Chapter Eighty-two
滋荣益气复神汤	Construction Nourishing, qi Boosting and Spirit Recovering Decoction	Chapter Seventy-six/Seventy-nine

12检